MRCP 1
Last Minute
Practice Questions
Second Edition

W Stephen Waring FRCP (Edin) PhD

Consultant Physician & Honorary Senior Lecturer
Acute Medical Unit
York Hospital
York

Philip D Ambery MBChB MRCP (UK) MFPM
Dip Pharm Med

Medical Director
GSK R&D and Honorary Clinical Fellow
Addenbrooke's Hospital
Cambridge

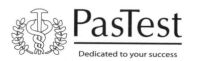
PasTest
Dedicated to your success

© 2006 PASTEST LTD
Egerton Court
Parkgate Estate
Knutsford
Cheshire
WA16 8DX

Telephone: 01565 752000

First Published 2006
Second Edition 2010

ISBN: 978 1905635 634
       1 905635 63X

A catalogue record for this book is available from the British Library.

The information contained within this book was obtained by the author from reliable sources. However, while every effort has been made to ensure its accuracy, no responsibility for loss, damage or injury occasioned to any person acting or refraining from action as a result of information contained herein can be accepted by the publishers or author.

PasTest Revision Books and Intensive Courses

PasTest has been established in the field of postgraduate medical education since 1972, providing revision books and intensive study courses for doctors preparing for their professional examinations.

Books and courses are available for the following specialties:

MRCGP, MRCP Parts 1 and 2, MRCPCH Parts 1 and 2, MRCPsych, MRCS, MRCOG Parts 1 and 2, DRCOG, DCH, FRCA, PLAB Parts 1 and 2.

For further details contact:

PasTest, Freepost, Knutsford, Cheshire WA16 7BR

Tel: 01565 752000   **Fax: 01565 650264**
www.pastest.co.uk   **enquiries@pastest.co.uk**

Text typeset and designed by Type Study, Scarborough, North Yorkshire

Printed and bound in the UK by CPI Antony Rowe, Chippenham, Wiltshire

CONTENTS

Introduction   v
Abbreviations   vii

1. Cardiology   1
   Questions and Answers

2. Clinical Pharmacology   47
   Questions and Answers

3. Clinical Sciences   113
   Questions and Answers

4. Dermatology   179
   Questions and Answers

5. Endocrinology   203
   Questions and Answers

6. Gastroenterology   249
   Questions and Answers

7. Haematology and Oncology   297
   Questions and Answers

8. Infectious Diseases   343
   Questions and Answers

9. Nephrology   389
   Questions and Answers

10. Neurology   429
    Questions and Answers

11. Ophthalmology   477
    Questions and Answers

12. Psychiatry   489
    Questions and Answers

13. Respiratory   515
    Questions and Answers

14. Rheumatology   559
    Questions and Answers

Index   609

CONTRIBUTORS

First Edition

Cardiology
Shani Esmail MB BChir BSc MRCP, Specialist Registrar in Cardiology,
York District Hospital, York

Respiratory Medicine
Elora Mukherjee MBBS MRCP, Senior House Officer, Renal Medicine,
King's College Hospital, London

Psychiatry
Gayle A. Christie MBChB BSc (Hons), Senior House Officer in Emergency Medicine,
St John's Hospital, Livingston, Edinburgh

INTRODUCTION

The MRCP(UK) diploma is a recognised entry qualification for higher specialist training in medicine and its related specialties. For many, the MRCP Part 1 examination is the first step towards obtaining the diploma. To be eligible to sit the MRCP Part 1 exam, applicants should normally have experience in medical employment for at least 12 months. Candidates sitting the MRCP Part 1 exam are expected to have a broad knowledge and understanding, including clinical sciences and features of common and important disorders. The MRCP Part 1 examines factual knowledge around a wide range of topics, and expects the candidate to be able to apply that knowledge to problem solving in the context of clinical scenarios presented in the examination paper.

The style of the MRCP Part 1 examination has evolved over recent years, and there have been a number of important changes. The number of questions has increased, and the 'best of five' format (one answer is chosen from five options) has gradually replaced the more traditional 'multiple choice' format. 'Negative marking' has been phased out and, in the current exam style, a correct answer will score +1, whereas no attempt or an incorrect answer will score 0. The exam is criterion-referenced, and a pass mark is set before each diet by experienced clinicians responsible for standard setting. These steps have been taken to create a more reliable assessment of candidates' abilities. Increasing assessment of knowledge as applied to theoretical clinical situations means that the exam has become more relevant to everyday medical practice.

The MRCP Part 1 examination is held three times per year, normally in January, May and September. It consists of two papers, each lasting 3 hours. Each paper has 100 questions in the 'best of five' question format (one answer is chosen from five options). Questions are chosen to represent each of the main specialty areas, and randomly distributed between both exam papers. The typical numbers of questions appearing in the exam for each specialty are shown below:

Clinical sciences*	25
Clinical pharmacology/therapeutics/toxicology	20
Cardiology	15
Clinical haematology/oncology	15
Respiratory medicine	15
Neurology	15
Nephrology	15
Rheumatology	15
Endocrinology	15
Gastroenterology	15
Infectious diseases, tropical medicine & STDs	15
Psychiatry	8
Dermatology	8
Ophthalmology	4
Total:	*200*

*Clinical science questions are made up of:

> Statistics, epidemiology, evidence-based medicine (5)
> Clinical biochemistry and metabolism (4)
> Clinical physiology (4)
> Immunology (4)
> Genetics (3)
> Clinical anatomy (3)
> Cell, molecular and membrane biology (2)

The best way to prepare for the exam will vary according to individual learning styles. It is crucial that candidates are familiar with all the topics outlined above, and that there are no major factual gaps. The knowledge tested in the MRCP Part 1 examination will probably be acquired from a number of different sources during General Professional Training, including ward-round teaching, Grand Rounds, Royal College symposia and local postgraduate educational programmes. Candidates should reinforce these learning opportunities by reading relevant materials in general textbooks and up-to-date scientific journals. In addition, a wide range of textbooks and online resources focused specifically on preparation for the MRCP Part 1 exam are currently available from PasTest. These can be an invaluable resource and allow candidates to become familiar with the style and format of the MRCP exam questions while guiding study towards an appropriate depth and breadth of knowledge.

Last Minute MRCP Part 1 Practice Questions gives candidates an opportunity to refresh their knowledge over the very broad range of topics included in the exam syllabus. The book contains 1000 questions written in 'best of five' examination style, and covers topics that are frequently encountered in the MRCP Part 1 exam. The large number of questions and answers provide an exceptional revision tool that is likely to be especially valuable to candidates nearing the exam date. The answers are given as an *aide mémoire* rather than an exhaustive summary of individual topics, and this will enable candidates to cover large numbers of questions more quickly.

Useful websites for further information are:

1. www.mrcpuk.org
   Further information on the MRCP Part 1 exam regulations and application process.
2. http://www.pastestonline.co.uk/
   Online revision source with practice papers (different questions from those appearing in the book range), including a free demo.

Good luck!

WSW
2010

ABBREVIATIONS

ACE	angiotensin-converting enzyme
ACTH	adrenocorticotropic hormone
ALP	alkaline phosphatase
ALT	alanine transaminase
ANCA	antineutrophil cytoplasmic antibody
APKD	adult polycystic kidney disease
APTT	activated partial thromboplastin time
ARDS	adult respiratory distress syndrome
ASCT	autologous stem cell transplantation
AST	aspartate transaminase
5-ASA	5-aminosalicylic acid
ASD	atrial septal defect
AWS	alcohol withdrawal syndrome
BDZ	benzodiazepine
BiPAP	bilevel positive airways pressure
CAPD	continuous ambulatory peritoneal dialysis
CMV	cytomegalovirus
CO	cardiac output
CABG	coronary artery bypass graft
COPD	chronic obstructive pulmonary disease
COX-1	cyclo-oxygenase-1
CPAP	continuous positive airways pressure
CSF	cerebrospinal fluid
CT	computed tomography
CTPA	computed tomography pulmonary angiography
DIC	disseminated intravascular coagulation
ECG	electrocardiography
ECT	electroconvulsive therapy
EEG	electroencephalography
EPS	extrapyramidal symptoms
ESR	erythrocyte sedimentation rate
ESRF	end-stage renal failure
FBN1	fibrillin 1
FEV	forced expiratory volume
FFP	fresh frozen plasma
FNAC	fine-needle aspiration cytology
FOC	faecal occult blood
FSH	follicle stimulating hormone
GABA	γ-aminobutyric acid
GFR	glomerular filtration rate
GGT	γ-glutamyl transpeptidase
GI	gastrointestinal
GLP-1	glucagon-like peptide 1
GTN	glyceryl trinitrate
GVHD	graft-versus-host disease
HAV	hepatitis A virus
hCG	human chorionic gonadotrophin

HELLP	haemolysis, elevated liver enzymes, low platelets
HSV	herpes simplex virus
HLA	human leukocyte antigen
HONK	hyperosmotic non-ketotic syndrome
HRT	hormone replacement therapy
HUS	haemolytic uraemic syndrome
IBS	irritable bowel syndrome
ICD	implantable cardiac defibrillator
ICP	intracranial pressure
INR	international normalised ratio
JVP	jugular venous pressure
KCO	CO transfer coefficient (= transfer factor divided by alveolar volume)
LDH	lactate dehydrogenase
LH	luteinising hormone
MAOI	monoamine oxidase inhibitor
MCV	mean corpuscular volume
MRI	magnetic resonance imaging
MUGA	multiple-gated acquisition
NAC	N-acetylcysteine
NMS	neuroleptic malignant syndrome
NO	nitric oxide
NOS	nitric oxide synthase
NSAIDs	non-steroidal anti-inflammatory drugs
PACS	partial anterior circulation stroke
$PaCO_2$	partial pressure of carbon dioxide
PaO_2	partial pressure of oxygen
PCR	polymerase chain reaction
PCWP	pulmonary capillary wedge pressure
PDA	patent ductus arteriosus
PET	positron emission tomography
PNH	paroxysmal nocturnal haemoglobinuria
PT	prothrombin time
PTH	parathyroid hormone
PTHrP	parathyroid hormone-related protein
PTSD	post-traumatic stress disorder
SARS	severe acute respiratory distress syndrome
SBE	subacute bacterial endocarditis
SBGH	sex hormone-binding globulin
SIADH	syndrome of inappropriate antidiuretic hormone
SLE	systemic lupus erythematosus
SPECT	single-photon emission computed tomography
SSRI	selective serotonin reuptake inhibitor
SVT	supraventricular tachycardia
SLE	systemic lupus erythematosus
TACS	total anterior circulation stroke
TB	tuberculosis
TCA	tricyclic antidepressant
TENS	transcutaneous electrical nerve stimulation
THS	thyroid-stimulating hormone

TIA	transient ischaemic attack
TNF	tumour necrosis factor
TPO	thyroid peroxidase
TRALI	transfusion-related acute lung injury
TRH	thyroid-releasing hormone
TTP	thrombotic thrombocytopenic purpura
VIP	vasoactive intestinal peptide
VMA	vanillyl mandelic acid
VSD	ventricular septal defect
VT	ventricular tachycardia
vWF	von Willebrand factor
VZV	varicella zoster virus

1. CARDIOLOGY

1.1 A 24-year-old traveller comes to the clinic. He is short of breath and has regular episodes of chest pain. His maximal right ventricular (RV) pressure is 112 mmHg, his maximal left ventricular (LV) pressure is 82 mmHg, and his LV O_2 saturation is 85%. What is the most likely finding on examination?

　　□ **A** An early diastolic murmur
　　☑ **B** Hypoxia which doesn't resolve on oxygen therapy
　　□ **C** Narrow, tented P waves on electrocardiography (ECG)
　　□ **D** Radio-femoral delay
　　□ **E** Tapping apex beat

1.2 A 64-year-old man collapsed in church complaining of chest pains. On examination his BP is 85/50 mmHg and he has very rapid palpitations. His ECG shows ventricular tachycardia with a rotating axis (*torsades de pointes*). Which of the following drugs is least likely to be associated with this arrhythmia?

　　□ **A** Digoxin
　　□ **B** Flecainide
　　□ **C** Risperidone
　　□ **D** Sotalol
　　☑ **E** Verapamil

1.3 A 62-year-old woman with manic depressive psychosis, who is on lithium, is sent to you for management of hypertension. Her BP is 160/85 mmHg. Which one of these agents would be least likely to have an adverse interaction with lithium?

　　□ **A** Amlodipine
　　□ **B** Bendroflumethiazide
　　☑ **C** Bisoprolol
　　□ **D** Enalapril
　　□ **E** Irbesartan

1.1   Answer: B

This man has a right-to-left shunt as a result of a longstanding ventricular septal defect (VSD). There is a pansystolic murmur, displaced apex and broad P waves.

1.2   Answer: E

Verapamil suppresses depolarisations and suppresses dispersion of repolarisation in the left ventricular wall. Other drugs which can predispose to *torsades* include macrolide antibiotics and antifungals such as ketoconazole.

1.3   Answer: C

Thiazides have an antidiuretic effect combined with lithium; ACE inhibitors increase lithium concentration and can promote toxicity in some patients. Calcium antagonists can provoke lithium neurotoxicity.

1.4 A 39-year-old smoker has sharp stabbing chest pain which is made worse by inspiration and by lying flat. His temperature is 38.2° C and you can hear a coarse rub at the left sternal edge. His ECG shows 1-mm ST elevation. What is the most appropriate treatment for him?

- [ ] **A** Aspirin
- [ ] **B** Clopidogrel
- [✓] **C** Diclofenac
- [ ] **D** Low molecular weight (LMW) heparin
- [ ] **E** rTPA (recombinant tissue plasminogen activator)

1.5 A 65-year-old woman with a history of type 2 diabetes and atrial fibrillation comes to the clinic. She has failed cardioversion and has an enlarged left atrium on echocardiography. How should she be managed?

- [ ] **A** Aspirin
- [ ] **B** Clopidogrel
- [ ] **C** Aspirin and dypridamole
- [✓] **D** Warfarin
- [ ] **E** Aspirin and clopidogrel

1.6 A 60-year-old man comes to the clinic for heart failure review. He is already taking adequate doses of furosemide, ramipril, bisoprolol and spironolactone. Over the past few months his heart failure has got so bad that he has been confined to the downstairs of his home and can only walk a few paces. On examination he has a blood pressure (BP) of 110/70 mmHg, significant bilateral crackles on auscultation and bilateral ankle oedema. His creatinine is 130 µmol/l, his ejection fraction is 29% and he has a QRS of 165 ms. What should you do next?

- [ ] **A** Arrange a single-chamber pacemaker
- [✓] **B** Arrange cardiac resynchronisation therapy
- [✗] **C** Implant a cardioverter/defibrillator
- [ ] **D** Increase his furosemide
- [ ] **E** Start digoxin

1.4 Answer: C

This man has symptoms and signs of acute pericarditis, most likely viral in origin. He should be told to rest and be given an appropriate NSAID for pain relief.

1.5 Answer: E

In this patient, who is at high risk of embolic disease, warfarinisation is recommended according to NICE guidance CG36.

1.6 Answer: B

This man fits the NICE criteria for cardiac resynchronisation therapy; studies suggest that he might derive significant symptomatic benefit. Digoxin is useful for symptoms of heart failure where other options are exhausted.

1.7 A 58-year-old woman with a history of breast cancer who is 12 months post-chemotherapy comes to the clinic with shortness of breath. She received a regime including transtuzumab. Her BP is 135/82 mmHg and her pulse is 92/min and regular. Her JVP is raised and she has bibasal crackles. What is the most likely diagnosis?

- [ ] **A** Carcinomatous pericardial effusion
- [x] **B** Chemotherapy-related cardiac failure
- [ ] **C** Lymphangitis carcinomatosa
- [ ] **D** Malignant pleural effusion
- [ ] **E** Radiation-related pulmonary fibrosis

1.8 A 62-year-old diabetic man had a bare metal stent inserted for inferior myocardial infarction. He re-presents with central chest pain and has new inferior ST depression. His troponin is negative. What is the most likely diagnosis?

- [ ] **A** Chronic stable angina
- [ ] **B** Coronary artery vasospasm
- [ ] **C** Embolism distal to the stent
- [x] **D** In-stent re-stenosis
- [ ] **E** New coronary artery disease distal to the stent

1.9 A 52-year-old man comes to the clinic with a history of type 2 diabetes (for which he takes metformin), hypertension and obesity, with a BMI of 34 kg/m² despite diet and exercise modification. Which of the following drugs might be most helpful in managing his obesity and diabetes?

- [x] **A** Exenatide
- [ ] **B** Orlistat
- [ ] **C** Rimonabant
- [ ] **D** Sibutramine
- [ ] **E** Thyroxine

1.7 Answer: B

Transtuzumab is known to cause congestive cardiac failure. It is thought that ErbB2 expression might be crucial in preventing the development of dilated cardiomyopathy.

1.8 Answer: D

In-stent re-stenosis is much commoner in patients with a history of diabetes. This finding precipitated the increased use of coated stents, but these appeared to be associated with an increased risk of late re-stenosis. This has led most recently to guidance being given that dual antiplatelet therapy with aspirin and clopidogrel should be given for an extended period in diabetics.

1.9 Answer: A

Exenatide has shown superior reductions in blood glucose to orlistat, with average reduction in weight of 5 kg during the first year of therapy.

1.10 A 74-year-old man who lives alone presents to the Emergency Department after a collapse in the supermarket. On examination he has a BP of 110/70 mmHg and a pulse of 62/min with second-degree heart block. While he is being monitored overnight he has two episodes of complete heart block, the longest lasting for 8 s. When you question him in the morning he tells you he has passed out on two other occasions in the past 6 months. He takes bisoprolol and ranitidine. Which of the following would be the best course of action?

- ✓ **A** Dual-chamber permanent pacing
- **B** Single-chamber permanent pacing
- **C** Stop bisoprolol
- **D** Stop bisoprolol and ranitidine
- **E** Stop ranitidine

1.11 A 72-year-old woman comes to the Emergency Department with nausea, central crushing chest pain and sweating. Her 12-lead ECG shows widespread ST elevation in the anterior leads. You diagnose an anterior myocardial infarction (MI) and prepare to move her to the Catheter Lab. Her pulse suddenly slows to 40/min complete heart block. She shows little response to atropine. Which one of the following could be the optimal treatment for this condition?

- **A** Adrenaline (epinephrine)
- **B** External pacing
- **C** Isoprenaline
- **D** Repeated atropine
- ✓ **E** Temporary pacing wire

1.12 A 72-year-old man with long-standing chronic obstructive pulmonary disease (COPD) comes to the clinic with shortness of breath and ankle swelling. He has a raised JVP and pitting oedema of his legs consistent with right heart failure. His BP is 152/89 mmHg. Which of the following will have most effect on his prognosis?

- ☒ **A** Bisoprolol
- **B** Furosemide
- ✓ **C** Home oxygen
- **D** Ramipril
- **E** Salmeterol/fluticasone inhaler

1.10   Answer: A

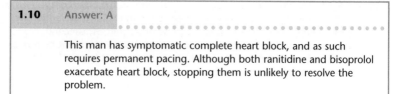

This man has symptomatic complete heart block, and as such requires permanent pacing. Although both ranitidine and bisoprolol exacerbate heart block, stopping them is unlikely to resolve the problem.

1.11   Answer: E

This woman has an anterior myocardial infarction, with complete heart block a very poor prognostic indicator. Unlike inferior MI, this is much less likely to resolve completely after re-perfusion.

1.12   Answer: C

This man has right heart failure secondary to severe COPD. His prognosis is very poor. Of the options given, home oxygen has the most significant impact on outcome.

1.13 A 72-year-old man is re-admitted 1 week after right hemicolectomy for colonic carcinoma. He has sweats and lethargy and on examination his temperature is 37.8 °C and he has a pansystolic murmur. Which of the following is likely to be the best antibiotic choice for him?

- A   Ciprofloxacin
- B   Flucloxacillin
- C   Gentamicin
- D   Metronidazole
- E   Penicillin

1.14 A 67-year-old man comes back to the hospital 6 months after aortic valve replacement. He feels washed out. He is apyrexial, his prosthetic valve is easily audible and he has mild left ventricular failure (LVF). His haemoglobin (Hb) is 9.7 g/dl with raised reticulocytes and haptoglobins. Faecal occult bloods (FOBs) are negative. Bilirubin is raised. Which of the following is the most likely diagnosis?

- A   Chronic gastrointestinal (GI) blood loss
- B   Obstructive jaundice
- C   Subacute bacterial endocarditis
- D   Valve haemolysis
- E   Warfarin-related haemolytic anaemia

1.15 A 56-year-old man is admitted with palpitations and chest discomfort. His ECG shows a broad-complex tachycardia. Which of the following suggest a supraventricular rather than a ventricular origin for the arrhythmia?

- A   AV dissociation
- B   Capture beats
- C   Fusion beats
- D   Slowing or termination following carotid sinus massage
- E   Ventricular concordance

1.13   Answer: D

Bacillus fragilis endocarditis is a rare complication of hemicolectomy; the bacterium is normally sensitive to metronidazole.

1.14   Answer: D

Valve haemolysis is a rare but recognised complication of mechanical valve replacement.

1.15   Answer: D

Supraventricular tachycardia (SVT) may be slowed or terminated by vagal manoeuvres (such as carotid sinus massage) or adenosine. The other answers all suggest ventricular tachycardia.

1.16 A 58-year-old man is admitted with palpitations and dizziness. An ECG shows a broad-complex tachycardia. Which is the most appropriate initial treatment?

- A Amiodarone
- ☑ B DC cardioversion
- C Digoxin
- D Temporary cardiac pacing
- E Verapamil

1.17 A 44-year-old woman is admitted after a sudden collapse. In the Emergency Department her ECG shows an appearance consistent with *torsades de pointes*. After initial resuscitation, normal sinus rhythm is restored, and a repeat ECG shows a prolonged QT interval. Which of the following is most likely to be responsible?

- A Adrenaline
- ☑ B Amiodarone
- C Atropine
- ☒ D Digoxin
- E Furosemide

1.18 A 26-year-old man is referred to Cardiology Outpatients with a history of palpitations and dizziness. His resting ECG shows a slurred upstroke to the QRS complex, and a 24-h ECG shows episodes of paroxysmal atrial fibrillation. Which of the following conditions is most likely to account for these findings?

- ☑ A Accessory pathway between the atria and ventricles
- B Lown–Ganong–Levine syndrome
- C Prolonged QT interval
- D Right bundle branch block
- E Structural heart disease

1.16   Answer: B

Scenario suggests ventricular tachycardia; in view of symptoms, treatment is as for ventricular fibrillation.

1.17   Answer: B

Other drugs commonly associated with prolonged QT interval are sotalol, quinidine and quinine, macrolide antibiotics, disopyramide, phenothiazines, terfenadine and other antihistamines. Non-drug causes include familial Romano–Ward and Jervell–Lange-Nielsen syndromes, ischaemic heart disease and metabolic disturbances.

1.18   Answer: A

This is the basis of Wolff–Parkinson–White syndrome, which results in short PR interval and widened QRS complex with a pathognomonic delta wave.

1.19 You review a 58-year-old woman in the Cardiology Outpatient Department 1 month after an acute anterior MI. An echocardiogram shows severe left ventricular systolic dysfunction, with an ejection fraction of 30%. Which of the following treatments is most likely to improve long-term survival?

A Digoxin

B Furosemide

C Glyceryl trinitrate

D Lisinopril ✓

E Spironolactone

1.20 Which of the following, when implemented after myocardial infarction, has been shown most convincingly to reduce the risk of further ischaemic cardiac events?

A Beta-carotene

B Cardiac rehabilitation ✓

C Diltiazem

D Hormone replacement therapy

E Warfarin

1.21 You have been asked to report ECGs requested by GPs to be performed in the ECG Department. One of these has a tall R wave in lateral lead V1. What is the most likely cause?

A Anterior myocardial infarction

B Duchenne muscular dystrophy ✓

C Left bundle branch block

D Left ventricular hypertrophy

E Wolff–Parkinson–White type B

1.19   Answer: D

Spironolactone can also reduce morbidity and mortality in addition to ACE inhibitor treatment. Digoxin has been shown to improve symptoms and reduce hospital admissions in chronic heart failure but is unlikely to improve survival.

1.20   Answer: B

This results in better compliance with medication in addition to ensuring patients are given appropriate lifestyle advice regarding exercise and diet.

1.21   Answer: B

This is a feature also found in right bundle branch block, right ventricular hypertrophy, posterior MI, dextrocardia, Wolff–Parkinson–White type A and hypertrophic cardiomyopathy.

1.22 You are reviewing a 66-year-old man in the Cardiology Outpatient Clinic, who has been taking amiodarone treatment for the past 8 months. Which of the following statements best describes the features of this drug?

- ☑ A Increases the plasma concentration of digoxin
- ☐ B Reduces the anticoagulant effect of warfarin
- ☐ C Short half-life and a small volume of distribution
- ☐ D Shortens the refractory period of cardiac tissue
- ☐ E Superior to implantable cardiac defibrillators in preventing sudden death

1.23 Which of the following features is most likely to be associated with the use of amiodarone?

- ☐ A Erythema nodosum
- ☐ B Gingival hyperplasia
- ☐ C Prolonged PR interval
- ☐ D Renal failure
- ☑ E Sodium-channel blockade

1.24 You are asked to help at a Paediatric Cardiology Clinic. An 11-month-old boy is referred with a history of failure to thrive and an episode of syncope. His mother mentions that he goes blue sometimes. On examination he is cyanosed and has finger clubbing. Which of the following is the most likely underlying diagnosis?

- ☐ A Atrial septal defect
- ☐ B Coarctation of the aorta
- ☐ C Congenital aortic stenosis
- ☐ D Patent ductus arteriosus (PDA)
- ☑ E Tetralogy of Fallot

1.25 Which of the following would most strongly support a diagnosis of tetralogy of Fallot?

- ☐ A Left ventricular hypertrophy and left axis deviation on ECG
- ☒ B Pulmonary plethora on chest X-ray (CXR)
- ☐ C Rib notching on CXR
- ☑ D Systolic thrill and pulmonary ejection systolic murmur
- ☐ E Wide fixed splitting of the second heart sound

1.22   Answer: A

The dose of digoxin must be reduced by around 50% to prevent toxicity. It potentiates the anticoagulant effect of warfarin. Amiodarone has a long half-life (30–110 days) and large volume of distribution and therefore a loading dose is needed.

1.23   Answer: E

Prolongs refractory period of cardiac tissue, so is considered a class III anti-arrhythmic agent, and prolongs QT interval. Inhibits potassium-, sodium- and calcium-channel activity, and exhibits α- and β-adrenergic antagonist properties. Adverse effects include skin photosensitivity, slate-grey or blue skin pigmentation, hypothyroidism and hyperthyroidism, ataxia, peripheral neuropathy, hepatitis and liver cirrhosis, pulmonary fibrosis and metallic taste.

1.24   Answer: E

The others all characteristically cause heart disease, but cyanosis would not be an expected feature.

1.25   Answer: D

Tetralogy of Fallot is the most common cause of cyanotic congenital heart disease and accounts for 10% of these patients. It usually presents after 6 months. Cardinal features are ventricular septal defect, right ventricular outflow tract obstruction, right ventricular hypertrophy and overriding aorta.

1.26 A 32-year-old woman presents to her GP with a history of palpitations. An ECG shows atrial fibrillation, and she is referred for echocardiography. This shows a small ostium secundum atrial septal defect (ASD). Which of the following findings is most typically associated with this condition?

- [ ] **A** Left axis deviation and right bundle branch block on ECG
- [ ] **B** Left ventricular hypertrophy
- [x] **C** Mitral valve prolapse
- [ ] **D** Oligaemic lung fields on CXR
- [x] **E** Wide fixed splitting of the first heart sound

1.27 A 56-year-old man presents to the Emergency Department after a blackout. On admission, he is found to be in complete heart block. What would you expect to see in the jugular venous pressure (JVP)?

- [x] **A** Cannon a-waves
- [ ] **B** Giant v-waves
- [ ] **C** Rapid y-descent
- [x] **D** Rise in the JVP with inspiration
- [ ] **E** Steep x-descent

1.28 A 55-year-old man presents with chest pain. His ECG shows ST depression and T-wave inversion in leads II, III and aVF. His troponin-T is abnormally high at 8 h after the onset of chest pain. Occlusion of which coronary vessel is most likely to account for his symptoms?

- [x] **A** Left anterior descending artery
- [ ] **B** Left circumflex artery
- [ ] **C** Left main stem artery
- [x] **D** Right coronary artery
- [ ] **E** Intermediate artery

1.26   Answer: C

Also associated with wide fixed splitting of the second heart sound. There may also be a pulmonary ejection systolic murmur and a mid-diastolic (tricuspid) murmur. Chest X-ray may show plethoric lung fields and prominent proximal pulmonary arteries. Right axis deviation and right bundle branch block may be seen in young patients.

1.27   Answer: A

The a-wave coincides with atrial contraction (so absent in atrial fibrillation). Cannon a-waves are caused by atrial contraction against a closed tricuspid valve, and are a feature of complete heart block (randomly occurring) and nodal or junctional rhythms (occur with every heartbeat). Large a-waves are seen in tricuspid stenosis, pulmonary hypertension and pulmonary stenosis.

1.28   Answer: D

The right coronary artery and its major branches supply the (i) inferior wall of the LV, (ii) posterior wall of the LV in most people via posterior descending branch, (iii) right ventricle via right ventricular branch, and (iv) sinus and AV nodes.

1.29 A 61-year-old man presents to the Emergency Department with features of an acute coronary syndrome. He goes on to have coronary angiography, which shows 95% ostial stenosis of the left anterior descending artery, which is amenable to angioplasty. Which of the following treatments is most likely to improve subsequent outcome when given at the time of the angioplasty?

- ☑ **A** Abciximab
- ☐ **B** Cefotaxime
- ☐ **C** Diclofenac
- ☐ **D** Streptokinase
- ☐ **E** Warfarin

1.30 A 48-year-old woman is referred to the Cardiology Outpatient Clinic with a history of exertional dyspnoea, orthopnoea and ankle swelling. An echocardiogram shows dilated right and left ventricles, severe global left ventricular systolic dysfunction and mitral regurgitation. Which of the following is most likely to explain these findings?

- ☑ **A** Alcohol excess
- ☐ **B** Carcinoid syndrome
- ☐ **C** Loeffler syndrome
- ☐ **D** Sarcoidosis
- ☐ **E** Previous radiotherapy

1.31 A 24-year-old man is referred to the Cardiology Clinic with a history of syncope. His brother died suddenly at 27 while playing football. What examination finding would most strongly suggest a diagnosis of hypertrophic cardiomyopathy?

- ☑ **A** Double apical impulse
- ☐ **B** Ejection click
- ☐ **C** Prominent v-wave in the JVP
- ☐ **D** Slow-rising pulse
- ☐ **E** Systolic murmur that increases in intensity with squatting

1.29 Answer: A

Abciximab is beneficial in some patients, eg those with intracoronary thrombus or after insertion of multiple stents. Antiplatelet therapy and stent insertion (including drug-eluting stents) are associated with improved outcome. Streptokinase and other thrombolytics have not been shown to improve outcome.

1.30 Answer: A

The history and echo findings are compatible with dilated cardiomyopathy. The others are more likely to cause a restrictive cardiomyopathy. Other recognised causes of dilated cardiomyopathy are ischaemic, hereditary, postpartum, hypertension, thiamine deficiency, viral infection (eg HIV, coxsackievirus), primary myopathies (eg Duchenne muscular dystrophy, myotonic myopathy, Friedreich's ataxia), thyroid disease and doxorubicin.

1.31 Answer: A

Double or multiple apical impulse, and the apex beat tends to be forceful. The pulse character tends to be jerky, with a rapid carotid upstroke. Other recognised features are prominent a-wave in JVP, late ejection systolic murmur that diminishes on squatting, palpable systolic thrill, fourth heart sound and mitral regurgitation.

1.32 Which of the following would be most helpful in the initial management of a young patient with suspected hypertrophic cardiomyopathy?

A 24-h Holter monitoring

B Carotid Doppler

C Exercising ECG

D Genetic testing

☑ E Transthoracic echocardiogram

1.33 You are asked to examine a 25-year-old woman who is 22 weeks pregnant. Which of the following statements best describes the haemodynamic alterations that can accompany pregnancy?

A Cardiac output falls by 30–40%

B Stroke volume falls during pregnancy

C Systolic blood pressure usually increases

☒ D Systemic and pulmonary vascular resistance increase

☑ E Total blood volume increases by around 40–50%

1.34 A 55-year-old man in shock undergoes Swan–Ganz catheterisation, which shows:

Cardiac index (normal reference):	1.7 (2.8–4.2 l/min/m²)
Pulmonary capillary wedge pressure: (PCWP)	20 (6–12 mmHg)
Systemic vascular resistance:	1850 (770–1500 dynes.s/cm²)
Mixed venous oxygen saturation:	47% (60–75%)

Which of the following treatments would be most appropriate in this situation?

A Hydrocortisone and chlorphenamine

B Intravenous antibiotics

C Intravenous diuretics

☒ D Intravenous fluids and noradrenaline

☑ E Inotropes and intra-aortic balloon pump insertion

1.32   Answer: E

Echocardiography can detect LVH, outflow tract obstruction and abnormal mitral valve motion. Exercise stress testing can provoke syncope, chest pain or breathlessness and poor BP response to exercise indicates risk of sudden death. Holter monitoring can be useful in detecting arrhythmias in some patients.

1.33   Answer: E

Cardiac output increases by up to 30–40%, and blood pressure falls due to a significant reduction in systemic vascular resistance. Other features are decreased pulmonary vascular resistance and increased stroke volume and heart rate.

1.34   Answer: E

Low cardiac index and high pulmonary capillary wedge pressure (PCWP) indicate cardiogenic shock. If thought due to ischaemic heart disease, coronary angiography and revascularisation should be considered.

1.35 You are asked to review a 72-year-old woman on the Coronary Care Unit (CCU), who was admitted with an inferior MI earlier that same day. She has become hypotensive (BP 85/50 mmHg) and clammy, and a bedside echo shows a dilated right ventricle. Urgent Swan–Ganz catheterisation shows raised CVP, reduced PCWP and low cardiac output (CO). Which of the following initial treatments is most appropriate?

- [ ] **A** Coronary angiography and possible angioplasty
- [ ] **B** Diuretics
- [ ] **C** Noradrenaline
- [x] **D** Rapid administration of fluids
- [ ] **E** Intravenous glyceryl trinitrate (GTN)

1.36 A 52-year-old man with diabetes and hyperlipidaemia is referred to Cardiology Outpatients with exertional chest tightness and dyspnoea. An exercise tolerance test is terminated at 2 min 15 s because of chest pain associated with ST depression and T-wave inversion in ECG leads V1–V4, I and AVL. Narrowing of which coronary artery is most likely to account for these features?

- [x] **A** Left anterior descending artery
- [ ] **B** Left circumflex artery
- [ ] **C** Left main stem artery
- [ ] **D** Posterior descending artery
- [ ] **E** Right coronary artery

1.37 A 58-year-old woman with known aortic stenosis is admitted to hospital for investigation of exertional chest tightness and breathlessness. Which of the following initial investigations would be most helpful?

- [x] **A** Cardiac catheterisation studies
- [ ] **B** Chest X-ray
- [ ] **C** Exercising ECG
- [ ] **D** Pulmonary function tests
- [x] **E** Repeat echocardiogram

1.35   Answer: D

The features suggest right ventricular infarction, complicating an inferoposterior MI. Intravascular volume should be expanded in order to increase RV preload and output and thereby optimise left ventricular filling pressures. Inotropic support and possible angioplasty of an occluded right coronary artery may also be helpful. Nitrates and diuretics would be potentially hazardous.

1.36   Answer: A

The ECG abnormalities predominantly involve the anterior and lateral walls of the left ventricle, which are normally supplied by the LAD.

1.37   Answer: E

This would allow assessment of disease progression (gradient across the aortic valve and aortic valve area), and determine LV function.

1.38 You review a 70-year-old man with mixed aortic valve disease in clinic. What pulse character is most characteristically associated with this condition?

- [ ] **A** Jerky pulse
- [ ] **B** Low-volume pulse
- [x] **C** Pulsus alternans
- [x] **D** Pulsus bisferiens
- [ ] **E** Pulsus paradoxus

1.39 A 57-year-old woman is referred to the Cardiology Outpatient Department with a history of exertional chest tightness and breathlessness. A resting ECG shows normal sinus rhythm. An exercise test is terminated because of chest pain associated with significant ST depression and T-wave inversion in the anteroseptal leads at 4 min 27 s. A subsequent coronary angiogram is reported as normal. What is the most likely explanation?

- [x] **A** Coronary microangiopathy
- [ ] **B** False-positive exercise tolerance test
- [ ] **C** Psychogenic chest pain
- [ ] **D** Variant angina
- [x] **E** Vincent's angina

1.40 A 48-year-old woman is referred to the General Medical Clinic with a history of fever, malaise, weight loss and arthralgia. Investigations show raised ESR, peripheral leukocytosis and mild haemolytic anaemia. There is a loud first heart sound and P2, and a murmur in early diastole. One week earlier, she noticed weakness of her left face and arm, which resolved over 36 h. What is the most likely underlying diagnosis?

- [x] **A** Left atrial myxoma
- [ ] **B** Mitral stenosis
- [ ] **C** Pulmonary thromboembolism
- [ ] **D** Subacute bacterial endocarditis
- [ ] **E** Systemic vasculitis

1.38   Answer: D

This pathognomonic finding manifests as a double peak. Pulsus alternans is alternating large- and small-volume pulses, due to severe heart failure. Pulsus paradoxus is an exaggerated fall in pulse volume on inspiration. A jerky pulse is associated with hypertrophic cardiomyopathy.

1.39   Answer: A

Coronary syndrome X is thought due to abnormal function of perforating myocardial vessels. Symptoms attributable to ischaemia and objective ECG signs indicate ischaemia. Symptoms with no ECG changes suggest a psychogenic cause, whereas ST depression in the absence of symptoms can be associated with a false-positive test.

1.40   Answer: A

Patients may be asymptomatic. Features can include murmurs mimicking mitral valve disease (can be postural), systemic embolisation, and constitutional symptoms of fever, malaise, weight loss and arthralgia. An early diastolic 'tumour plop' is characteristic of atrial myxoma however. Diagnosis is usually confirmed by echocardiography.

1.41 You review a 66-year-old woman with persistent atrial fibrillation in the Cardiology Outpatient Department. She has previously been intolerant of warfarin due to a severe blistering rash over her torso, and you are considering the use of ximelagatran. Which of the following statements best describes the effects of this drug?

- A   Glycoprotein IIb/IIIa receptor antagonist
- B   It has a more delayed onset than warfarin
- C   Liver enzyme disturbance occurs in around 5% of patients
- D   Selective inhibition of COX-2
- E   Selective inhibition of factor Xa

1.42 A 56-year-old man from Pakistan presents with progressive abdominal and ankle swelling, fatigue and dyspnoea. Pulse is 100/min and irregular in rate. The JVP is elevated and rises further with inspiration. Apex beat is impalpable, and heart sounds are barely audible. Chest X-ray shows a rim of pericardial calcification. What is the most likely cause of his symptoms?

- A   Acute myocardial infarction
- B   Acute pericarditis
- C   Constrictive pericarditis
- D   Mitral stenosis
- E   Tricuspid regurgitation

1.43 You are asked to review a 60-year-old man on the cardiothoracic ward 24 h after coronary bypass grafting. He has become breathless, and feels dizzy and faint. BP is 90/65 mmHg and pulse rate 120/min. His JVP is elevated, and apex beat is impalpable. On auscultation, heart sounds are softly audible and lung fields are clear. An ECG shows an alternans pattern. What is the most likely diagnosis?

- A   Cardiac tamponade
- B   Constrictive pericarditis
- C   Pulmonary embolism
- D   Right ventricular infarction
- E   Septic shock

1.41   Answer: C

Prodrug of the oral thrombin inhibitor melagatran. It has rapid onset of effect (within 1 h), a wider therapeutic window than warfarin and does not require therapeutic drug monitoring. Hepatotoxicity occurs in 4–7% of patients.

1.42   Answer: C

Typically presents with ascites and peripheral oedema. JVP signs include prominent x- and y-descents, and Kussmaul's sign. Calcification suggests tuberculous pericarditis. It is often difficult to distinguish clinically between constrictive pericarditis and restrictive cardiomyopathy.

1.43   Answer: A

A small amount of pericardial fluid, eg < 200 ml, can cause cardiac tamponade if it accumulates quickly, whereas up to 2 l can be accommodated if it develops slowly. Symptoms are secondary to reduced cardiac output. Symptoms include chest discomfort, cough, dysphagia, hoarseness or hiccups. Kussmaul's sign is often positive. Treatment is urgent pericardiocentesis.

1.44 A 62-year-old smoker presents to the Emergency Department with a 10-h history of chest pain. An ECG shows ST elevation in the anterior and septal leads, and both troponin-T and creatine kinase concentrations are raised. Which one of the following is most likely to improve survival within the first 24 h of symptom onset?

- ☐ A Atenolol
- ☐ B Diltiazem
- ☐ C Glyceryl trinitrate
- ☑ D Lisinopril
- ☑ E Oxygen

1.45 You review a 61-year-old woman with dilated cardiomyopathy in the Cardiology Outpatient Clinic. She has severe left ventricular systolic dysfunction. Which of the following is most likely to improve long-term survival?

- ☐ A Angiotensin II
- ☐ B Digoxin
- ☐ C Milrinone
- ☐ D Prolonged bedrest
- ☑ E Spironolactone

1.46 A 70-year-old man with ischaemic heart disease and severe heart failure (ejection fraction 25%) presents to the Emergency Department with breathlessness and chest discomfort. His ECG shows a broad-complex tachycardia. He has a short-lived arrest due to ventricular fibrillation in the Emergency Department that is reversed by resuscitation. Which of the following treatment strategies is most likely to improve his long-term survival?

- ☑ A Automated implantable cardiac defibrillator
- ☐ B Amiodarone
- ☐ C Flecainide
- ☐ D Permanent pacemaker insertion
- ☐ E Propafenone

1.44 Answer: D

Most of the mortality benefit conferred by ACE inhibitor treatment is derived within the first 24 h post-infarction. Therefore, treatment should not be delayed unnecessarily. Beta-blockers also improve survival by reducing arrhythmic deaths. Nitrates and opiates confer symptomatic relief only.

1.45 Answer: E

As with many positive inotropes, milrinone increases mortality in heart failure. ACE inhibitors, angiotensin II receptor antagonists and β-blockers improve survival in patients with severe heart failure.

1.46 Answer: A

Implantable cardiac defibrillators (ICDs) reduce mortality in heart failure patients who have had ventricular tachycardia (VT) or ventricular fibrillation (VF). Biventricular pacing can improve haemodynamic symptoms in patients unresponsive to medical therapy that have broad QRS complexes on ECG. Amiodarone reduces mortality in heart failure patients who have had ventricular arrhythmias, but ICDs appear more effective. Flecainide and propafenone may precipitate arrhythmias in ischaemic heart disease.

1.47 A 60-year-old man is referred by his GP with a history of breathlessness, hoarseness and dysphagia. On examination, he has a collapsing pulse and an early diastolic murmur over the left lower sternal edge. His BP is 180/70 mmHg. His chest X-ray shows a widened mediastinum. Which of the following best explains his presenting features?

- ☑ **A** Aortic dissection
- ☐ **B** Aortic regurgitation
- ☐ **C** Mitral stenosis
- ☐ **D** Oesophageal cancer
- ☑ **E** Thoracic aortic aneurysm

1.48 You are reviewing the biochemistry results of a newly admitted patient in the Acute Medical Admissions Unit. These show: sodium 134 mmol/l, potassium 6.1 mmol/l, urea 21 mmol/l, creatinine 403 μmol/l, bicarbonate 11 mmol/l. What corresponding abnormality is most likely to be seen on the patient's ECG?

- ☐ **A** Narrow QRS complexes
- ☐ **B** Short PR interval
- ☐ **C** Tall P waves
- ☐ **D** Tall R wave in V1
- ☑ **E** Tall T waves

1.49 An 18-year-old patient with newly diagnosed hypertension is referred to the Cardiovascular Risk Clinic. Her GP has suggested a diagnosis of aortic coarctation in the referral letter. Which one of the following features would most strongly support this diagnosis?

- ☒ **A** Anterior notching of the ribs on plain chest X-ray
- ☐ **B** Asthma in childhood
- ☐ **C** Female gender
- ☑ **D** Presence of ventricular septal defect
- ☐ **E** Systolic blood pressure higher in right leg than right arm

1.47   Answer: E

Widened mediastinum is a feature of aortic aneurysmal enlargement (not a feature of dissection), retrosternal goitre, mediastinal lymphadenopathy or thymoma. Wide pulse pressure and murmur indicate aortic incompetence (possibly secondary). Hoarseness and dysphagia are due to mechanical compression of the recurrent laryngeal nerve and oesophagus.

1.48   Answer: E

Tall 'tented' T waves are an early feature of hyperkalaemia. Later features include prolonged PR interval, reduced P-wave amplitude and prolonged QRS duration.

1.49   Answer: D

Two to five times more common in males, accounts for 7% of congenital heart defects. Posterior rib notching is caused by increased collateral blood flow via intercostal arteries (anterior intercostal arteries do not lie in the costal grooves). Associated with bicuspid aortic valve (and aortic stenosis and aortic regurgitation), patent ductus arteriosus, ventricular septal defect (VSD), Turner syndrome, berry aneurysms and renal abnormalities.

1.50 A 26-year-old asylum seeker presents to the Emergency Department with a history of breathlessness, fatigue and haemoptysis. On examination she has finger clubbing and is centrally cyanosed. Her JVP is raised and there is a loud P2 on auscultation and added third and fourth heart sounds. A soft systolic murmur and diastolic murmur are heard over the second left intercostal space. Her ECG shows right axis deviation and peaked P waves, and chest X-ray shows cardiomegaly, bilateral hilar enlargement and peripheral pruning of the pulmonary arteries. What is the most likely diagnosis?

 A Eisenmenger syndrome

☐ B PDA

☐ C Primary pulmonary hypertension

☑ D Severe mitral stenosis

☐ E Tuberculosis

1.51 You review a 60-year-old man with ischaemic heart disease in the Cardiology Outpatient Department. He is concerned that his breasts have enlarged. Which of the following medications is most likely to have caused this?

☐ A Candesartan

☐ B Carvedilol

☐ C Furosemide

☑ D Spironolactone

☐ E Warfarin

1.52 You are doing a CCU ward round and review a new patient who was admitted overnight. He has an intra-aortic balloon pump in place. Which of the following statements regarding this device is correct?

☐ A Heparin should be avoided due to risk of haemorrhage

☐ B Increases afterload and left ventricular work

☑ C Increases coronary perfusion pressure in diastole

☐ D Useful in the management of severe aortic regurgitation

☐ E Useful in type B aortic dissection

1.50 Answer: A

Features are irreversible pulmonary hypertension accompanied by reversal of a left-to-right shunt. It is more commonly a complication of VSD and PDA than ASD. Eisenmenger's can be complicated by infective endocarditis, cerebral abscess, paradoxical embolisation, arrhythmias and sudden death, heart failure and pneumonia.

1.51 Answer: D

Other commonly recognised drug causes of gynaecomastia are digoxin, cimetidine, cyproterone acetate, oestrogens, ketoconazole, phenothiazines and cannabis use.

1.52 Answer: C

Intra-aortic balloon pump is inflated and deflated in time with the cardiac cycle, provides haemodynamic support and improves coronary blood flow. It is indicated in cardiogenic shock and refractory unstable angina. It is contraindicated in aortic dissection, aortic aneurysm, aortic insufficiency and severe peripheral vascular disease.

1.53 A 55-year-old apparently healthy man is referred to the Cardiology Clinic. A routine insurance medical ECG shows left bundle branch block (LBBB). Which of the following would be most likely to cause this?

- A   Aortic valve disease
- D   Cardiomyopathy
- ☒ C   Ischaemic heart disease
- ☑ D   Left ventricular hypertrophy
- E   Normal variant

1.54 You review a 72-year-old woman with mitral stenosis in the Cardiology Clinic. Which of the following most strongly indicates a diagnosis of mild mitral stenosis?

- A   Graham Steell murmur
- B   Loud P2
- C   Right ventricular heave
- ☒ D   Short interval between S2 and the opening snap
- ☑ E   Valve area > 1.5 cm²

1.55 Which of the following statements best describes the pathophysiology of acute rheumatic fever?

- A   Caused by *Trypanosoma cruzi*
- ☑ B   Exaggerated immune response to group A streptococcal infection
- C   Infection on the endocardial surface of the heart
- D   Infection with the spirochaete *Borrelia burgdorferi*
- E   Results from cardiotoxin production by *Corynebacterium diphtheriae*

1.56 A 54-year-old woman presents with syncope, chest discomfort and dyspnoea. On examination her blood pressure is 85/50 mmHg, respiratory rate 24/min and pulse 120/min and regular. Oxygen saturation is 82% on air, and chest X-ray is normal. ECG shows a sinus tachycardia, right bundle branch block and right axis deviation. Arterial blood gases show a type 1 pattern of respiratory failure. What is the most likely diagnosis?

- A   Acute left ventricular failure
- B   Acute pneumonia
- C   Cardiogenic shock
- ☑ D   Pulmonary embolism
- E   Septic shock

1.53 Answer: D

LBBB is never physiological; the other listed items are recognised causes, but unlikely in the absence of cardiovascular symptoms or signs. Other causes include myocarditis, valve replacement and right ventricular pacemaker.

1.54 Answer: E

The other answers are features of severe mitral stenosis. A loud P2 and right ventricular heave indicate pulmonary hypertension, and a Graham Steell murmur indicates pulmonary regurgitation. Severe mitral stenosis is associated with a valve area < 1.0 cm^2 and moderate mitral stenosis with a valve area of 1.0–1.5 cm^2.

1.55 Answer: B

Streptococcal antigens closely resemble glycoprotein in human cardiac tissue. *Borrelia burgdorferi* causes Lyme disease, *Trypanosoma cruzi* causes Chagas' disease, and *Corynebacterium diphtheriae* liberates cardiotoxin (myocarditis recognised complication of all three infections).

1.56 Answer: D

Often the ECG and chest X-ray are normal (> 25% for each). The most common ECG abnormality is sinus tachycardia; other features include right axis deviation, right bundle branch block and an S1-Q3-T3 morphological pattern.

1.57 Which of the following investigations would be most helpful for confirming a diagnosis of suspected acute pulmonary thromboembolism?

- A   Blood cultures
- B   CT pulmonary angiography (CTPA)
- C   D-Dimers
- D   Swan–Ganz catheterisation
- E   Ventilation-perfusion (V/Q) scanning

1.58 A 58-year-old man presents to the Emergency Department with a history of flu-like symptoms, fever and right-sided weakness. On examination, temperature is 38 °C, respiratory rate 18/min and pulse 92/min and regular. His JVP is not raised, there is no peripheral oedema and heart sounds are normal. An early diastolic murmur is audible at the lower left sternal edge. His chest is clear. He has a right spastic hemiparesis and dysphasia. Urinalysis shows blood ++ and protein ++. Fundoscopy shows a retinal haemorrhage with a pale centre. Which of the following investigations would be most likely to establish the underlying diagnosis?

- A   Carotid Doppler
- B   CT scan of thorax
- C   Fasting glucose
- D   Repeated blood cultures
- E   Urine culture

1.59 Which of the following is most characteristically found as a complication of subacute bacterial endocarditis?

- A   Ash-leaf macules
- B   Focal proliferative glomerulonephritis
- C   Heberden's nodes
- D   Nail pitting
- E   Polycythaemia

1.57   Answer: B

CTPA reliably diagnoses proximal clot, although it might not identify small peripheral emboli. Serum D-dimers can be useful but there is a high false-positive rate. V/Q scanning is less useful in acutely unwell patients, and is easiest to interpret in the absence of lung disease.

1.58   Answer: D

The most likely unifying diagnosis is infective endocarditis, and this is best established by demonstration of bacteraemia. About 10% of patients with endocarditis have culture-negative endocarditis.

1.59   Answer: B

Characterised by asymptomatic haematuria, proteinuria and renal impairment. Occasionally results in nephrotic syndrome and renal failure. Infective endocarditis may be associated with Janeway lesions, not ash-leaf macules (tuberous sclerosis). Anaemia is a recognised feature.

1.60 You are asked for advice regarding coronary artery bypass grafting (CABG) by one of your patients in the Cardiology Outpatient Clinic. Which of these statements is most accurate with regard to the procedure?

- A 50% of patients report an improvement in angina symptoms
- B 90% of saphenous vein grafts are patent after 10 years
- C CABG improves prognosis in patients with left main stem or triple-vessel coronary artery disease
- D Long-term patency of venous grafts is superior to that of arterial grafts
- E Repeat CABG is associated with similar operative mortality to the first operation

1.61 You are examining the JVP of a patient on the Cardiology Ward, and note that there are large v-waves. Which of the following statements best fits the description of v-waves?

- A Coincide with atrial contraction
- B Can indicate tricuspid incompetence
- C Occur in mitral stenosis
- D Recognised feature in complete heart block
- E Usually associated with a collapsing pulse character

1.62 A 52-year-old man with atypical chest pain has been referred for exercise stress testing. He is unable to exercise sufficiently (he has severe osteoarthritis of his right knee). Which of the following would be the most appropriate alternative investigation?

- A Cardiac electron-beam CT scanning
- B Doppler echocardiography
- C Multiple-gated acquisition (MUGA) scan
- D Myocardial perfusion scanning during pharmacological stress
- E Tilt testing

1.63 Which of the following statements is correct in relation to management of coarctation of the aorta?

- A Balloon angioplasty is a recognised treatment
- B Correction can worsen lower limb blood flow
- C Dacron grafts should normally be avoided
- D Recurrence is a rare complication of surgical repair
- E Site involved is usually proximal to the right common carotid artery

1.60   Answer: C

When compared with medical therapy. It also improves long-term survival in patients with two-vessel disease that includes the left anterior descending artery. Around 50–60% of saphenous grafts and 90% of left internal mammary grafts are patent at 10 years. Re-do coronary artery bypass graft (CABG) carries a 2- to 3-fold increased risk compared with the first operation.

1.61   Answer: B

v-waves are caused by a rise in right atrial pressure due to bulging of the tricuspid valve towards the atrium during systole. Giant v-waves can indicate tricuspid regurgitation, which might also be associated with pulsatile hepatomegaly.

1.62   Answer: D

Dobutamine stress echocardiography is another means, and both modalities have equivalent sensitivity and specificity for diagnosing coronary artery disease and assessing prognosis.

1.63   Answer: A

Coarctation recurs in 5–10% of cases following surgical repair. Most common site is immediately distal to the origin of the left subclavian artery; can present with hypertension, heart failure or intermittent claudication. Severity is assessed by echocardiography, magnetic resonance imaging (MRI) and aortography. Coarctation may be complicated by hypertension, left ventricular failure, endocarditis and aortic dissection.

1.64 A 58-year-old woman is admitted for investigation of severe chest pain radiating to the back. On examination, you can hear a soft early diastolic murmur. Which of the following would be most helpful for establishing a diagnosis?

- A Barium swallow
- ✓ B Contrast CT chest
- C Plain chest X-ray
- D Right heart catheterisation studies
- E Transthoracic echocardiography

1.65 A 33-year-old woman presents with sharp left-sided chest pain and is found to have a pericardial rub and widespread ST-segment elevation on her ECG. What treatment is most likely to be helpful?

- A Diuretic therapy
- ✓ B Ibuprofen
- C Pericardiocentesis
- D Pericardiectomy
- E Warfarin

1.66 You are asked to give advice on a 42-year-old patient in whom the radial pulse volume feels very different between inspiration and expiration. Which of the following conditions is most likely to be associated with this physical sign?

- A Dehydration
- B Diabetes
- C Hay fever
- D Heart failure
- ✓ E Uncontrolled asthma

1.67 A 61-year-old man with known aortic valve stenosis is found to have a peak gradient of 78 mmHg by echocardiogram, and underlying left ventricular function is normal. Before undertaking aortic valve repair, invasive angiography is arranged. What information will be most likely to influence his subsequent management?

- A Aortic regurgitation
- B Aortic valve gradient
- C Co-existing mitral valve disease
- ✓ D Coronary artery stenosis
- E High right heart pressures

1.64 Answer: B

The history and examination findings strongly suggest thoracic aortic dissection and aortic incompetence. Contrast CT chest will establish the diagnosis and determine the extent of any associated aneurysm (determines medical or surgical management).

1.65 Answer: B

Treatment aims to reverse any underlying cause, and to give symptomatic relief. Non-steroidal anti-inflammatory drugs (NSAIDs) are highly effective, but associated with significant adverse effects.

1.66 Answer: E

Pulsus paradoxus is an exaggeration of the normal fall in pulse pressure that occurs during inspiration (usually expiratory–inspiratory pressure > 20 mmHg), and is also found in constrictive pericarditis, cardiac tamponade, severe COPD and massive pulmonary embolus.

1.67 Answer: D

In patients with significant coronary artery disease, coronary artery bypass grafting can be undertaken at the same time as aortic valve replacement. Echocardiography is a sufficient means of assessing left ventricular function and aortic valve gradient in most cases.

1.68 You are examining a 56-year-old man in the Coronary Care Unit and you notice that his JVP is slightly elevated, and rises further during deep inspiration. What is the most likely underlying cause of this physical sign?

- A Alcoholic cardiomyopathy
- B Cardiac tamponade
- C Congestive cardiac failure
- D Myocardial infarction
- E Uraemic pericarditis

1.69 A 68-year-old man is referred to the Cardiology Clinic by his GP, who thought he could hear a murmur. On auscultation, you hear an added fourth heart sound and no additional murmurs. What is the most likely underlying cause?

- A Amyloidosis
- B Atrial fibrillation
- C Hypertension
- D Ischaemic heart disease
- E Thyrotoxicosis

1.70 A 46-year-old man is brought to the Emergency Department after collapsing at home. His ECG shows a broad-complex tachycardia, with heart rate around 170/min. Which of the following characteristics most strongly suggests an underlying diagnosis of ventricular tachycardia?

- A Administration of adenosine restores sinus rhythm
- B Cardiac axis remains normal
- C Fusion beats are seen
- D Previous myocardial infarction 18 months before
- E QRS 106 ms

1.71 Which of the following conditions is most likely to cause prolongation of the QT interval on a resting 12-lead ECG?

- A Hyperkalaemia
- B Hypermagnesaemia
- C Hyperthyroidism
- D Hypocalcaemia
- E Hyponatraemia

1.68   Answer: B

Normally, right atrial pressure falls during inspiration. Kussmaul's sign arises when the right heart chambers are unable to accommodate increased blood flow due to restriction. Other recognised causes are constrictive pericarditis and restrictive cardiomyopathy.

1.69   Answer: C

A fourth heart sound is always pathological. It occurs in early diastole in association with atrial contraction (hence not a recognised feature in atrial fibrillation). Other recognised causes are left ventricular hypertrophy, hypertrophic cardiomyopathy, cardiac amyloid deposition (less common than hypertension!).

1.70   Answer: D

Ventricular tachycardia (VT) is more likely than supraventricular tachycardia (SVT) in patients with a history of ischaemic heart disease, if the QRS duration is > 140 ms, if the cardiac axis is grossly abnormal and if there is concordance of electrical activity across the ECG lateral leads.

1.71   Answer: D

Other recognised causes are ischaemic heart disease, hypokalaemia, hypomagnesaemia, hypothermia, hypothyroidism, mitral valve prolapse, and a number of different drugs.

1.72 Which of the following treatments would be most appropriate in a patient with *torsades de pointes* secondary to ischaemic heart disease?

- A Amiodarone
- B Digoxin
- C Adrenaline
- D Intravenous calcium administration
- E Overdrive pacing

1.73 Which of the following features is most strongly associated with an underlying diagnosis of tetralogy of Fallot?

- A Ejection murmur loudest on expiration
- B Left ventricular hypertrophy on an ECG
- C Methaemoglobinaemia
- D Polycythaemia
- E Pulmonary congestion

1.74 Which of the following statements is most correct with respect to atrial septal defects?

- A Left-to-right shunt ratio should only be corrected in symptomatic patients
- B Ostium primum defects are associated with leftward cardiac axis deviation
- C Pulmonary oedema and congestive cardiac failure
- D Risk of endocarditis is not increased
- E Systemic hypertension is a recognised complication

1.72 Answer: E

Isoprenaline can be used as a temporary measure if pacing is not available. Intravenous magnesium may also be helpful.

1.73 Answer: D

Clinical features include cyanosis, finger clubbing, parasternal (right ventricular) heave, pulmonary systolic murmur (and thrill). The ECG may show right axis deviation and changes of right atrial and ventricular hypertrophy. Chest X-ray shows oligaemic lung fields. Complications include polycythaemia, thromboembolism, endocarditis, cerebral abscess and heart failure.

1.74 Answer: B

Ostium secundum defects are more typically associated with right axis deviation; both are associated with right axis deviation. Recognised complications of ASD are pulmonary hypertension, right ventricular failure, tricuspid regurgitation, atrial fibrillation or flutter, stroke and (rarely) infective endocarditis. Left-to-right shunt ratio > 2:1 should be corrected regardless of symptoms.

2. CLINICAL PHARMACOLOGY

2.1 You review a 74-year-old woman with type 2 diabetes. She has a creatinine of 190 μmol/l and the GP is wondering which treatment agent would be best for her in view of her renal failure. Which one of the following agents is most appropriate?

- A Chlorpropamide
- B Glibenclamide
- ☑ C Gliclazide
- D Metformin
- E Tolbutamide

2.2 You are reviewing the mode of action of agents for the treatment of osteoporosis. Which one of the following is thought to act predominantly by inhibition of the RANK ligand?

- ☒ A Alendronate
- ☑ B Denosumab
- C Etidronate
- D Strontium
- E Teriparatide

2.3 A man with a history of epilepsy comes to the clinic with severe epigastric pain and vomiting. An amylase is measured at 1032 IU/l. Which of the following agents is most likely to be responsible?

- A Gabapentin
- B Lamotrigine
- C Phenytoin
- ☑ D Sodium valproate
- E Vigabatrin

2.1 Answer: C

Gliclazide is metabolised predominantly by the liver; all the others need dose reduction or are contraindicated in renal failure.

2.2 Answer: B

RANK-ligand inhibition blocks pre-osteoclast differentiation and inhibits osteoclast activity.

2.3 Answer: D

Sodium valproate is well known as a drug associated with acute pancreatitis.

2.4   You are reviewing a 72-year-old man who has been started on warfarin for persistent atrial fibrillation despite attempted cardioversion. Which of the following fruit juices is most likely to cause significant interaction with warfarin?

- ☐ A   Apple juice
- ☑ B   Cranberry juice
- ☐ C   Grapefruit juice
- ☐ D   Orange juice
- ☐ E   Tomato juice

2.5   A 56-year-old obese man attends the clinic. He has raised levels of urinary free cortisol. What is the primary mechanism by which free cortisol levels are regulated?

- ☐ A   Hepatic metabolism
- ☐ B   Metabolism in fat
- ☐ C   Metabolism in muscle
- ☑ D   Protein conjugation
- ☒ E   Urinary excretion

2.6   A 62-year-old man has recently started medication for hypertension. He comes to the clinic 3 months later to complain because his dentist tells him that the medication he is taking has caused unsightly hypertrophy of his gums. Which of the following medications is most likely to have been responsible?

- ☐ A   Atenolol
- ☐ B   Doxazosin
- ☑ C   Nifedipine
- ☐ D   Ramipril
- ☐ E   Valsartan

2.4 Answer: B

A CSM warning was issued which recommended that cranberry juice should not be consumed by people being treated with warfarin. Others including grapefruit juice may also interact with drugs such as warfarin.

2.5 Answer: D

Around 95% of cortisol is protein-bound at any one time, and changes in protein composition may have a major impact on free cortisol concentrates.

2.6 Answer: C

Calcium antagonists, phenytoin and ciclosporin are all known to cause gum hypertrophy.

Clinical pharmacology answers

2.7 A 17-year-old girl with a body mass index (BMI) of 14 kg/m^2 and anorexia is admitted for feeding. Which of the following electrolytes are you most concerned about with respect to re-feeding syndrome?

- ☐ **A** Chloride
- ☑ **B** Phosphate
- ☐ **C** Potassium
- ☐ **D** Selenium
- ☐ **E** Sodium

2.8 A 54-year-old man attends the clinic. He has chronic atrial fibrillation, hypertension and erectile dysfunction. He complains that his vision is often blue. Which of the following medications is most likely to be associated with blue vision?

- ☐ **A** Alprostadil
- ☒ **B** Digoxin
- ☐ **C** Ramipril
- ☑ **D** Sildenafil
- ☐ **E** Warfarin

2.9 A 70-year old man with rheumatoid arthritis comes to the Emergency Department. He has acute loss of vision in his left eye. Examination reveals slightly increased ocular pressure in the right eye, with a marked increase in the left eye with corneal clouding. Both eyes display cupping of the optic disc and partial pupil dilatation. Which of the following is the most likely cause?

- ☑ **A** Amitriptyline
- ☐ **B** Captopril
- ☐ **C** Hydroxchloroquine
- ☒ **D** Metformin
- ☐ **E** Prednisolone

2.7   Answer: B

Hypophosphataemia can lead to significant problems, including muscle weakness, decreased cardiac output and arrhythmias.

2.8   Answer: D

Phosphodiesterase 5 (PDE-5) inhibitors used at high dose also have some crossover with PDE-6, which is involved in the functioning of retinal photoreceptors.

2.9   Answer: A

Tricyclics are associated with increased risk of acute glaucoma. Hydroxychloroquine mimics chronic open angle glaucoma; prednisolone causes it.

2.10 A 72-year-old man with a history of atrial fibrillation and heart failure and is warfarinised. He also has chronic renal failure, with a recent creatinine level of 185 μmol/l. He presents on this occasion with acute gout. Which of the following treatments is most suitable?

A Allopurinol

☑ B Colchicine

C Diclofenac

D Predinsolone

E Rasburicase

2.11 You are reviewing case reports about psychiatric disturbance in response to an anti-influenza medication. In total there have been 95 reports in the UK. Which of the following is the most prompt means of determining if this is a casual relationship?

A A further randomised controlled trial

☑ B A nested case–control study

C A prospective cohort study

☑ D Database analysis

E Examination of licensing studies

2.12 A 64-year-old man comes to the clinic with muscle pain and fatigue. He has a history of dyslipidaemia controlled with simvastatin and COPD, for which he has recently started antibiotics from his GP. His creatine kinase is elevated at 405 IU/l. Which of the following antibiotics is most likely to be responsible?

A Cefalexin

B Ciprofloxacin

☑ C Clarithromycin

D Co-amoxiclav

E Penicillin

2.10 Answer: B

This will not affect renal failure or worsen heart failure, and rarely increases the international normalised ratio (INR).

2.11 Answer: B

For rare events such as these, a nested case–control study is the fastest initial way to investigate the relationship.

2.12 Answer: C

Clarithromycin is an inhibitor of CYP450-3 and so can cause rhabdomyolysis in conjunction with simvastatin.

2.13 A 38-year-old woman is diagnosed with a phaeochromocytoma. She has episodic hypertension and headaches, with a BP approaching 170/110 mmHg on occasions. Which of the following is the most important target with respect to lowering of the blood pressure?

- [ ] **A** ACE inhibition
- [✓] **B** Alpha blockade
- [ ] **C** Angiotensin-receptor blockade
- [ ] **D** Beta blockade
- [ ] **E** Calcium-channel blockade

2.14 A 29-year-old woman with a history of epilepsy is pregnant with her first child. She currently takes phenytoin for management of her epilepsy. What should she do with respect to her medication?

- [ ] **A** Change to carbamazepine
- [ ] **B** Change to gabapentin
- [✗] **C** Change to lamotrigine
- [ ] **D** Change to valproate
- [✓] **E** Stick with her current medication at the lowest dose possible

2.15 A 72-year-old man is admitted by ambulance after his daughter found him collapsed. He has written a suicide note; his wife died recently. On admission his BP is 80/60 mmHg, with a pulse of 38/min. Which of the following is the most appropriate intervention?

- [ ] **A** Intramuscular adrenaline
- [ ] **B** Intravenous atropine
- [✓] **C** Intravenous glucagon
- [ ] **D** Intravenous insulin
- [ ] **E** Temporary pacing

2.13 Answer: B

Alpha blockade with phenoxybenzamine is the crucial first step in managing phaeochromocytoma-associated hypertension.

2.14 Answer: E

A Cochrane review from 2004 found little evidence to differentiate between agents.

2.15 Answer: C

The suspicion is that he has taken a ß-blocker overdose, and glucagon would therefore be the most appropriate therapy. Large doses (eg 10–15 mg) are often required.

2.16 A 17-year-old boy is reviewed. He complains of thirst and polyuria and tells you that he always needs to have water close at hand to drink. He has recently begun treatment for acne. His sodium is elevated at 149 mmol/l, urea 11 mmol/l, creatinine 165 µmol/l, glucose 4.1 mmol/l, calcium 2.2 mmol/l. Which of the following antibiotics is the most likely cause?

diabetes insipidus

- ☐ **A** Ciprofloxacin
- ☐ **B** Clarithromycin
- ☑ **C** Doxycycline
- ☐ **D** Flucloxacillin
- ☐ **E** Penicillin

2.17 A 70-year-old man is admitted with an INR of 9.4. He is warfarinised for atrial fibrillation and has been using a Chinese herbal medication. He also has a history of peptic ulceration and had one admission 5 years ago for a GI bleed. How should you manage his anticoagulation?

- ☐ **A** Continue his warfarin at a lower dose
- ☒ **B** Stop his warfarin
- ☐ **C** Stop his warfarin and give fresh frozen plasma (FFP)
- ☐ **D** Stop his warfarin, give FFP and vitamin K
- ☑ **E** Stop his warfarin and give vitamin K

2.18 A man with type 2 diabetes is admitted with acute epigastric pain and severe vomiting. His amylase is 1250 IU/l. He is taking a number of medications to control his blood sugar. Which one of the following is thought to have an association with this clinical picture?

- ☐ **A** Acarbose
- ☑ **B** Exenatide
- ☒ **C** Gliclazide
- ☐ **D** Insulin
- ☐ **E** Rosiglitazone

2.16 Answer: C

Tetracyclines can cause diabetes inspidus.

2.17 Answer: E

Where there are risk factors for bleeding, guidance suggests giving 0.5–1 mg vitamin K and discontinuing warfarin for a period.

2.18 Answer: B

Glucagon-like peptide 1 (GLP-1) agents are thought to have an association with acute pancreatitis.

2.19 A new anti-diabetic agent which has better HbA1c-lowering capacity than its direct alternative is launched. The difference over a 6-month trial was 0.2%. Cost-effectiveness data suggest a quality-adjusted life-year (QALY) increment of 0.13. Which of the following is true?

- [ ] **A** The new agent is significantly more cost-effective
- [ ] **B** The new agent has significantly more effectiveness clinically
- [x] **C** The new agent is statistically significantly more effective
- [ ] **D** The new agent should not be used in the NHS
- [ ] **E** The new agent will not be recommended by NICE

2.20 What type of agent usually requires therapeutic drug monitoring?

- [ ] **A** Those with a large volume of distribution
- [ ] **B** Those with a low side-effect profile
- [ ] **C** Those with efficacy at a low dose
- [ ] **D** Those with a broad therapeutic window
- [x] **E** Those with a narrow therapeutic window

2.21 Which of the following statements regarding the mechanism of action of non-steroidal anti-inflammatory drugs (NSAIDs) is correct?

- [ ] **A** Can be used to treat patent foramen ovale
- [x] **B** Inhibit production of prostaglandins and thromboxane
- [ ] **C** Inhibition of cyclo-oxygenase-1 (COX-1) is responsible for most of their anti-inflammatory effects
- [ ] **D** They have analgesic but not antipyretic properties
- [ ] **E** They may improve blood pressure response to thiazide diuretics

2.22 Which of the following statements is true of drugs with a wide volume of distribution (V_d)?

- [ ] **A** Maximum V_d is around 50 l in a 70-kg man
- [ ] **B** Most have short plasma half-lives
- [ ] **C** They are subject to rapid renal clearance
- [x] **D** They tend to be lipophilic
- [ ] **E** Typically they are largely confined to the circulating compartment

2.19   Answer: C

From the information given, as we have no idea of price, the only conclusion we can draw is on the statistical difference between therapies.

2.20   Answer: E

In agents with a narrow therapeutic window the dose range between efficacy and significant toxicity is narrow.

2.21   Answer: B

COX-2 is induced in the presence of inflammation; inhibition is responsible for some analgesic, antipyretic and anti-inflammatory properties. COX-1 inhibition causes toxic effects, especially gastrointestinal. NSAIDs cause salt and water retention and limit the effectiveness of diuretic treatment.

2.22   Answer: D

Drugs with a wide volume of distribution are highly bound to tissues and proteins, and circulate in low concentrations. Half-life tends to be long, and clearance low. It is a theoretical volume that can vastly exceed actual bodily volume, eg amiodarone V_d is 200–300 l.

2.23 You review a 46-year-old man in the Medical Outpatient Department. He has a past history of ulcerative colitis, and has been taking sulfasalazine for more than 5 years. Which of the following statements regarding aminosalicylates is correct?

- A Balsalazide is contraindicated in patients with sulphonamide allergy
- B Mesalazine is not effective in treating acute exacerbations of colitis
- C Microcytic anaemia is a recognised complication of sulfasalazine treatment
- ☑ D Sulfapyridine is subject to hepatic acetylation
- E Sulfasalazine can be given by the oral route of administration only

2.24 A 47-year-old woman has returned to the UK after a 2-week holiday to Spain with her family. She has been suffering crampy abdominal pain for 3 days, associated with fever and profuse watery diarrhoea. Which of the following statements is correct regarding infective diarrhoea?

- A Antispasmodic treatment is particularly effective in children
- B Ciprofloxacin will shorten duration of symptoms in most cases
- C Loperamide has 80–90% oral bioavailability
- ☑ D Paralytic ileus is a recognised adverse effect of codeine phosphate
- E Yoghurt containing lactobacilli prevents gastroenteritis

2.25 You are asked to review a 68-year-old man in the Outpatient Department. Three months ago he developed a painful vesicular rash over the right side of his lower chest wall. The rash completely resolved more than 6 weeks ago, but he is still suffering pain and the area is extremely sensitive to minimal stimulation. You suspect that he has developed post-herpetic neuralgia. Which of the following is true regarding this condition?

- A Aciclovir treatment reduces the risk of neuralgia after herpes zoster
- B Around 50% of patients develop neuralgia after herpes zoster
- ☑ C Corticosteroids can reduce the duration of post-herpetic neuralgia
- ☒ D Post-herpetic neuralgia persists for several years in most patients
- E Simple analgesics are adequate after neuralgia is established

2.23 Answer: D

Sulfasalazine is a combination of sulfapyridine and 5-aminosalicylic acid (5-ASA), given orally or rectally. Mesalazine (5-ASA), balsalazide (5-ASA prodrug) and olsalazine (5-ASA dimer) avoid sulphonamide adverse effects, which include megaloblastic anaemia, hypersensitivity reactions and Stevens–Johnson syndrome.

2.24 Answer: D

Antispasmodics and anti-emetics are rarely effective in children, but may be useful adjuncts in adults. Most simple gastroenteritis is viral, and antibiotics are reserved for bacterial gastroenteritis with systemic features. *Lactobacillus* preparations have not been shown to prevent gastroenteritis. Loperamide has poor oral bioavailability, and its anti-motility action is a local effect on gut opiate receptors. Codeine phosphate has a predominantly central effect.

2.25 Answer: C

10% of patients develop neuralgia after herpes zoster, which can last for several months to years. Aciclovir and valaciclovir do not reduce the risk of neuralgia but reduce the duration of symptoms. Simple analgesia is usually ineffective, and low-dose amitriptyline, gabapentin and transcutaneous electrical nerve stimulation (TENS) may be helpful.

2.26 A 64-year-old man is taking multiple medications. He attends his GP with sudden onset of pain and inflammation affecting the first metatarsophalangeal joint of his right foot. The GP suspects acute gout. Which of the following is most likely to precipitate acute gout?

- ☐ **A** Atenolol
- ☐ **B** Hydrocortisone
- ☐ **C** Lisinopril
- ☑ **D** Low-dose aspirin
- ☒ **E** Triamterene

2.27 You see a 24-year-old woman who is referred to the Outpatient Department for investigation of an urticarial rash. She has a history of mild asthma and seasonal hay fever. Which of the following statements regarding possible treatments is correct?

- ☐ **A** Drowsiness may not become apparent for 48–72 h after treatment
- ☒ **B** Most antihistamines have additional anti-nicotinic properties
- ☐ **C** Non-sedating antihistamines do not interact with alcohol
- ☐ **D** Oral corticosteroids are the treatment of choice
- ☑ **E** Sedating antihistamines relieve itch more effectively than non-sedating ones

2.28 A 28-year-old woman is brought to the Emergency Department after a suspected drug overdose. The ambulance crew brought two empty amitriptyline packets that were found at the scene. On examination, she smells strongly of alcohol and has reduced conscious level. Which of the following features would most strongly suggest that an alternative or additional drug had been ingested?

- ☐ **A** Dry mucous membranes
- ☐ **B** Extensor plantar responses
- ☑ **C** Miosis
- ☐ **D** Prolonged QRS duration on an ECG
- ☐ **E** Sinus tachycardia

2.26   Answer: D

Low-dose aspirin inhibits renal tubular secretion of urate, so overall urate clearance is lower. Angiotensin-converting enzyme (ACE) inhibitors and angiotensin II receptor antagonists are uricosuric. Triamterene is a potassium-sparing diuretic and has little effect on urate. Thiazides reduce urate clearance, and loop diuretics cause a small increase in urate due to haemoconcentration.

2.27   Answer: E

Drowsiness can diminish after several days' treatment. Alcohol may interact with both sedative and non-sedative antihistamines. Most have additional antimuscarinic properties. Sedation appears to aid relief from itch.

2.28   Answer: C

Tricyclic overdose typically causes tachycardia, mydriasis, abnormal neurology (can be hyperreflexia, extensor plantars or absent reflexes) and dry mouth due to antimuscarinic effects. Prolonged QRS duration indicates increased risk of arrhythmia or seizure. Miosis suggests opiate ingestion.

2.29 A 47-year-old man presents to the Emergency Department alleging to have taken 28 500-mg paracetamol tablets 10 h earlier. He is complaining of vague abdominal pain and nausea. Which of the following statements regarding his clinical management is most appropriate?

☐ **A** Acute alcohol intake increases risk of paracetamol-induced liver toxicity

☐ **B** Cimetidine increases the risk of paracetamol-induced liver toxicity

☐ **C** Measure paracetamol level immediately to determine need for N-acetylcysteine (NAC) treatment

☐ **D** Measure paracetamol level in 4 h to determine treatment

☑ **E** Start NAC immediately and await paracetamol level

2.30 A 31-year-old woman is brought to the Emergency Department late at night by a friend who was worried that she may have taken a deliberate drug overdose. On examination, she is drowsy but rousable and smells strongly of alcohol. Pupils are widely dilated and eye movements appear normal. Heart rate is 112/min, blood pressure 108/76 mmHg, reflexes are brisk and symmetrical and there is sustained ankle clonus. Ingestion of which of the following drugs is most likely to account for these features?

☐ **A** Doxazosin

☐ **B** Ecstasy

☑ **C** Imipramine

☐ **D** Metamphetamine

☐ **E** Temazepam

2.31 Isoniazid undergoes hepatic acetylation, which is subject to genetic variation. Which of the following statements regarding isoniazid metabolism is correct?

☐ **A** Around 5% of the UK population are rapid acetylators

☒ **B** Rapid acetylators are more prone to neuropathy

☐ **C** Rapid acetylators need careful dose reduction to avoid adverse effects

☐ **D** Slow acetylators are more prone to hepatitis

☑ **E** Slow acetylators show greater therapeutic response

2.29 Answer: E

Potentially fatal paracetamol ingestion (> 12 g in previously healthy adult) more than 8 h earlier necessitates immediate NAC while awaiting paracetamol concentrations. Acute alcohol ingestion may be protective, whereas chronic alcohol intake increases risk through up-regulation of P450 enzyme activity. Cimetidine is a P450 enzyme inhibitor.

2.30 Answer: C

Doxazosin is unlikely to alter conscious level directly. Ecstasy and amphetamines might also cause hyperreflexia and tachycardia, but they are characteristically associated with agitation and arousal.

2.31 Answer: E

Around 50% of the UK population are rapid acetylators: low isoniazid levels, poor response to treatment and tuberculosis (TB) relapses. Slow acetylators: higher isoniazid levels and greater risk of neuropathy. Hepatitis is due to a metabolite, and is more common in rapid acetylators.

2.32 Genetic polymorphism is a major determinant of drug metabolism in humans. Metabolism of which of the following drugs is *not* significantly influenced by genetic polymorphism?

A Hydralazine

B Isoniazid

C Norfloxacin

D Procainamide

E Sulfasalazine

2.33 A 47-year-old female patient presents to the Emergency Department alleging to have taken a drug overdose. She has reduced conscious level, gross ataxia and there is bruising over all of her limbs. There is coarse nystagmus on left and right lateral gaze. Overdose of which of the following drugs might account for her clinical condition?

A Atenolol

B Carbamazepine

C Digoxin

D Furosemide

E Sertraline

2.34 A 23-year-old woman attends her GP and describes a number of allergic episodes that have followed ingestion of peanuts. These had been characterised by facial flushing, headache, wheeze and nausea. Which of the following statements is correct in relation to treatment of allergy?

A Bronchospasm usually develops 3–4 h after allergen exposure

B Desensitisation to foodstuff allergens is generally effective

C Diagnosis is typically established using skin tests

D Patients with asthma have greater likelihood of anaphylaxis

E Pollen extract desensitisation is usually effective in allergic hay fever

2.32   Answer: C

The others are metabolised by acetylation, including the sulfapyridine component of sulfasalazine.

2.33   Answer: B

Carbamazepine and phenytoin overdose cause prominent cerebellar toxicity, often mistaken for alcohol intoxication. Repeated doses of activated charcoal should be considered, with ECG monitoring and correction of electrolyte abnormalities.

2.34   Answer: D

Bee and wasp allergen and grass and tree pollen extracts can be used for desensitisation, but carry a risk of anaphylaxis. Used in patients who do not respond to antihistamines. Desensitisation to foodstuffs and animal dander is ineffective. Diagnosis depends on detailed history; skin tests may be unreliable.

2.35   A patient is taking multiple medications, and presents to the Emergency Department with reduced conscious level. The ambulance crew found a number of empty medicine packets at the scene, and a drug overdose is suspected. For which of the following drugs would measurement of plasma drug concentrations be most useful?

- [ ] **A** Amlodipine
- [x] **B** Digoxin
- [ ] **C** Furosemide
- [ ] **D** Gabapentin
- [ ] **E** Isoniazid

2.36   A 56-year-old woman with a long history of bipolar disorder is admitted to the Medical Assessment Unit with a 48-h history of progressive confusion and slurred speech. On examination, she has reduced conscious level, and initial investigations show: sodium 123 mmol/l, potassium 3.6 mmol/l, urea 3.4 mmol/l and creatinine 108 µmol/l. Serum osmolality is 236 mOsm/kg and urinary osmolality 261 mOsm/kg. Which of the following is most likely to account for these abnormalities?

- [ ] **A** Carbamazepine-induced hyponatraemia
- [x] **B** Carbamazepine-induced syndrome of inappropriate ADH
- [ ] **C** Diuretic abuse
- [ ] **D** Lithium-induced diabetes insipidus
- [ ] **E** Psychogenic polydipsia

2.37   A 37-year-old woman attends the Medical Outpatient Department after experiencing a number of short-lived episodes of anxiety, associated with palpitations, sweating, choking sensation and numbness of both upper limb extremities. Physical examination and routine investigations are normal. You diagnose panic attacks as the underlying cause of her symptoms. Which of the following is true regarding pharmacological treatment of this condition?

- [ ] **A** 5–10% of patients relapse within 12 months of drug discontinuation
- [x] **B** Diazepam use can lead to dependence
- [ ] **C** Only a short-term course of treatment is necessary in most patients
- [ ] **D** Paroxetine rapidly relieves panic with agoraphobia
- [ ] **E** Tricyclic antidepressants are of no benefit in this condition

2.35   Answer: B

Levels can guide the need for antidote or inform prognosis. For monitoring to be useful there should be a close relationship between plasma concentration and drug effects or toxicity. Digoxin concentrations determine the need for Fab antibody antidote.

2.36   Answer: B

Carbamazepine is a recognised cause of syndrome of inappropriate antidiuretic hormone (SIADH) due to excess ADH secretion, while chlorpropamide and rifampicin increase renal tubular sensitivity to ADH. Hyponatraemia does not explain low serum osmolality and inappropriately high urine osmolality.

2.37   Answer: B

Benzodiazepines have rapid onset, but should be reserved for short-term treatment to avoid dependence and tolerance. Selective serotonin reuptake inhibitors (SSRIs) and tricyclic antidepressants (TCAs) have slower onset of action and exacerbate symptoms. Around 30–75% of patients relapse within 6–12 months of drug discontinuation, and long-term treatment may be needed.

2.38 You are on call overnight, and called to review a 56-year-old man with a past history of schizophrenia. During the past 4 h he has become increasingly agitated, and he is becoming impulsive and violent towards the ward staff. Which of the following would be the most appropriate initial sedative treatment in this emergency situation?

☒ A High-dose intramuscular chlorpromazine

☐ B High-dose rectal diazepam

☐ C Intramuscular haloperidol in high doses

☑ D Intravenous haloperidol and lorazepam in standard doses

☐ E Oral risperidone

2.39 You see a 46-year-old man in the Medical Outpatient Department for investigation of an infected leg ulcer. He has a past history of alcohol excess, and is currently taking disulfiram 100 mg daily. Which of the following drugs is most likely to adversely interact with disulfiram and should be avoided?

☐ A Atenolol

☐ B Captopril

☐ C Metformin

☑ D Theophylline

☐ E Valsartan

2.40 A 64-year-old woman attends the Medical Outpatient Department complaining of recurrent cough. She is taking a number of medications, which you feel might be responsible. Which of the following drugs is most likely to cause a cough that resolves after drug withdrawl?

☐ A Amiodarone

☐ B Bleomycin

☐ C Methotrexate

☑ D Perindopril

☐ E Sulfasalazine

2.38   Answer: D

Combination of intravenous or intramuscular haloperidol (or oral risperidone) with intravenous or intramuscular lorazepam (or rectal diazepam) has a synergistic effect. Intravenous administration allows rapid onset of effect, but the intramuscular route may be less hazardous in the acute situation.

2.39   Answer: D

Disulfiram inhibits hepatic aldehyde-NAD reductase, causing accumulation of acetaldehyde after ethanol ingestion: flushing, nausea and vomiting. A similar reaction occurs due to interaction with metronidazole. Disulfiram causes non-specific P450 inhibition so phenytoin and theophylline toxicity are more likely.

2.40   Answer: D

ACE inhibitors are associated with cough in up to 30%. This is reversible in > 80% of cases, and in the remainder is likely to have been present before treatment. The other drugs listed are characteristically associated with pulmonary fibrosis.

2.41 A 30-year-old woman with essential hypertension presents to the Antenatal Clinic at 6 weeks after conception. She is currently taking nifedipine MR 10 mg daily, and her BP is consistently high, averaging 168/104 mmHg. Which of the following additional antihypertensive medications would be most appropriate for controlling her blood pressure?

- A Atenolol
- B Bendroflumethiazide
- C Lisinopril
- ☑ D Methyldopa
- E Valsartan

2.42 You review a 48-year-old man with a renal transplant who has been taking several medications for immunosuppression and blood pressure control. His renal function is normal, but his serum potassium has risen to 6.4 mmol/l. Which one of the following drugs is *least* likely to have caused hyperkalaemia?

- A Candesartan
- ☒ B Ciclosporin A
- ☑ C Nifedipine
- D Ramipril
- E Sirolimus

2.43 A 45-year-old man presents to the Emergency Department within 1 h of ingesting 40 tablets of slow-release theophylline. Which of the following statements regarding treatment of this patient is correct?

- ☒ A Alkaline diuresis reduces theophylline toxicity
- B Ipecacuanha is the best method to reduce gut absorption
- C Metabolic alkalosis indicates a poor prognosis
- D Oral activated charcoal is ineffective in reducing gut absorption
- ☑ E The degree of hypokalaemia is a marker of severity of poisoning

2.41 Answer: D

Methyldopa is not known to be harmful in pregnancy. Beta-blockers can cause intrauterine growth retardation. ACE inhibitors (and probably angiotensin II receptor antagonists) are teratogenic, while thiazides can cause neonatal thrombocytopenia.

2.42 Answer: C

Hyperkalaemia is a particular problem when renal function has declined and serum concentrations of ciclosporin, tacrolimus or sirolimus have increased. Therapeutic drug monitoring is required to prevent nephrotoxicity and hyperkalaemia.

2.43 Answer: E

Theophylline toxicity causes hypokalaemia, metabolic acidosis, arrhythmia and seizures. Oral activated charcoal is particularly useful and repeated treatment may be needed to enhance elimination. Haemodialysis can be used to assist clearance in severe toxicity. Ipecacuanha is now redundant in most overdose situations.

2.44   A 22-year-old man is brought to the Emergency Department having been found convulsing in the street at 4 am. He is agitated, has dilated pupils, heart rate is 132/min and BP 178/112 mmHg. Which of the following is most likely to account for these clinical features?

- ☐ **A** Amitriptyline
- ☐ **B** Chlorpromazine
- ☑ **C** Cocaine
- ☐ **D** Co-codamol (paracetamol + codeine)
- ☐ **E** Methadone

2.45   You are asked to review a 21-year-old university student in the Medical Outpatient Department. She has suffered recurrent migraine attacks over the past 3 years, which render her unable to concentrate on her studies for several days each time. Which of the following statements is correct regarding migraine prophylaxis?

- ☑ **A** Amitriptyline prevents migraine but is commonly associated with antimuscarinic effects
- ☐ **B** Pizotifen is commonly associated with agitation and weight loss
- ☐ **C** Prophylactic therapy avoids the need for symptomatic treatment
- ☐ **D** Prophylaxis should be used if migraine occurs at least every 6 months
- ☒ **E** Propranolol is preferred to atenolol due to lack of cardioselectivity

2.46   When considering the use of haemodialysis to assist drug elimination in a patient with chronic renal impairment, which of the following properties of the drug would make haemodialysis most effective?

- ☐ **A** High drug-receptor affinity
- ☐ **B** Highly lipophilic drug
- ☐ **C** Large volume of distribution
- ☑ **D** Low degree of plasma protein binding
- ☒ **E** Short drug elimination half-life

2.44   Answer: C

Amitriptyline is associated with tachycardia and dilated pupils, and conscious level tends to be reduced. Chlorpromazine, codeine and methadone tend to be sedative, and reduce conscious level.

2.45   Answer: A

Pizotifen can cause drowsiness and weight gain. Prophylaxis reduces migraine frequency and severity, and is used when there are more than one or two attacks per month. Propranolol is lipid-soluble, and therefore has better central nervous system (CNS) penetration.

2.46   Answer: D

Haemodialysis is most effective in clearing drugs with a low volume of distribution, ie confined largely to the circulating component. These tend to be water-soluble drugs that are not highly bound to tissue proteins. Dialysis is most useful where the half-life would ordinarily be long.

2.47 A 64-year-old woman presents to hospital 12 h after ingestion of 6 g quinine sulphate. Which of the following would be expected as a feature of drug toxicity?

- [ ] **A** Flaccid hemiparesis
- [x] **B** Hyperacusis
- [x] **C** Horizontal nystagmus
- [ ] **D** Intractable vomiting
- [ ] **E** Thrombocytosis

2.48 You are asked to review the prescription chart of a 56-year-old woman in the High Dependency Unit who suffered a pathological fracture of her left neck of femur 3 days ago. She is complaining of severe hip and groin pain, and headache. Which of the following statements is correct in relation to analgesic therapy?

- [x] **A** Bisphosphonates can relieve bone pain due to metastases
- [ ] **B** Carbamazepine is effective in treating acute bony pain
- [ ] **C** Corticosteroids worsen headache in raised intracranial pressure (ICP) due to fluid retention
- [ ] **D** NSAIDs should be avoided due to bleeding risk at the injury site
- [x] **E** Slow-release morphine should be initiated

2.49 A 30-year-old man with a history of rheumatoid arthritis is being investigated for infertility, and is keen to avoid taking any medications that would reduce his sperm count. Which of the following drugs is most likely to cause oligospermia?

- [ ] **A** Gold
- [ ] **B** Hydroxycobalamin
- [ ] **C** Penicillamine
- [ ] **D** Prednisolone
- [x] **E** Sulfasalazine

2.47 Answer: C

Quinine causes nausea, vomiting, tremor, tinnitus and deafness. Blurred vision may progress to blindness within a few hours. Tachycardia, arrhythmias, hypotension, intravascular haemolysis and acute renal failure, seizures and coma are also recognised features.

2.48 Answer: A

Carbamazepine and gabapentin can be effective for neuropathic pain; corticosteroids can relieve pain due to neuropathy, raised intracranial pressure and bony metastases. NSAIDs are effective for inflammatory bone pain, although the risk of gastrointestinal bleeding is increased. Opiates may be needed, and initiated with short-acting preparations.

2.49 Answer: E

Sulfasalazine causes oligospermia, reduced sperm motility and increased sperm morphological abnormalities. The effects are mediated at a late stage in sperm maturation, and are usually reversible on drug withdrawal. The sulphapyridine moiety is thought to be responsible.

2.50 A 65-year-old man is brought to the Emergency Department having been found unconscious in the street at 2 am. On examination, he is localising to painful stimuli, and there is no evidence of head injury or meningism. Initial investigations showed: sodium 145 mmol/l, potassium 3.4 mmol/l, venous bicarbonate 16 mmol/l, urea 10.4 mmol/l, creatinine 142 µmol/l, glucose 5.4 mmol/l and serum osmolality 318 mOsm/kg. Which of the following is most likely to account for these initial findings?

- ☐ A Ethylene glycol ingestion
- ☑ B Lactic acidosis
- ☐ C Long-standing sleep apnoea
- ☐ D Rhabdomyolysis
- ☐ E Diclofenac toxicity

2.51 A 58-year-old non-diabetic woman was found to have BP 168/94 mmHg, proteinuria +++, and serum creatinine 172 µmol/l. Renal biopsy revealed membranous glomerulonephritis, and treatment with lisinopril was started. Which of the following changes is most likely to occur as a result of this treatment?

- ☐ A Increased serum low-density lipoprotein (LDL) cholesterol concentration
- ☐ B Increased serum magnesium concentration
- ☒ C Reduced serum creatinine concentration
- ☑ D Reduced serum potassium concentration
- ☑ E Reduced urinary protein excretion

2.52 A 46-year-old farm-worker attended the Emergency Department after a deliberate overdose of organophosphate pesticide. He was treated initially with atropine. Which one of the following clinical features can most reliably be used to assess his response to atropine?

- ☑ A Bronchorrhoea
- ☐ B Heart rate
- ☐ C Peripheral pulse volume
- ☐ D Pupil size
- ☐ E Systolic blood pressure

2.50   Answer: B

The data suggest a metabolic acidosis; lactate should be measured. NSAID ingestion and rhabdomyolysis are typically associated with hyperkalaemia. Calculated osmolality is close to the actual measured osmolality, excluding significant circulating concentrations of ethylene glycol, methanol or alcohol. Long-standing type 2 respiratory failure can cause a metabolic alkalosis.

2.51   Answer: E

ACE inhibitor treatment will improve blood pressure and reduce the decline in glomerular filtration rate (GFR), but creatinine is unlikely to fall. Serum potassium may increase, particularly if there is renovascular insufficiency.

2.52   Answer: A

Organophosphates and nerve agents bind to acetylcholinesterase, thereby exaggerating the effects of acetylcholine (ACh) at nicotinic and muscarinic synapses. Classically, patients will have excess salivation and lacrimation, bronchorrhoea, and miosis, but effects on pupil size, heart rate and blood pressure are highly variable.

2.53 A 32-year-old woman presented to the Emergency Department 6 h after taking 30 g of paracetamol. Which one of the following factors most strongly predicts an increased risk of paracetamol-induced hepatotoxicity?

- ☑ **A** Anorexia nervosa
- ☐ **B** Cimetidine ingestion with the paracetamol
- ☐ **C** Gilbert's disease
- ☐ **D** Recreational cannabis use
- ☐ **E** Regularly smoking 20 cigarettes per day

2.54 A 26-year-old woman presented 9 h after a mixed overdose of paracetamol, diazepam and ethanol. She was drowsy, mildly dehydrated, and complaining of mild nausea. Treatment with intravenous *N*-acetylcysteine was started and, 20 min later, she developed breathlessness and facial flushing and developed a tachycardia of 140/min. What is the most likely explanation for this reaction?

- ☐ **A** Acute left ventricular failure
- ☐ **B** Allergic reaction to paracetamol
- ☑ **C** Anaphylactoid reaction to NAC
- ☐ **D** Overdose of NAC has been administered
- ☐ **E** The patient has received NAC previously

2.55 You review the analgesia prescription for a 69-year-old woman with breast carcinoma and painful bony metastases. She has been taking regular oral modified-release morphine, and has required additional morphine solution for breakthrough pain. Which of the following pharmacokinetic factors is most important in deciding the dose and frequency of morphine to be administered?

- ☑ **A** Half-life
- ☐ **B** Patient body mass index (BMI)
- ☐ **C** Serum creatinine concentration
- ☐ **D** The extent of first-pass metabolism
- ☐ **E** Volume of distribution

2.53   Answer: A

Anorexia, chronic alcohol excess and HIV infection are associated with malnourishment and glutathione depletion; hepatic enzyme induction (eg chronic alcohol intake, carbamazepine, phenytoin and rifampicin) is associated with more rapid formation of toxic metabolites. Chronic cigarette smoking has a weak hepatic enzyme-inducing effect.

2.54   Answer: C

Anaphylactoid reactions occur in around 15% of patients treated with NAC, and are usually self-limiting. Infusion should be temporarily discontinued, and treatment administered if needed (antihistamine, corticosteroids). NAC treatment can be recommenced in most cases.

2.55   Answer: A

Short-acting preparations should be used initially, and then modified-release preparations introduced after analgesic requirements are established. The other factors listed can be indicative of half-life, but are less important.

2.56 A 42-year-old man is diagnosed as having rheumatoid arthritis, and you are considering starting treatment with the disease-modifying anti-rheumatic drug (DMARD), sulfasalazine. A history of allergy to which one of the following drugs would be a contraindication to the use of sulfasalazine?

- [ ] A Amiodarone
- [x] B Co-trimoxazole
- [ ] C Lisinopril
- [ ] D Penicillin
- [ ] E Valaciclovir

2.57 A 22-year-old woman with poorly controlled asthma presented to the Emergency Department with wheeze and breathlessness. Peak flow rate was 150 l/min, and she was treated with intravenous hydrocortisone and nebulised salbutamol. Her clinical condition improved within 20 min. Which one of the following statements regarding her therapy is correct?

- [ ] A Hydrocortisone inhibits adenosine release
- [ ] B Hydrocortisone upregulates β_2 receptors in the lung
- [ ] C Increased heart rate after salbutamol is due to its β_1-agonist effects
- [ ] D Rapid response is due to additive effect of hydrocortisone and salbutamol
- [x] E Pharmacological effects of hydrocortisone take at least 6 h

2.58 Exposure to which one of the following agents is most likely to cause significant toxic effects within 1 h?

- [ ] A Amitriptyline
- [x] B Glue solvents
- [ ] C Lithium
- [ ] D Paracetamol
- [ ] E Warfarin

2.56   Answer: B

Co-trimoxazole (trimethoprim and sulfamethoxazole). Allergic reactions to sulphonamide are more likely than to trimethoprim, and suggests a high risk of allergic reaction to the sulfapyridine component of sulfasalazine. Therefore, an alternative aminosalicylic acid preparation should be used.

2.57   Answer: E

The anti-inflammatory effects of corticosteroids do not manifest for several hours after administration, but they should be given early in severe exacerbations of COPD or asthma. Salbutamol is a pure β_2 agonist. Tachycardia is due to functional crossover between β_1 and β_2 receptors, and due to peripheral vaodilatation.

2.58   Answer: B

Solvents (eg toluene) are readily absorbed through skin or by inhalation, leading to rapid onset of airway irritation, bronchospasm and asphyxiation. Systemic effects include nausea, reduced conscious level, and arrhythmia. Toxic effects of lithium are characteristically delayed while the drug accumulates intracellularly.

2.59 Compared with naproxen, which statement regarding celcoxib is true?

☐ **A** Anti-inflammatory effects are greater

☒ **B** Concomitant diuretic treatment can be given more safely

☐ **C** It acts by inhibiting a different enzyme pathway

☑ **D** It has a lower level of antiplatelet activity

☐ **E** There is a lower risk of hepatic adverse effects

2.60 A 60-year-old man describes a history of chest pain on exertion, and is diagnosed with angina. He is prescribed sublingual glyceryl trinitrate (GTN) as required. Which one of the following is *not* a mechanism by which GTN gives symptomatic relief?

☐ **A** Activation of guanylate cyclase

☐ **B** Dilation of collateral coronary vessels

☐ **C** Dilation of major peripheral veins

☒ **D** Formation of nitric oxide

☑ **E** Inhibition of calcium channels

2.61 You are asked to review a 24-year-old woman in the Medical Outpatient Department. She had attended the Emergency Department several weeks earlier complaining of anxiety symptoms, restlessness and poor concentration. Physical examination, routine blood tests, including thyroid function tests, and a resting ECG were normal, and she was given a short-term supply of diazepam. Which of the following is correct with regard to drug treatment of generalised anxiety disorder?

☑ **A** Beta-blockers are useful for controlling somatic symptoms of anxiety

☒ **B** Benzodiazepines should be avoided in chronic anxiety

☐ **C** Buspirone has anxiolytic properties mediated by the benzodiazepine receptor

☐ **D** Restlessness and disturbed sleep usually respond well to propranolol

☐ **E** Short-acting benzodiazepines do not increase the risk of falls in elderly patients

2.59	Answer: D

Antiplatelet activity is thought to be mediated predominantly through blockade of the COX-1 pathway.

2.60	Answer: E

GTN is metabolised by endothelium to liberate nitric oxide (NO). NO is rapidly degraded, so its effects are mediated close to its site of formation. It acts on vascular smooth muscle to cause relaxation and vasodilatation.

2.61	Answer: A

Benzodiazepines are useful for short-term control of anxiety but carry a risk of dependence and withdrawal phenomena. Sedative effects are enhanced by alcohol. Buspirone is an anxiolytic with longer duration of onset than benzodiazepines, and withdrawal is less likely to occur. Somatic symptoms (eg tachycardia) can respond well to β-blockers.

2.62   A 72-year-old woman presents to the Emergency Department having been thought to have accidentally taken an overdose of her normal medications. BM glucose is 1.8 mmol/l. Which of the following is most likely to cause hypoglycaemia in overdose?

☐ **A** Digoxin

☐ **B** Enalapril

☐ **C** Furosemide

☒ **D** Metoprolol

☒ **E** Paracetamol

2.63   A 22-year-old male student is admitted via the Emergency Department having been found unconscious by his flatmate. Initial investigations show: sodium 140 mmol/l, potassium 4.0 mmol/l, calcium 1.8 mmol/l, bicarbonate 12 mmol/l, and albumin 42 mmol/l. Ingestion of which of the following drugs is most likely to have caused these laboratory findings?

☐ **A** Amitriptyline

☐ **B** Ecstasy (MDMA)

☒ **C** Ethylene glycol

☐ **D** Heroin

☐ **E** Paracetamol

2.64   A 72-year-old man with disseminated prostatic carcinoma is taking regular modified-release oral morphine and regular paracetamol, with standard-release morphine for breakthrough pain. He is complaining of worsening rib and thoracic spine pain, associated with severe nausea, and you wish to adjust his drug regimen. Which of the following interventions would be most appropriate?

☐ **A** Add carbamazepine and reduce the dose of morphine

☐ **B** Add dexamethasone and reduce the dose of morphine

☒ **C** Add ibuprofen and reduce the dose of morphine

☐ **D** Substitute a once-daily morphine formulation

☒ **E** Substitute diamorphine given by continuous subcutaneous infusion

2.62 Answer: E

Hypoglycaemia is a recognised feature of paracetamol overdose, thought to be due to impaired glycogenolysis. A low BM recording should always be confirmed by a laboratory venous glucose measurement.

2.63 Answer: C

Ethylene glycol ingestion is associated with severe metabolic acidosis, hypocalcaemia, renal failure, seizures, arrhythmia and coma. Treatment is with ethanol (to compete for metabolism and reduce toxic metabolite formation) and haemodialysis to assist elimination of ethylene glycol and its metabolites.

2.64 Answer: C

NSAID treatment is effective for inflammatory bone pain. More flexible pain control can be achieved by combined long- and short-acting oral morphine preparations than by continuous administration (bioavailability also more predictable). Carbamazepine can be effective in neuropathic pain, and dexamethasone is useful for headache associated with raised intracranial pressure (ICP).

2.65 Which of the following is a recognised feature of cyclophosphamide treatment?

- [ ] **A** Absorbed poorly from the gut
- [ ] **B** Dermal photosensitivity
- [x] **C** Haemorrhagic cystitis
- [ ] **D** Hirsutism
- [ ] **E** Inhibition of folic acid

2.66 You see a 48-year-old man in the Medical Outpatient Department and note that he is receiving flupentixol as a depot preparation. Which one of the following statements regarding depot antipsychotic medications is correct?

- [ ] **A** Associated with poorer bioavailability than oral preparations
- [ ] **B** Around 20% of patients with schizophrenia receive depot preparations
- [ ] **C** Can easily be titrated to control adverse effects
- [ ] **D** Drug release can be delayed by up to several months
- [x] **E** They allow a greater remission rate than oral preparations

2.67 You see a 46-year-old in the Emergency Department on a Saturday night. He smells strongly of alcohol, and has slurred speech and unsteady gait. He is uncooperative with physical examination but there are no abnormal cardiac, respiratory or abdominal findings, and an ECG and chest X-ray are normal. You suspect from his demeanour that he regularly drinks alcohol to excess, and are concerned about the possibility of alcohol withdrawal syndrome (AWS). Which of the following is most accurate regarding AWS?

- [ ] **A** Alpha-blockers are useful in reducing symptom severity
- [ ] **B** Chlordiazepoxide is anxiolytic but does not reduce the risk of seizure
- [x] **C** Oral thiamine is recommended to prevent neuropathy
- [x] **D** Suicidal ideation is a recognised feature
- [ ] **E** Wernicke's encephalopathy can occur due to pyridoxine deficiency

2.65   Answer: C

Acrolein, a metabolite, causes this serious adverse effect. Mesna reacts with the metabolite, and prevents urothelial toxicity. Methotrexate exerts a folate antagonist effect, which can be avoided by administration of folinic acid.

2.66   Answer: E

Depot preparations are associated with high remission rates and assured compliance (used in 60% of patients in Europe). A disadvantage is the inability to down-titrate dose in the event of adverse effects. Drug release can be delayed by up to several weeks.

2.67   Answer: D

Thiamine is a co-factor for carbohydrate metabolism, and deficiency can be precipitated by dextrose administration (intravenous Pabrinex should be administered to prevent this). Diazepam and chlordiazepoxide are effective in symptom control in reducing courses, and reduce seizure risk.

2.68 A 34-year-old man presents 36 h after an intentional overdose of paracetamol, alcohol and fluoxetine. Which of the following tests would be most helpful in determining the prognosis?

☐ **A** Platelet count

☑ **B** Prothrombin time

☐ **C** Serum alanine transaminase

☐ **D** Serum alkaline phosphatase

☐ **E** Serum creatinine

2.69 You are asked to see a 28-year-old woman who is pregnant. She has been complaining of cough and fever for 3 days, and on respiratory examination is found to have crackles at the left lung base. You decide to prescribe a short course of antibiotics. Which of the following should be *avoided*?

☐ **A** Cefotaxime

☐ **B** Co-amoxiclav

☑ **C** Co-trimoxazole

☐ **D** Erythromycin

☐ **E** Metronidazole

2.70 A 34-year-old woman has developed cellulitis 2 weeks after giving birth to a healthy baby girl. There is marked erythema and tenderness of skin overlying the medial aspect of her left breast, and you wish to prescribe a course of antibiotics. She is breastfeeding her child. Which of the following drugs would it be most important to *avoid*?

☐ **A** Co-amoxiclav

☐ **B** Erythromycin

☐ **C** Flucloxacillin

☑ **D** Metronidazole

☒ **E** Trimethoprim

2.68 Answer: B

At 36 h after ingestion, it is unlikely that there will be a significant risk due to fluoxetine. Prothrombin time and alanine transaminase (ALT) are indicative of hepatocellular damage after paracetamol ingestion. Platelet count, ALT, renal function and lactate influence clinical management, but do not reliably inform prognosis.

2.69 Answer: C

Co-trimoxazole is potentially teratogenic, due to the anti-folate effects of trimethoprim. Sulphonamides confer a risk of neonatal haemolysis and methaemoglobinaemia. The others, including penicillin, are regarded as safe. Metronidazole is teratogenic in animals, but appears safe in humans.

2.70 Answer: D

Significant amounts of metronidazole are secreted in breast milk, which can alter neonatal gut flora to cause significant diarrhoea. Clarithromycin should be avoided, but erythromycin is only secreted in small amounts and appears safe. Penicillins and trimethoprim are secreted in breast milk in small amounts but appear safe.

2.71 Which one of the following drugs taken by a mother poses the greatest risk to her breastfed infant?

 A Aspirin

☒ B Diclofenac

☐ C Dipyridamole

☐ D Heparin

☐ E Warfarin

2.72 A 59-year-old woman presented to hospital 4 h after an alleged drug overdose. Initial investigations showed: sodium 139 mmol/l, potassium 6.3 mmol/l and urea 6.2 mmol/l. Ingestion of which one of the following drugs is most likely to have caused this metabolic abnormality?

☐ A Amitriptyline

☑ B Digoxin

☐ C Salbutamol

☐ D Theophylline

☐ E Verapamil

2.73 Which of the following poses the greatest risks to the developing fetus when taken by the mother in therapeutic doses?

☐ A Carbidopa

☑ B Carbimazole

☐ C Cefalexin

☐ D Cimetidine

☐ E Ciprofloxacin

2.74 A 34-year-old woman is undergoing antenatal screening and found to have consistently high blood pressure, averaging 164/82 mmHg. You wish to commence antihypertensive treatment. Which of the following is regarded as most safe?

☐ A Bendroflumethiazide

☐ B Bisoprolol

☑ C Methyldopa

☐ D Nifedipine

☐ E Perindopril

2.71 Answer: A

Aspirin poses the risk of Reye syndrome; high maternal doses of aspirin can impair neonatal platelet function (greater sensitivity). Dipyridamole is present in small amounts in breast milk, and requires some caution. The others are generally regarded as safe.

2.72 Answer: B

Other features include nausea, vomiting, xanthopsia, arrhythmia, seizures and coma. Toxic features (particularly arrhythmia) are more likely in the presence of hypokalaemia. Theophylline toxicity is associated with hypokalaemia and metabolic acidosis, and salbutamol causes dose-dependent hypokalaemia.

2.73 Answer: B

Risks of neonatal goitre and hypothyroidism. Ciprofloxacin and other quinolones usually avoided because animal studies have shown arthropathy.

2.74 Answer: C

Thiazide diuretics can cause neonatal thrombocytopenia, whereas β-blockers cause intrauterine growth retardation. Calcium-channel blockers can inhibit labour and are teratogenic in animals. ACE inhibitors and angiotensin II receptor antagonists are associated with oligohydramnios.

2.75 Which of the following drugs should be used with particular caution in very elderly patients?

- [ ] **A** Amoxicillin
- [x] **B** Enalapril
- [ ] **C** Low-dose aspirin
- [ ] **D** Quinine
- [x] **E** Ranitidine

2.76 Which one of the following drugs is significantly more likely to cause adverse effects in elderly rather than in young adults, when used in normal therapeutic doses?

- [ ] **A** Co-amoxiclav
- [ ] **B** Erythromycin
- [ ] **C** Omeprazole
- [x] **D** Temazepam
- [ ] **E** Thyroxine

2.77 A 64-year-old man is referred to the Outpatient Clinic for investigation of falls. On examination, he has features suggesting Parkinson's disease. Which of the following would be most effective as a potential treatment?

- [x] **A** Carbidopa
- [ ] **B** Dopamine
- [ ] **C** Lithium
- [ ] **D** Methyldopa
- [x] **E** Selegeline

2.75 Answer: B

In older patients with impaired renal blood flow, NSAIDs, ACE inhibitors and angiotensin receptor antagonists reduce efferent arteriolar tone and can cause a dramatic reduction in glomerular filtration.

2.76 Answer: D

Drugs with sedative properties are likely to cause greater effects in elderly patients, and caution is required, eg benzodiazepines, antidepressants, antipsychotics, due to inefficiency of the blood–brain barrier and cerebral atrophy.

2.77 Answer: E

Selegeline can be used as monotherapy or in addition to L-dopa. Carbidopa is a peripheral dopa decarboxylase inhibitor that is ineffective in the absence of L-dopa. Dopamine is broken down before crossing the blood–brain barrier; methyldopa is primarily an antihypertensive.

2.78 You see a 76-year-old woman in the Outpatient Department. She has had parkinsonism for a number of years, successfully treated with co-beneldopa (L-dopa and benserazide), one capsule three times daily. However, she has recently noticed that her mobility has become progressively worse just before each dose. Which of the following changes to her medications would be most appropriate?

- ☐ A Add bromocriptine
- ☐ B Discontinue co-beneldopa and commence L-dopa
- ☒ C Discontinue co-beneldopa and commence selegeline
- ☐ D Increase dose to two capsules three times per day
- ☑ E Maintain usual daily amount but switch to modified-release preparation

2.79 You review an 81-year-old man in the Medical Outpatient Department. He has been suffering from recurrent falls and reduced mobility. He had been started on L-dopa by his GP 4 weeks ago for suspected Parkinson's disease, but had not noted any significant improvement. On examination, his seated BP was 148/84 mmHg, and 116/80 mmHg on standing. Which of the following statements is correct?

- ☐ A Bromocriptine is a more appropriate treatment than L-dopa
- ☐ B Fludrocortisone treatment should be introduced
- ☐ C His blood pressure drop on standing indicates autonomic neuropathy
- ☐ D Lack of response to L-dopa excludes Parkinson's disease
- ☑ E L-Dopa should be combined with an extracerebral decarboxylase inhibitor

2.80 Which of the following drugs would it be most important to avoid, where possible, in patients with severe renal impairment?

- ☐ A Amoxicillin
- ☑ B Metformin
- ☐ C Omeprazole
- ☐ D Paracetamol
- ☐ E Simvastatin

2.78 Answer: E

'End of dose deterioration' can be addressed by switching to long-acting formulations, or by adding adjunctive treatment, eg entacapone. This avoids potential adverse effects of increasing the total daily dose.

2.79 Answer: E

Dopamine agonists (eg bromocriptine, cabergoline, ropinirole) are less appropriate in elderly patients due to potential neuropsychiatric adverse effects. Postural hypotension is a common adverse effect of L-dopa, but is less common in combination with a peripheral dopa decarboxylase inhibitor.

2.80 Answer: B

Metformin can cause lactic acidosis, especially in patients with renal impairment. The adverse effects of simvastatin (hepatitis and myositis) are more likely in patients with renal impairment, and it should be used with caution.

2.81   A 46-year-old woman is admitted to hospital for treatment of severe gastroenteritis and dehydration. Which one of the following drugs would be most likely to account for a sudden deterioration in her renal function?

- ☐ A   Ceftriaxone
- ☑ B   Ciprofloxacin
- ☐ C   Erythromycin
- ☐ D   Metronidazole
- ☒ E   Oral vancomycin

2.82   A 56-year-old man has been receiving warfarin for recurrent deep venous thrombosis, and his INR has been stable at 2.4–2.8 for the past 8 months. He presents to the Emergency Department pale, hypotensive and tachycardic after suffering abdominal pain and melaena. He had been started on antibiotic therapy 5 days earlier for a suspected respiratory tract infection. Which of the following drugs is most likely to have increased his risk of bleeding?

- ☐ A   Amoxicillin
- ☑ B   Ciprofloxacin
- ☐ C   Metronidazole
- ☐ D   Oxytetracycline
- ☐ E   Rifampicin

2.83   A 42-year-old woman is admitted to the Emergency Department with severe colicky abdominal pain, nausea and vomiting. You diagnose left-sided ureteric colic and possible pyelonephritis. Which of the following is correct regarding symptomatic treatment?

- ☐ A   Azapropazone causes less GI irritation than ibuprofen
- ☑ B   Diclofenac is associated with a 10-fold increased risk of aplastic anaemia
- ☐ C   Meptazinol causes greater respiratory depression than morphine
- ☐ D   Morphine provides rapid relief of pain and nausea
- ☒ E   Pethidine is associated with tachycardia and hypertension

2.81 Answer: B

Severe dehydration increases the risk of ciprofloxacin-induced crystalluria, especially when high doses are used.

2.82 Answer: B

Ciprofloxacin is an enzyme inhibitor, so the INR and bleeding risk will increase. Metronidazole has weak hepatic enzyme inhibiting properties. Other important enzyme inhibitors are erythromycin, cimetidine and allopurinol. Rifampicin is an enzyme inducer that is likely to cause a fall in INR.

2.83 Answer: B

Azapropazone appears to be associated with the greatest risk of GI irritation, and ibuprofen the lowest risk amongst NSAIDs. Meptazinol is a partial agonist, thought to cause less respiratory depression. Opiates provide effective pain relief, but cause nausea and haemodynamic effects (tachycardia and hypotension), partly due to histamine release.

2.84 You are asked to review a 56-year-old woman who was admitted 3 days earlier for treatment of severe community-acquired pneumonia. Her liver biochemistry tests were normal on admission to hospital, but now show: bilirubin 58 μmol/l, alanine transaminase 52 IU/l, alkaline phosphatase 256 IU/l, γ-glutamyl transpeptidase (GGT) 54 IU/l and albumin 41 g/l. Which one of the following drugs is most likely to have caused these abnormalities?

- [ ] **A** Amoxicillin
- [ ] **B** Ciprofloxacin
- [ ] **C** Clarithromycin
- [x] **D** Co-amoxiclav
- [x] **E** Trimethoprim

2.85 A 45-year-old businesswoman has returned to the UK from a 6-month business trip to Pakistan. Two weeks earlier, she had suffered fever, breathlessness and cough, and was commenced on treatment. Her blood tests show: bilirubin 52 μmol/l, alanine transaminase 196 IU/l, alkaline phosphatase 76 IU/l, GGT 64 IU/l and albumin 37 g/l. Which one of the following drugs is most likely to have caused these abnormalities?

- [ ] **A** Ciprofloxacin
- [ ] **B** Co-amoxiclav
- [ ] **C** Erythromycin
- [ ] **D** Ethambutol
- [x] **E** Rifampicin

2.86 A 17-year-old girl presented to the Emergency Department 2 h after deliberately taking a paracetamol overdose. A 4-h serum paracetamol level was 260 mg/l and intravenous NAC administration was commenced. One hour later, she became nauseated, and was found to have facial flushing and an urticarial rash over her trunk and back. You suspect an anaphylactoid reaction to the NAC treatment. Which of the following statements is correct?

- [ ] **A** Anaphylactoid reactions occur in 2–5% of patients treated with NAC
- [ ] **B** Antihistamines must be administered early
- [ ] **C** Corticosteroid treatment should be routinely administered
- [x] **D** NAC treatment should be discontinued and not re-commenced
- [ ] **E** Nebulised salbutamol can improve the clinical condition

2.84   Answer: D

The pattern of biochemical abnormalities is consistent with biliary obstruction or cholestatic jaundice. Also recognised as an adverse effect of erythromycin and, rarely, ciprofloxacin.

2.85   Answer: E

The biochemical abnormalities are consistent with hepatitis. Rifampicin, isoniazid, pyrazinamide and rifabutin can all cause hepatotoxicity. Ethambutol can cause visual disturbances, especially in patients with renal impairment.

2.86   Answer: E

Stopping the infusion is often all that is required. Antihistamine may be necessary, and corticosteroids are indicated only if the reaction is severe. Nebulised bronchodilators should be used if bronchospasm is significant. NAC can often be recommenced at a lower rate.

2.87 A 56-year-old man has been treated for asthma for 8 years, and is taking regular theophylline and inhaled beclometasone, and salbutamol when required. Four days ago he suffered increased cough and fever, and was commenced on an antibiotic. He is now complaining of severe nausea and headache, and plasma theophylline concentration is found to be 186 µmol/l (therapeutic range 55–110 µmol/l). Which of the following drugs is most likely to have precipitated the theophylline toxicity?

- A   Amoxicillin
- ☑ B   Ciprofloxacin
- C   Co-amoxiclav
- D   Metronidazole
- E   Penicillin V

2.88 Which of the following statements is correct regarding the development of potential new drugs?

- A   Further development is abandoned if no therapeutic effects are seen in phase I studies
- B   Head-to-head comparison with existing therapy occurs only in phase IV studies
- ☑ C   Oral bioavailability can be examined in phase I studies
- D   Phase I studies typically involve 100–500 patients
- ☒ E   Phase IV studies must be completed before a marketing licence is given

2.89 You are involved in the conduct of a study to investigate the effects of a new treatment for septic shock in patients admitted to an intensive therapy unit (ITU). Which of the following statements is correct regarding the conduct of such a study?

- ☒ A   A double-blind, randomised, placebo-controlled design must be used
- B   Consent need not be sought because most patients will be unconscious
- C   If suitability for inclusion is in doubt then patients should be enrolled to increase statistical power
- D   It is usually acceptable to withhold standard care during a clinical trial
- ☑ E   Next of kin can provide consent on behalf of the patient

2.87 Answer: B

Theophylline is metabolised by the liver, and has a narrow therapeutic range. Ciprofloxacin is an enzyme inhibitor, so that theophylline metabolism is delayed and clearance reduced. Others include erythromycin, allopurinol and omeprazole.

2.88 Answer: C

Phase I studies (including 'first in human') determine safety, and usually involve healthy volunteers. Data from single and multiple administration dose-escalation studies can be used to determine pharmacokinetics. Efficacy is determined in phases II and III, often against a comparator. Phase IV studies are often undertaken post-marketing.

2.89 Answer: E

Where possible, informed consent should be sought. If appropriate, this can be obtained from the next of kin or appointed guardian, and an independent arbitrator can oversee in cases of doubt. It would be exceptional for standard therapy to be withheld, particularly in a critical care environment.

2.90 You are supervising a single ascending dose phase I study in healthy subjects. On reviewing the safety data after the second dose tier, you note that one of eight subjects had an elevated alanine transaminase (145 IU/l) at 24 h after dose administration. Which of the following statements is correct?

- [ ] **A** Development of the drug should be abandoned
- [ ] **B** Further dose escalation should be halted
- [x] **C** Interpretation depends on clinical and laboratory safety variables and pharmacokinetic data
- [ ] **D** The study blinding code must be broken
- [ ] **E** The subject in question must have received active drug

2.91 A 62-year-old woman has been taking the same dose of digoxin for 8 years for chronic atrial fibrillation. She attends the Emergency Department with a short history of nausea, vomiting and visual disturbance, and is found to have a serum digoxin level of 3.4 nmol/ml (therapeutic range 1.1–2.5 nmol/l). Introduction of which of the following drugs is most likely to have precipitated digoxin toxicity?

- [ ] **A** Atenolol
- [ ] **B** Doxazosin
- [x] **C** Omeprazole
- [ ] **D** Ramipril
- [x] **E** Verapamil

2.92 A 52-year-old man attends the Medical Outpatient Department for investigation of anaemia. Initial investigations show: bilirubin 58 µmol/l, Hb 8.7 g/dl and mean cell volume (MCV) 101 fl. Which of the following drugs is most likely to account for these abnormalities?

- [ ] **A** Amiodarone
- [ ] **B** Hydralazine
- [x] **C** Methyldopa
- [x] **D** Methotrexate
- [ ] **E** Thyroxine

2.90   Answer: C

It is not uncommon for abnormal liver function tests to occur, sometimes > 2× upper limit of normal, even after placebo administration (hence need for placebo arm in early phase I). The study code need only be broken if the adverse effect is regarded as serious and possibly study drug-related.

2.91   Answer: E

Verapamil and nifedipine impair renal clearance of digoxin. Verapamil, diltiazem and β-blockers enhance atrioventricular (AV) nodal blockade but do not significantly increase digoxin concentrations.

2.92   Answer: C

The investigations indicate anaemia, mild macrocytosis and hyperbilirubinaemia, which strongly suggest haemolysis. Urobilinogen on urinalysis is also recognised. Methyldopa and penicillin cause antibody-mediated warm autoimmune haemolytic anaemia (WAHA).

2.93 You are reviewing data regarding development of a novel compound for the treatment of asthma. Drug 'A' is a more potent bronchodilator than drug 'B'. Which of the following statements regarding drug 'A' is correct?

- A Causes the same response as drug 'B' at any given dose
- B It causes a greater clinical response
- C It is more efficacious
- D It is associated with fewer adverse effects
- ☑ E Lower concentrations can cause the same effects as drug 'B'

2.94 A 13-year-old girl presents with a history of severe headache and nausea. She undergoes a lumbar puncture examination, and cerebrospinal fluid (CSF) microscopy is strongly suggestive of viral meningitis. You are asked to prescribe analgesia in view of her persisting headache. Which of the following statements is correct?

- ☑ A Combined codeine-paracetamol preparations are more effective than paracetamol alone
- B High-dose aspirin would be a suitable treatment
- C Non-steroidal anti-inflammatory drugs are effective
- D Paracetamol should be avoided in this condition
- E Short-acting opiate treatment is preferred

2.95 A 34-year-old woman attends the Emergency Department having suffered intermittent and severe left-sided headaches over the past 10 days. She suffered similar symptoms around 3 years ago and was investigated at another hospital. You suspect that she is suffering from cluster headaches. Which of the following is true regarding the pharmacological treatment of cluster headache?

- A Alcohol excess can increase the risk of a further headache cluster
- ☑ B Inhalation of 100% oxygen can abort the headache
- C Oral ergotamine treatment is highly effective
- D Prophylactic treatment has no clear role in management
- E Symptoms do not respond to NSAIDs

2.93 Answer: E

Potency is an expression of drug efficacy with regard to the administered dose/tissue concentration. Both drugs might be equally efficacious, and no comment can be made regarding clinical utility.

2.94 Answer: A

Combinations of codeine or dihydrocodeine with paracetamol have marginally greater analgesic efficacy than paracetamol alone. Aspirin has better anti-inflammatory effects but is contraindicated in patients < 16 years of age, due to the risk of Reye syndrome. Opiates increase nausea, so use sparingly.

2.95 Answer: B

Oral ergotamine is too slow-acting. Although access is limited, 100% oxygen is effective treatment. Parenteral dihydroergotamine or serotonin-1 (5-HT$_1$) agonists have rapid onset. Alcohol precipitates headache during cluster, but does not evoke clusters when in remission. Prophylactic treatment includes lithium, verapamil and pizotifen. Chronic paroxysmal hemicrania variant responds well to indometacin.

2.96 You are reviewing the clinical trial literature regarding tamoxifen, a partial oestrogen agonist. Which of the following statements regarding partial agonists is correct?

☐ **A** Higher doses are needed to achieve the same response as a pure receptor agonist

☐ **B** They competitively antagonise the effects of pure receptor antagonists

☐ **C** They do not exhibit any dose–response relationship

☑ **D** They have a lower E_{max} than pure receptor agonists

☐ **E** They show binding affinity but no intrinsic efficacy

2.97 Which of the following is *most* likely to be a feature of buprenorphine treatment?

☐ **A** Causes greater respiratory depression in overdose than morphine

☒ **B** Effects are not reversed by naloxone

☑ **C** It has a lower potential for dependence than morphine

☐ **D** It is < 5% bound to plasma proteins

☐ **E** Plasma half-life is around 18 hours

2.98 Which of the following statements best describes the role of local Drug and Therapeutics Committees?

☐ **A** Cheaper drugs are always recommended as first-line treatments

☐ **B** Decide optimum treatment on the basis of the monthly prescription cost

☐ **C** Determine the safety and efficacy of new drugs

☑ **D** Evaluate the clinical effectiveness and cost-effectiveness of drugs

☐ **E** Primarily ration delivery of effective treatments

2.99 Adverse drug effects and drug interactions place individual patients at risk, and add an additional healthcare burden for the NHS. What proportion of patients is admitted to acute medical units in the UK wholly or partly as a result of adverse drug effects?

☐ **A** 0.01%

☐ **B** 0.3%

☑ **C** 3%

☐ **D** 15%

☐ **E** 40%

| 2.96 | Answer: D |

Agonists, antagonists and partial agonists all exhibit binding affinity. Agonists have full intrinsic efficacy, antagonists have none, and partial agonists are intermediate. Partial agonists will have lower E_{max} than agonists, regardless of whether the dose can competitively inhibit the effects of a full agonist.

| 2.97 | Answer: C |

Buprenorphine is a mixed agonist-antagonist that behaves as an opiate partial agonist. It is less effectively reversed by naxolone. It has less potential for dependence and withdrawal syndromes and can be a useful adjunct in opiate withdrawal programmes. Plasma protein binding is > 95%, and the half-life is 2–3 hours.

| 2.98 | Answer: D |

Regulatory authorities (eg MHRA) determine quality and safety of new drugs. Drug and Therapeutics Committees are interested in ensuring that clinically effective and cost-effective treatments are used appropriately in clinical practice.

| 2.99 | Answer: C |

The proportion may be significantly higher, although studies suggest that acute hospital attendances directly attributable to adverse effects of medications is thought to be 2–12%.

2.100 One of your patients asks for some general advice regarding laxative treatment for simple constipation. Which one of the following statements is correct regarding treatment of simple constipation?

- ☐ **A** Bisacodyl acts as a faecal softener
- ☒ **B** Ispaghula husk should be avoided in patients with diverticular disease
- ☑ **C** Lactulose is a disaccharide that is not absorbed from the gut
- ☐ **D** Magnesium salts act as stool bulking agents
- ☐ **E** Senna typically takes 48–72 h to take effect

2.101 Use of which of the following recreational drugs is likely to present with features of agitation and hyponatraemia?

- ☐ **A** Benzodiazepines
- ☐ **B** Cannabis
- ☐ **C** Cocaine
- ☑ **D** Ecstasy
- ☐ **E** Heroin

2.102 A patient comes to the surgery complaining of muscle pain. You note that he has familial mixed hyperlipidaemia and is currently taking atorvastatin and fenofibrate in combination. He has recently been prescribed some antiobiotics by a locum. His creatine kinase is elevated at 490 IU/l. Which of the following antibiotics is most likely to be responsible?

- ☑ **A** Clarithromycin
- ☐ **B** Amoxicillin
- ☐ **C** Olfloxacin
- ☐ **D** Metronidazole
- ☐ **E** Ciprofloxacin

2.100 Answer: C

Stimulant laxatives, eg bisacodyl and senna, act within 6–12 h. Bulking agents, such as ispaghula husk, can take 48–72 h to take effect, and are useful in patients with stomas, diverticulosis and irritable bowel sydrome. Osmotic laxatives increase water in the large bowel, including phosphate enemas, magnesium and sodium salts, and lactulose.

2.101 Answer: D

This may be one of the mechanisms by which ecstasy increases the risk of seizures. Other characteristic effects include euphoria or dysphoria, restlessness, hyperthermia, coma and multi-organ failure.

2.102 Answer: A

Atorvastatin is metabolised by CYP-3A4, which is inhibited by clarithromycin, which is therefore the most likely to have led to the increased myopathy reported here. Patients taking a statin and fibrate in combination are particularly prone to the problem.

Clinical pharmacology answers

3. CLINICAL SCIENCES

3.1 A 58-year-old patient with long-standing diabetes comes to the clinic with a swollen, deformed right ankle. He says that he is finding it difficult to walk because the ankle aches. He has diabetic peripheral neuropathy. On examination the ankle is warm, swollen and deformed. His ESR is measured at 8 mm/h. Which of the following is the most likely diagnosis?

☑ **A** Charcot's arthropathy

☐ **B** Gout

☐ **C** Infective arthritis

☐ **D** Osteoarthritis

☐ **E** Reiter syndrome

3.2 A patient comes to the clinic with nephrotic syndrome. Which of the following is the most likely finding?

☐ **A** High serum calcium

☐ **B** Increased high-density lipoprotein (HDL) cholesterol

☒ **C** Increased infections due to low gammaglobulin

☑ **D** Increased non-HDL cholesterol

☐ **E** Raised prothrombin time (PT) and activated partial thromboplastin time (APTT)

3.3 A new drug is launched which acts on tumour necrosis factor alpha (TNFα). Which one of the following is true of TNFα?

☐ **A** It acts on only one target cell

☐ **B** It is a 422-amino-acid protein

☐ **C** Low levels are associated with rheumatoid arthritis

☑ **D** Raised levels are associated with increased insulin resistance

☐ **E** TNFα is produced only by fat cells

3.1 Answer: A

Proven neuropathy with a relatively painless, deformed joint and normal ESR makes Charcot's the most likely diagnosis.

3.2 Answer: D

Nephrotic syndrome leads to protein loss, although infections are not particularly common. Lipoprotein changes lead to increased non-HDL cholesterol levels.

3.3 Answer: D

Raised levels are associated with insulin resistance and a number of inflammatory conditions.

3.4 A lady presents with advanced breast cancer. Treatment is planned with an ErbB2 inhibitor. Which one of the following is most commonly recognised as an adverse effect?

A Constrictive pericarditis

B Diarrhoea

C Dilated cardiomyopathy

D Haemorrhagic cystitis

E Pulmonary fibrosis

3.5 A 20-year-old man presents to the Neurology Department with symptoms of Parkinson's. Which of the following is the usual inheritance pattern of juvenile Parkinson's disease?

A Autosomal dominant

B Autosomal recessive

C X-linked dominant

D X-linked recessive

E X-linked recessive with genetic anticipation

3.6 You are reviewing the action of rituximab and its data in rheumatoid arthritis. Which of the following best describes the action of rituximab?

A An anti-CD3

B An anti-CD8

C An anti-CD20

D An anti-CD26

E An anti-CD21

3.7 Which one of the following best describes the mechanism of action of osteoprotogenerin?

A It decreases osteoblast activity

B It increases osteoblast activity

C It increases osteoclast activity

D It decreases osteoclast activity

E It is produced by osteoclasts

3.4   Answer: C

ErbB2 expression prevents the development of dilated cardiomyopathy.

3.5   Answer: B

Parkinson's is very rare in under-40s, but the very early-onset form is an autosomal recessive disorder.

3.6   Answer: C

Rituximab is an anti-CD20 agent; CD-20 is expressed on B lymphocytes.

3.7   Answer: D

Osteoprotogenerin is produced by osteoblasts and decreases osteoclast formation and activity.

3.8 A 50-year-old man presents with increased skin pigmentation, type 2 diabetes mellitus, chronic liver disease and erectile dysfunction. On which chromosome is the underlying defect most likely to be found?

☐ A Chromosome 4
☑ B Chromosome 6
☐ C Chromosome 8
☐ D Chromosome 11
☐ E Chromosome 12

3.9 You are asked to take part in the study of a new treatment for type 1 diabetes; it is an anti-CD3 monoclonal antibody. Where is the CD3 receptor found?

☐ A On B lymphocytes
☒ B On β cells
☐ C On eosinophils
☐ D On macrophages
☑ E On T lymphocytes

3.10 GLP-1 is a small-bowel hormone. Which one of the following correctly describes one of the actions of GLP-1?

☐ A It has proved effects in regenerating human β cells
☐ B It increases blood glucose
☒ C It increases glucagon levels
☑ D It increases insulin levels
☐ E It speeds up gastric emptying

3.11 A couple had a child who was thought to have died of Wiskott–Aldrich syndrome. Which of the following would most likely suggest an alternative diagnosis?

☐ A Eczema
☐ B Haematological malignancy
☑ C High platelets
☐ D Low platelets
☒ E IgM deficiency

3.8   Answer: B

The *HFE* gene is found on chromosome 6, which encodes HFE protein, also known as human haemochromatosis protein.

3.9   Answer: E

CD3 monoclonals are T lymphocyte-specific.

3.10   Answer: D

Beta-cell regeneration is theoretical at the moment.

3.11   Answer: C

Wiskott–Aldrich syndrome is associated with low platelets.

3.12 Which of the following is most likely to occur in patients with chronic hypertriglyceridaemia?

- [ ] **A** Acute cholecystitis
- [ ] **B** Diabetes insipidus
- [x] **C** Eruptive xanthomata
- [ ] **D** Hypothyroidism
- [ ] **E** Nephrotic syndrome

3.13 A mother is undergoing tissue matching in an attempt to give a kidney to her son. She is being matched for class II antigens. Which of the following is a class II human leukocyte antigen (HLA) antigen?

- [ ] **A** HLA-A
- [ ] **B** HLA-B
- [ ] **C** HLA-C
- [x] **D** HLA-DP
- [ ] **E** HLA-G

3.14 You are asked to review a family in which the male members are affected by a genetic disorder but the female members are not. Which of the following is an X-linked recessive disorder?

- [ ] **A** Achondroplasia
- [x] **B** Becker's muscular dystrophy
- [x] **C** Gilbert's disease
- [ ] **D** Marfan syndrome
- [ ] **E** Neurofibromatosis

3.15 A 32-year-old woman presents with renal stones. Which of the following is the commonest type of renal stone?

- [x] **A** Calcium phosphate
- [ ] **B** Cystine stones
- [ ] **C** Silicate
- [ ] **D** Struvite
- [ ] **E** Uric acid

3.12   Answer: C

Eruptive xanthomata and pancreatitis occur more commonly in patients with hypertriglyceridaemia.

3.13   Answer: D

HLA-DP, -DQ and -DR are class II antigens.

3.14   Answer: B

Muscular dystrophies are generally inherited in an X-linked recessive manner.

3.15   Answer: A

Calcium-containing renal stones are the commonest type. Struvite stones occur with *Proteus* infection.

3.16 A woman undergoes a second renal transplant. Unfortunately she suffers acute rejection, thought to be due to anti-HLA antibodies. Which type of immunoglobulin are anti-HLA antibodies?

- ☐ A IgA
- ☐ B IgD
- ☐ C IgE
- ☑ D IgG
- ☒ E IgM

3.17 Which of the following muscles normally serves to abduct the larynx?

- ☐ A Cricothyroid
- ☐ B Lateral cricoarytenoid
- ☐ C Oblique arytenoid
- ☑ D Posterior cricoarytenoid
- ☐ E Transverse arytenoid

3.18 A man presents with an episode of haematemesis. An endoscopy shows extensive peptic ulceration. He was admitted for a similar event 6 months earlier and started on high-dose omeprazole. Which hormone would you measure?

- ☐ A Cholecystokinin
- ☑ B Gastrin
- ☐ C Glucagon-like peptide 1 (GLP-1)
- ☐ D Secretin
- ☐ E Somatostatin

3.19 A 32-year-old woman presents with primary pulmonary hypertension. Which of the following is most implicated in primary pulmonary hypertension?

- ☐ A Angiotensin I
- ☐ B Angiotensin II
- ☑ C Endothelin
- ☐ D Oxytocin
- ☒ E Vasopressin

3.16   Answer: D

IgG antibodies lead to acute rejection.

3.17   Answer: D

The others all cause adduction; the cricothyroid muscle also lengthens the larynx.

3.18   Answer: B

Gastrin is associated with increased secretion of gastric acid.

3.19   Answer: C

Endothelin-receptor antagonists are an important therapy option for primary pulmonary hypertension.

3.20 A man who is admitted with chest pain is found to have a raised troponin. Which of the following best describes the location of troponin in the cardiac myocyte?

A Adjacent to the thick myofilaments

B Adjacent to the thin myofilaments

C Free within the cytoplasm

D In the mitochondria

E In the T tubules

3.21 You are responsible for quality control for the biochemistry lab. Which of the following is likely to be a lab error?

A pH 7.38, PaO_2 13.2 kPa, $PaCO_2$ 3.9 kPa, bicarbonate 17 mmol/l

B pH 7.15, PaO_2 13.8 kPa, $PaCO_2$ 3.0 kPa, bicarbonate 24 mmol/l

C pH 7.42, PaO_2 12.8 kPa, $PaCO_2$ 5.2 kPa, bicarbonate 22 mmol/l

D pH 7.35, PaO_2 9.6 kPa, $PaCO_2$ 7.0 kPa, bicarbonate 32 mmol/l

E pH 7.45, PaO_2 13.5 kPa, $PaCO_2$ 3.4 kPa, bicarbonate 18 mmol/l

3.22 A 27-year-old woman comes to the hospital for a scan; she is 24 weeks pregnant. The child's father has haemophilia A and the fetus is male. What is the chance that the child has haemophilia A?

A 0%

B 10%

C 20%

D 50%

E 100%

3.23 A 29-year-old woman is 24 weeks pregnant with a male fetus. Her father has haemophilia A. Her partner is in good health. What is the chance of the child having haemophilia A?

A 100%

B 75%

C 50%

D 25%

E 0%

3.20   Answer: B

Troponin binds to actin, forming an actin–tropomyosin complex.

3.21   Answer: B

The pH is low, but the $PaCO_2$ is low and the bicarbonate in the normal range. The low pH would normally be explained by either a respiratory acidosis (high $PaCO_2$) or metabolic acidosis (low bicarbonate).

3.22   Answer: A

The child's X chromosome comes from the mother, who is normal. She is unlikely to be a carrier of haemophilia.

3.23   Answer: C

The mother has one affected X chromosome, which comes from her father.

3.24 A 27-year-old man who has fragile X syndrome is having a child. His partner has cerebral palsy but is not known to suffer from any inherited disorder. What is the chance of a daughter being a carrier for fragile X?

- ☒ **A** 0%
- ☐ **B** 25%
- ☐ **C** 33%
- ☐ **D** 50%
- ☑ **E** 100%

3.25 A woman with chronic myeloid leukaemia is Phildelphia chromosome-positive. You're aware this represents expression of the BCR-ABL fusion protein. What does the *BCR-ABL* gene code for?

- ☐ **A** Alkaline phosphatase
- ☐ **B** Epidermal growth factor
- ☐ **C** Serine protease
- ☑ **D** Tyrosine kinase
- ☐ **E** Xanthine oxidase

3.26 Which of the following statements is most accurate with respect to hepcidin?

- ☐ **A** High levels cause iron overload in haemochromatosis
- ☐ **B** It increases iron absorption from the gut
- ☒ **C** It is a 55-kDa glycoprotein
- ☑ **D** Levels are increased in anaemia of chronic disease
- ☐ **E** Most circulating hepcidin is of dietary origin in humans

3.27 Which of the following is the most commonly recognised feature of relapsing polychondritis?

- ☑ **A** Airway compromise from tracheolaryngeal disease is an important cause of mortality
- ☐ **B** Co-exisiting autoimmune or connective tissue disease is rare
- ☐ **C** It is usually inherited in an autosomal dominant pattern
- ☐ **D** Non-cartilaginous tissue is the predominant site of involvement
- ☐ **E** Treatment is with long-term antibiotics

3.24 Answer: E

The inheritance pattern most closely resembles X-linked dominant with variable penetrance.

3.25 Answer: D

Tyrosine kinase induces massive granulocytic expansion.

3.26 Answer: D

Involved in iron metabolism: enterocyte iron absorption and macrophage iron cycling. High levels are associated with anaemia of chronic disease, low levels with iron overload (eg in haemochromatosis).

3.27 Answer: A

Cartilage is classically affected, resulting in collapse of the nasal bridge, cardiac valve dysfunction and hearing loss. Diagnosis is via auricular cartilage biopsy. Treatment is with high-dose steroids and cytotoxic agents.

3.28 Which of the following statements best describes the long-term management of nephrotic syndrome?

   A Antibiotics are required routinely

   B Anticoagulation is not required routinely

   C Diuretics should be avoided

   D Lipid-lowering drugs are ineffective in this disorder

   E Salt restriction is an important measure

3.29 von Willebrand factor (vWF) is an important protein in maintaining cardiovascular integrity. Which of the following best describes the features of von Willebrand's disease?

   A Bleeding time is prolonged, vWF is increased, factor VIII is reduced

   B Bleeding time is prolonged, vWF is reduced, factor VIII is reduced

   C Bleeding time is prolonged, vWF is reduced, factor VIII is increased

   D Bleeding time is reduced, vWF is reduced, factor VIII is increased

   E Bleeding time is reduced, vWF is reduced, factor VIII is reduced

3.30 A GP refers a patient with α-galactosidase A deficiency to the Medical Outpatients Department for investigation of renal impairment. Which of the following is most accurate with regard to this condition?

   A Corneal microdeposits suggest an alternative diagnosis

   B Diagnosis is confirmed by skin biopsy

   C End-stage renal failure is a rare complication

   D Inheritance is autosomal dominant

   E Treatment involves administration of α-galactosidase

3.31 A Turkish man presents to the Emergency Department with a painful genital ulcer. On examination, he also has conjunctival injection and you consider a diagnosis of Behçet's disease. Which of the following is most strongly supportive of this diagnosis?

   A Anterior uveitis

   B Erythema nodosum

   C HLA-B51 positivity

   D Positive pathergy test

   E Recurrent genital and oral ulceration

3.28 Answer: E

Salt restriction is important in managing oedema. In severe oedema a low sodium diet and large doses of combination diuretics may be required.

3.29 Answer: B

vWF is a carrier protein for factor VIII, and forms bridges between platelets and collagen, so allowing platelets to adhere to damaged vessel walls. Bleeding is often superficial bruising or mucosal bleeds (epistaxis/gastrointestinal/menorrhagia).

3.30 Answer: E

Renal failure is often apparent by the fifth decade. There is deposition of glycospinolipids in liver, kidney, nerve cells and blood cells, and inheritance is X-linked recessive.

3.31 Answer: C

There is a strong association with HLA-B51, although not essential for the diagnosis. Note that pathergy is a hypersensitivity reaction at the site of minor trauma.

3.32 Which one of the following features is *least* likely to be found in Werner syndrome (MEN I) and might suggest an alternative diagnosis?

- A Autosomal dominant inheritance pattern
- B Gastrinoma
- C Medullary carcinoma of thyroid
- D Pituitary tumours
- E Primary hyperparathyroidism

3.33 Which of the following most strongly suggests a diagnosis of Sipple syndrome (MEN II) in a patient with high serum calcium?

- A Autosomal recessive inheritance pattern
- B Marfanoid habitus
- C Multinodular goitre
- D Pancreatic cyst on CT scan
- E Primary hyperparathyroidism

3.34 Which of the following features most strongly suggests a diagnosis of Wilson's disease?

- A Autosomal dominant pattern of inheritance
- B Cerebellar incoordination
- C Lens dislocation
- D Serum copper levels are increased
- E Urinary copper levels are reduced

3.35 Which of the following conditions is most likely to be a feature of Wilson's disease in adults?

- A Alcoholic liver disease
- B Hypercalcaemia
- C Low serum bicarbonate
- D Raised reticulocyte count
- E Wilms' tumor

3.32   Answer: C

MEN I: primary hyperparathyroidism, pituitary tumours, pancreatic tumours.

3.33   Answer: B

Other features include medullary carcinoma of the thyroid, mucosal neuromata, phaeochromocytoma and primary hyperparathyroidism (the latter is too common to support a MEN syndrome in the absence of other abnormalities).

3.34   Answer: D

Defect in synthesis of caeruloplasmin prevents excretion of copper through bile (normal route). Therefore there is increased serum copper/urine copper and hepatic copper content. Reduced serum caeruloplasmin levels.

3.35   Answer: D

Recognised features are haemolysis, hepatocellular carcinoma, parkinsonism and renal tubular acidosis. Wilms' tumor or nephroblastoma is a childhood urological malignancy and not related to Wilson's disease.

3.36 A young man presents to you with dysdiadochokinesia and an ataxic gait. There is no vertigo or hearing loss. Which one of the following is most likely?

- [ ] **A** Acoustic neuroma
- [ ] **B** Myasthenia gravis
- [ ] **C** Neurofibromatosis type 2
- [✓] **D** von Hippel–Lindau syndrome
- [ ] **E** von Recklinghausen's disease

3.37 Tuberous sclerosis is a rare neurological condition with a number of clinical manifestations. Which of the following is most likely to be a feature of the condition?

- [ ] **A** Acne vulgaris
- [ ] **B** Hypertension
- [✗] **C** Marfanoid body habitus
- [✓] **D** Peri-ungual fibroma
- [ ] **E** Torticollis

3.38 Which of the following is *least* likely to be a feature of Peutz–Jeghers syndrome?

- [ ] **A** Autosomal dominant pattern of inheritance
- [ ] **B** Bowel obstruction due to intussusception
- [ ] **C** Malignant transformation of gastrointestinal polyps
- [ ] **D** Peri-oral mucocutaneous pigmentation
- [✓] **E** Vitamin B_{12} deficiency

3.39 A 38-year-old man presents with diarrhoea and evidence of malabsorption. There is no history of travel abroad and you suspect coeliac disease and arrange a jejunal biopsy. Which of the following findings most strongly supports this diagnosis?

- [ ] **A** CLO test-positive
- [ ] **B** Granulomata
- [ ] **C** Inclusion bodies seen after silver staining
- [ ] **D** Lymphocyte infiltration of the sub-villus margin
- [✓] **E** Sub-total villus atrophy on microscopy

3.36   Answer: D

Autosomal dominant inheritance. A combination of retinal and intra-cranial haemangioblastomas, typically cerebellar.

3.37   Answer: D

Tuberous sclerosis is a classic triad of mental retardation, epilepsy and cutaneous manifestations (shagreen patches/ash-leaf macules/peri-/subungual fibromas/adenoma sebaceum). Peripheral calcification of cerebral tissue can occasionally be seen on plain skull X-ray.

3.38   Answer: E

GI tract involvement includes polyps which may undergo malignant change, and regular review is required, with polypectomy where necessary.

3.39   Answer: E

Sub-total villus atrophy on jejunal biopsy is also seen with viral gastroenteritis, giardiasis, hypogammaglobulinaemia, and soya milk and cow's milk protein intolerance.

3.40 Which of the following disorders is correctly paired with the corresponding genetic abnormality responsible?

- A Down syndrome – trisomy 12
- B Fragile X syndrome – 46,XYY
- ☒ C Klinefelter syndrome – 46,XXY
- D Testicular feminisation syndrome – 46,XXY
- ☑ E Turner syndrome – 45,X

3.41 Which of the following statements best describes the role of mast cells?

- A Activated by complement but not by physical injury
- B Derived from eosinophils
- C Do not contain lytic enzymes
- ☑ D Release histamine
- E Stimulate IgG-mediated responses

3.42 Which of the following features is most commonly recognised as a manifestation of immune thrombocytopenic purpura?

- A Diarrhoea
- B Hypothermia
- C Liver failure
- ☑ D Neurological involvement
- E Raised white cell count

3.43 Which of the following disorders is most likely to show genetic anticipation?

- A Charcot–Marie–Tooth disease
- ☒ B Duchenne muscular dystrophy
- ☑ C Friedreich's ataxia
- D Hereditary spherocytosis
- E Wilson's disease

3.40   Answer: E

Fragile X is a trinucleotide repeat disorder, where CGG repeats at least 30 times over. XYY syndrome results in males who tend to be more aggressive and antisocial.

3.41   Answer: D

Mast cells are basophilic cells that express IgE, and can be stimulated by a number of triggers to cause inflammatory and immune responses.

3.42   Answer: D

Classic features are fever, microangiopathic haemolytic anaemia, neurological involvement and renal failure. Diarrhoea is more commonly associated with TTP.

3.43   Answer: C

Genetic anticipation is a phenomenon where successive generations develop disease earlier and severity increases. Other examples are Huntington's disease, myotonic dystrophy and spinocerebellar ataxia.

3.44 Which of the following statements is most correct with respect to the process of apoptosis?

- [ ] **A** Apoptosis is a random process
- [✓] **B** Caspases are proteases involved in apoptosis
- [ ] **C** It is a pro-inflammatory event
- [ ] **D** Macrophages play an important early role
- [ ] **E** There is local lymphocyte infiltration

3.45 Which of the following conditions would *not* be expected to cause macrocytosis, suggesting an alternative diagnosis?

- [ ] **A** Alcohol abuse
- [ ] **B** Hypothyroidism
- [ ] **C** Pregnancy
- [ ] **D** Reticulocytosis
- [✓] **E** Turner syndrome

3.46 Which of the following disorders is most likely to cause the appearance of macrocytes on a peripheral blood film?

- [✓] **A** Anaemia of chronic disease
- [ ] **B** Iron deficiency anaemia
- [✗] **C** Lead poisoning
- [ ] **D** Sideroblastic anaemia
- [ ] **E** Thalassaemia trait

3.47 Which of the following appearances on a peripheral blood film most strongly suggests a diagnosis of vitamin B$_{12}$ deficiency?

- [ ] **A** Bite cells
- [ ] **B** Foam cells
- [ ] **C** Howell–Jolly bodies
- [✓] **D** Hypersegmented neutrophils
- [ ] **E** Smear cells

3.44 Answer: B

In contrast to necrosis, where there is cell destruction, apoptosis is not an inflammatory process. Cells undergo compaction of chromatin and cytoplasmic budding, forming apoptotic bodies, which eventually undergo phagocytosis. *TP53* is a tumour suppressor gene that causes apoptosis.

3.45 Answer: E

Pregnancy is a physiological cause of macrocytosis.

3.46 Answer: A

Anaemia of chronic disease is usually associated with a normal mean cell volume (MCV), and the appearance of normocytes, microcytes and macrocytes on a blood film.

3.47 Answer: D

Bite cells suggest glucose-6-phosphate dehydrogenase (G6PD) deficiency, foam cells suggest Gaucher's disease, Howell–Jolly bodies suggest hyposplenism, and smear cells suggest chronic lymphocytic leukaemia.

3.48 Which of the following mechanisms is believed to be most important in the development of systemic lupus erythematosus (SLE)?

- [ ] A Hypogammaglobulinaemia
- [✓] B Immune complex formation
- [ ] C Mast cell degranulation
- [ ] D Suppression of cytokine release
- [ ] E T-cell autoantibody production

3.49 Which one of the following statements best describes the features of pseudohypoparathyroidism?

- [✓] A A syndrome of end-organ resistance to parathyroid hormone
- [ ] B DiGeorge syndrome is a congenital form
- [ ] C Grand mal convulsions secondary to basal calcification
- [ ] D McCune–Albright syndrome affects only men
- [ ] E Parathyroid failure can be due to infective causes

3.50 Which of the following is most likely to be a feature of DiGeorge syndrome?

- [ ] A Chromosome 24 defect
- [ ] B Intussusception is common
- [ ] C Maldevelopment arising from second and third branchial arches
- [✓] D Thymic hypoplasia
- [ ] E Transient hypermagnesaemia

3.51 A 58-year-old man presents with bitemporal hemianopia, prompting suspicion of a chiasmal lesion. Which one of the following hormones is most likely to be preserved in the setting of a compressive lesion arising from the anterior pituitary?

- [✓] A Antidiuretic hormone (ADH)
- [ ] B Adrenocorticotropic hormone (ACTH)
- [ ] C Growth hormone
- [ ] D Gonadotrophins
- [ ] E Thyroid-stimulating hormone (TSH)

3.48 Answer: B

B-cell activation results in autoantibody formation and hypergammaglobulinaemia. T-cell regulation of immune responses is also disrupted.

3.49 Answer: A

Pseudohypoparathyroidism is due to resistance rather than parathyroid failure. Albright's hereditary osteodystrophy is the typical phenotype (short stature, short metacarpals, low IQ). Grand mal convulsions occur secondary to hypocalcaemia.

3.50 Answer: D

Mnemonic 'CATCH 22':

C – Cleft palate and other facial anomalies (micrognathia, abnormal ears)
A – Antibody responses impaired (IgA/IgG)
T – Thymic hypoplasia – third and fourth branchial arches = T-cell deficiency
C – Congenital cardiac defects
H – Hypocalcaemic tetany
22 – Located on chromosome 22

3.51 Answer: A

ADH (vasopressin) and oxytocin are released from the posterior pituitary. The others (and dopamine) are produced by the anterior pituitary.

3.52   Which of the following is *least* likely to be involved by a lesion affecting the cavernous sinus?

☑ **A**   Cranial nerve VI

☐ **B**   Internal carotid artery

☐ **C**   Oculomotor nerve

☐ **D**   Trigeminal nerve

☒ **E**   Trochlear nerve

3.53   A 31-year-old man presents with arthritis and back pain. Examination reveals pigmentation of the ear cartilage, and a plain X-ray spine shows intervertebral disc calcification. Which of the following is most correct regarding the underlying diagnosis?

☑ **A**   Autosomal recessive inheritance pattern

☒ **B**   Maple syrup odour from urine

☐ **C**   Neuropsychiatric manifestations common

☐ **D**   Overproduction of homogentisic acid oxidase

☐ **E**   Subperiosteal bone resorption is a recognised feature

3.54   Which of the following features is most characteristic of porphyria cutanea tarda?

☒ **A**   Autosomal dominant inheritance

☑ **B**   Photosensitivity with rash and bullae are common findings

☐ **C**   Reduced porphobilinogen deaminase activity

☐ **D**   Responds well to phenytoin

☐ **E**   Urine turns dark-orange on standing

3.55   Which one of the following would most often be expected in acute intermittent porphyria?

☐ **A**   Autosomal recessive inheritance pattern

☐ **B**   Good response to high-protein diet

☐ **C**   Increased porphobilinogen deaminase activity

☐ **D**   Male predominance

☑ **E**   Neuropsychiatric involvement

3.52   Answer: A

The sixth cranial nerve (abducens) lies just outside the cavernous sinus and is particularly vulnerable to compression in the setting of raised intracranial pressure.

3.53   Answer: A

Alkaptonuria (ochronosis) is a deficiency of enzyme homogentisic acid oxidase, resulting in deposition of alkapton in cartilaginous tissues. Urine turns brown/black on standing. Maple syrup urine is an independent inborn error of amino acid metabolism.

3.54   Answer: B

Porphyria cutanea tarda is caused by reduced porphobilinogen decarboxylase activity. Urine colour is normal. It is inherited but the pattern of symptom inheritance is variable. Treatment is with venesection and chloroquine.

3.55   Answer: E

Treatment is supportive, including a high carbohydrate diet. Gonadotropin-releasing hormones may prevent attacks, and antidepressants can be effective in some cases.

3.56 Deficiency of which of the following enzymes is thought responsible for phenylketonuria?

- ☐ **A** Alanine transaminase
- ☐ **B** Cystathionine β synthase
- ☐ **C** Homogentisic acid oxidase
- ☑ **D** Phenylalanine hydroxylase
- ☐ **E** Tyrosine hydroxylase

3.57 A 49-year-old woman presents to you with a calcium concentration of 3.8 mmol/l, and you commence treatment with intravenous saline while trying to determine the underlying cause. Which of the following medications is most likely to contribute to hypercalcaemia?

- ☐ **A** Aspirin
- ☐ **B** Atenolol
- ☒ **C** Bendroflumethiazide
- ☐ **D** Gliclazide
- ☑ **E** Theophylline

3.58 Which of the following complement deficiencies is most commonly associated with SLE?

- ☐ **A** C1-esterase deficiency
- ☐ **B** C5–C9 deficiency
- ☑ **C** Deficiency of the classical pathway
- ☐ **D** Deficiency of factor H
- ☐ **E** Isolated C3 deficiency

3.59 Which of the following statements is most accurate with regard to immunoglobulins?

- ☐ **A** IgA normally activates the classical complement pathway
- ☑ **B** IgE is expressed by both mast cells and basophils
- ☐ **C** IgG does not cross the placenta
- ☐ **D** IgM concentrations are high at birth but fall during the first year of life
- ☒ **E** IgM deficiency affects 10–15% of all adults

3.56 Answer: D

Alkaptonuria results from homogentisic acid oxidase deficiency, and homocystinuria results from cystathionine β synthase deficiency.

3.57 Answer: C

Theophylline is a recognised cause of hypercalcaemia, but less important.

3.58 Answer: C

Of note, deficiency of factor H (decay accelerating factor) and membrane inhibitor of reactive lysis results in paroxysmal nocturnal haemoglobinuria. An acquired defect with spontaneous lysis of red cells.

3.59 Answer: B

IgM is very effective against bacteria and is the main immunoglobulin of the primary immune system. It is undetectable at birth; adult levels are attained by 12 months.

3.60 A 51-year-old man presents to the General Medical Outpatient Clinic with blurred vision. He has facial muscle atrophy, frontal balding and distal limb muscle weakness, and he tells you there is a genetic predisposition to muscle weakness in his family. What is the most likely underlying diagnosis?

- A Duchenne muscular dystrophy
- B Facio-scapulo-humeral dystrophy
- C Huntington's disease
- D Myasthenia gravis
- ☑ E Myotonic dystrophy

3.61 A 15-year-old boy walks into the clinic accompanied by his mother. He is generally performing well at school, except that he has been unable to cope with sports activities. He has required help when standing from the floor on a number of occasions, and has been seen to use his hands to climb up his legs. On examination, there is marked proximal muscle wasting, particularly in the lower extremities, accompanied by hypertrophy of his calf muscles. Resting ECG is normal. What is the most likely diagnosis?

- ☑ A Becker's muscular dystrophy
- B Duchenne muscular dystrophy
- C Facio-scapulo-humeral dystrophy
- D Limb girdle dystrophy
- E Thomsen's disease

3.62 A 27-year-old man attends clinic complaining of severe cramp while trying to exercise, usually after only a few moments. There is no evidence of muscle wasting and neurological examination is normal. Full blood count and routine electrolytes including lactate are normal. Urine dipstick shows myoglobinuria, and no protein or glucose. What is the most likely diagnosis?

- ☒ A Hypokalaemic periodic paralysis
- B Eaton–Lambert syndrome
- ☑ C McArdle syndrome
- D MELAS (mitochondrial myopathy, encephalopathy, lactic acidosis and stroke)
- E Rhabdomyolysis

3.60   Answer: E

Inherited as an autosomal dominant disorder associated with CTG trinucleotide repeat, and displaying genetic anticipation. Affects males and females equally; cardiac involvement includes heart block; and congenital myotonic dystrophy is a recognised cause of respiratory arrest. Subcapsular cataracts are a common long-term complication.

3.61   Answer: A

X-linked recessive, resulting in dystrophin deficiency. The scenario describes the characteristic 'Gower's sign' while attempting to stand. The fact he has walked in to clinic effectively excludes Duchenne's, where disability is severe by age 10.

3.62   Answer: C

Autosomal recessive disorder, lack of skeletal muscle myophosphorylase, causing easy fatiguability. A characteristic finding is the lack of lactate rise with exercise.

3.63 A 17-year-old thin male, who has been wearing a plaster cast after an ankle fracture, presents with foot drop after the cast is removed. Which of the following features most strongly suggest a common peroneal nerve palsy?

☑ **A** Absent sensation over the dorsum of the foot, foot drop, lack of eversion

☐ **B** Absent sensation over the dorsum of the foot, foot drop, lack of inversion

☐ **C** Absent sensation over the dorsum of the foot, foot drop, peroneal muscle wasting

☐ **D** Normal sensation over the dorsum of the foot, foot drop, lack of eversion

☐ **E** Normal sensation over the dorsum of the foot, foot drop, lack of inversion

3.64 A 49-year-old man of Mediterranean origin presents to the Emergency Department with mild jaundice. His initial investigations show Hb 9.1 g/dl. Which of the following findings most strongly suggests an underlying diagnosis of glucose-6-phosphate dehydrogenase deficiency?

☐ **A** Coombs' test positive

☐ **B** Deranged liver biochemistry

☐ **C** Family history in a second-degree relative

☑ **D** Haemolysis after exposure to aspirin

☐ **E** Smear cells on blood film

3.65 A 48-year-old woman presents with symptoms of nasal regurgitation, especially after taking fluids. Her voice has a nasal intonation. On examination there is evidence of lower limb muscle wasting, increased tone in the upper limbs and a wasted, fibrillating tongue. What is the most likely diagnosis?

☐ **A** Alzheimer's disease

☑ **B** Motor neurone disease

☐ **C** Parkinsonism

☐ **D** Spastic paraparesis

☐ **E** Vascular dementia

3.63 Answer: A

On the other hand, lack of ankle inversion is caused by L5 nerve root lesions.

3.64 Answer: D

Exposure to fava beans or drugs (aspirin, dapsone, quinolones) can cause haemolysis in G6PD deficiency. Heinz bodies are a characteristic feature. Positive Coombs' test suggests autoimmune haemolytic anaemia.

3.65 Answer: B

There are features of lower and upper motor neurone degeneration. Progressive bulbar palsy involves lower cranial nerves, resulting in dysarthria, dysphagia and nasal regurgitation of fluids. Cerebellar signs, extrapyramidal signs, dementia and sphincter involvement are rare.

3.66 Which of the following tissue staining methods would be most appropriate in confirming the presence of *Cryptococcus* spp. in CSF in a patient presenting with features of meningitis?

☒ A   Congo red

☐ B   Perl's stain

☐ C   Rubeonic stain

☑ D   Silver stain

☐ E   Ziehl–Neelsen

3.67 Which one of the following clinical characteristics is most likely to be found in a patient with congenital syphilis?

☐ A   Accessory nipple

☐ B   Cataracts

☐ C   Cleft palate

☑ D   Interstitial keratitis

☒ E   Phocomelia

3.68 A mother with long-standing well-controlled SLE gives birth to a baby with complete heart block. Which of the following antibody tests is most likely to be positive in the newborn?

☐ A   ANA

☐ B   Anti-double-stranded DNA

☐ C   Anti-La antibodies

☑ D   Anti-Ro antibodies

☒ E   Anti-RNP antibodies

3.69 Which of the following organisms is most commonly associated with development of gas gangrene?

☐ A   *Clostridium botulinum*

☐ B   *Clostridium novyi*

☑ C   *Clostridium perfringens*

☐ D   *Clostridium septicum*

☐ E   *Clostridium tetani*

3.66   Answer: D

Congo red for amyloidosis, Perl's stain for iron deposition
(haemochromatosis), Ziehl–Neelsen for *Mycobacterium tuberculosis.*
Silver stain can also be used to identify *Pneumocystis carinii.*

3.67   Answer: D

Other features include inner ear deafness and saddle nose deformity.
Cataracts are a feature of galactosaemia and intrauterine measles, but
not of congenital syphilis. Hutchinson's triad consists of interstitial
keratitis, Hutchinson's incisors and deafness.

3.68   Answer: D

ANA is increased in drug-induced lupus, anti-dsDNA is a feature of
SLE, and anti-RNP is a feature of mixed connective tissue disease
(overlap syndromes).

3.69   Answer: C

Also known as *Clostridium welchii.* Less common causes are
Clostridium septicum and *Clostridium novyi.*

3.70 Which of the following features is most strongly suggestive of hypertrophic obstructive cardiomyopathy?

☑ **A** Asymmetrical septal hypertrophy

☐ **B** Dilated left ventricle

☐ **C** Left ventricular aneurysm

☐ **D** Right ventricular dilatation

☐ **E** Right ventricular hypertrophy

3.71 A 22-year-old man presents with progressive ataxia. Examination shows bilateral pes cavus, scoliosis, absent ankle reflexes with extensor plantars. What is the most likely underlying diagnosis?

☐ **A** Cervical spondylosis

☑ **B** Friedreich's ataxia

☐ **C** Motor neurone disease

☐ **D** Multiple sclerosis

☐ **E** Tabes dorsalis

3.72 Which of the following statements most correctly describes the features of *Pseudomonas* spp.?

☒ **A** Capsulated bacteria

☐ **B** Gentamicin resistance is common

☐ **C** Gram-positive bacillus

☑ **D** Greenish-blue pigmentation in culture

☐ **E** Route of transmission is normally by direct inoculation

3.73 Which of the following disorders is *least* likely to be caused by production of an autoantibody (ie autoimmune disease)?

☐ **A** Addison's disease

☑ **B** Cryptogenic fibrosing alveolitis

☐ **C** Graves' disease

☐ **D** Hashimoto's thyroiditis

☐ **E** Myasthenia gravis

3.70 Answer: A

There is left ventricular hypertrophy and septal hypertrophy, causing almost complete obliteration of the left ventricle; dilatation is not generally recognised.

3.71 Answer: B

A trinucleotide repeat disorder of autosomal recessive inheritance. Characterised by spinocerebellar tract degeneration, and cardiomyopathy.

3.72 Answer: D

This is a Gram-negative bacillus, normally sensitive to gentamicin and quinolone antibiotics. Burns victims and patients with interstitial lung disease and cystic fibrosis are at greatest risk.

3.73 Answer: B

The exact aetiology is unclear. The other disorders are all mediated by autoantibodies, and there is often clustering of multiple autoimmune conditions, eg vitiligo, Addison's disease and autoimmune thyroid disease.

3.74 Which of the following disorders is a characteristic feature of Still's disease?

☐ A Foot drop

☐ B Heart block

☑ C Lymphadenopathy

☐ D Parotid swelling

☐ E Polycythaemia

3.75 'Saturday night palsy' resulting in wrist drop is characteristically caused by a lesion affecting which nerve?

☐ A Axillary

☐ B Median

☐ C Nerve to serratus anterior

☑ D Radial

☐ E Ulnar

3.76 Which of the following disorders is most likely to be associated with a raised concentration of α-fetoprotein (AFP)?

☐ A Choriocarcinoma

☑ B Hepatoma

☐ C Pregnancy

☐ D Seminoma

☐ E Teratoma

3.77 Which one of the following hormones belongs to the amine group?

☐ A Aldosterone

☐ B Cortisol

☑ C Catecholamine

☒ D Retinoic acid

☐ E Testosterone

3.74   Answer: C

Other features also include pyrexia, splenomegaly and serositis.

3.75   Answer: D

Usually caused by compression of the radial nerve at the level of the upper humerus. Usually reversible, but palsy can be permanent if the period of compression is prolonged.

3.76   Answer: B

Beta-hCG is produced from the trophoblast layer of non-germ-cell tumours, and is characteristically raised in the other disorders listed (A, C, D, E).

3.77   Answer: C

The remainder are steroids.

3.78   Which of the following best describes the action of corticosteroids?

☑ **A**   Act on DNA to alter gene expression

☐ **B**   Bind to extracellular cytosolic receptors

☐ **C**   Close relationship between plasma levels and intracellular effects

☒ **D**   Stimulate cGMP secondary messengers

☐ **E**   Trigger intracellular cAMP

3.79   Which of the following disorders is thought to be mediated via a G-protein defect?

☐ **A**   Graves' disease

☑ **B**   Hypoparathyroidism

☐ **C**   Osteoporosis

☐ **D**   Relapsing polychondritis

☒ **E**   Vitamin D-resistant rickets   150 − 120

3.80   Investigations show: sodium 145 mmol/l, potassium 5.0 mmol/l, creatinine 178 µmol/l, urea 9.0 mmol/l, bicarbonate 20 mmol/l, chloride 100 mmol/l and glucose 11 mmol/l. Based on these blood results, what is the calculated anion gap?

☐ **A**   15 mmol/l

☐ **B**   20 mmol/l

☐ **C**   25 mmol/l

☒ **D**   30 mmol/l

☐ **E**   35 mmol/l

3.81   Investigations in an apparently healthy 20-year-old man show: sodium 136 mmol/l, potassium 4.0 mmol/l, creatinine 156 µmol/l, urea 6.0 mmol/l, bicarbonate 18 mmol/l, chloride 102 mmol/l and glucose 10 mmol/l. What is the calculated serum osmolarity?

☐ **A**   156 mOsm/kg

☐ **B**   172 mOsm/kg

☑ **C**   296 mOsm/kg

☐ **D**   302 mOsm/kg

☐ **E**   312 mOsm/kg

$$2 \times (Na + K) + ur + glucose$$

3.78   Answer: A

Bind to intracellular receptors to exert effects on DNA transcription
without triggering an intracellular cascade of second messengers.
cAMP, cGMP and IP3 second messengers are important for hormones
that bind to extracellular receptors.

3.79   Answer: B

Others include acromegaly and night-blindness.

3.80   Answer: D

Anion gap = [(Na$^+$ + K$^+$) – (HCO$_3^-$ + Cl$^-$)], normal range =
10–18 mmol/l.

3.81   Answer: C

Calculated plasma osmolarity: [2 × (Na$^+$ + K$^+$) + urea + glucose].
A significantly higher result from measured osmolality suggests the
presence of an unmeasured osmotic agent, eg ethylene glycol.
Normal = 275–295 mOsm/kg.

3.82 The chromosomes associated with a large number of genetic disorders are known. Which of the following chromosomes is thought to contain the gene responsible for Edwards syndrome?

- A Chromosome 7
- B Chromosome 13
- **C Chromosome 18**
- D Chromosome 21
- E Chromosome 22

3.83 Which of the following features is most strongly suggestive of cholesterol atheroembolism in a patient with a vasculitic skin rash overlying both feet?

- A Acute renal failure
- B Eosinophilia
- **C Livedo reticularis**
- D Raised ESR
- **E Recent angiography procedure**

3.84 Which one of the following disorders is most likely to be associated with a *negative* anti-neutrophil cytoplasmic antibody (ANCA) test?

- A Churg–Strauss
- **B Goodpasture's**
- **C Henoch–Schönlein purpura**
- D Microscopic polyangiitis
- E Wegener's granulomatosis

3.85 Which one of the following microscopic findings is most likely to be present in a healthy individual with no renal disease?

- A Granular casts
- **B Hyaline casts**
- C Red cell casts
- D Tubular casts
- E White cell casts

3.82 Answer: C

Williams syndrome is associated with chromosome 7, Patau syndrome with chromosome 13, DiGeorge syndrome with chromosome 22 and Down syndrome with chromosome 21.

3.83 Answer: E

The other items are recognised features. Spontaneous atheroembolism is comparatively rare, whereas it usually follows some invasive vascular procedure.

3.84 Answer: C

ANCA titres correlate with disease activity in the other conditions.

3.85 Answer: B

Tamm–Horsfall protein (hyaline casts) is not pathological. Red cell casts are found in glomerulonephritis, granular casts suggest haemoglobin traversing the glomerular membrane, white cell casts suggest acute pyelonephritis, and tubular casts are found in acute tubular necrosis (ATN).

3.86 Which of the following is true concerning amyloid-related diseases?

- [ ] **A** Alzheimer's disease is not associated with true amyloid deposits
- [x] **B** Amyloid A protein is seen in familial Mediterranean fever
- [ ] **C** Beta-2 microglobin is found in lymphoma-associated amyloidosis
- [ ] **D** Congo red stain shows amyloid as a charcoal-black appearance
- [x] **E** Serum amyloid P is unhelpful in clinical practice

3.87 A 43-year-old woman is referred to the General Medical Clinic for assessment of weakness affecting elbow flexion in her left arm. On examination, there is grade 4 power of left elbow flexion. Reflexes in the upper limbs are normal and symmetrical. What is the likely cause?

- [x] **A** Biceps muscle injury
- [ ] **B** Brachial plexus injury
- [ ] **C** C5,6 nerve root compression
- [ ] **D** Cervical radiculopathy
- [ ] **E** Radial nerve contusion

3.88 A 32-year-old man fell down a flight of stairs 2 days ago while intoxicated. He did not report any loss of consciousness. Since that time, he has been aware of difficulty moving his left shoulder. On examination, there is profound weakness of left shoulder abduction. What is the most likely cause for these findings?

- [ ] **A** Atlanto-axial subluxation
- [ ] **B** Axillary nerve compression
- [x] **C** C4,5 nerve root compression
- [ ] **D** C6,7 nerve root compression
- [x] **E** Deltoid muscle contusion

3.89 A 36-year-old woman with long-standing severe rheumatoid arthritis has noticed increasing difficulty with dressing. On examination, she is found to have significant weakness of left elbow supination. Which of the following explanations is most appropriate?

- [ ] **A** Axillary nerve lesion
- [x] **B** C5,6 nerve root lesion
- [ ] **C** C8 nerve root lesion
- [ ] **D** Median nerve lesion
- [ ] **E** Ulnar nerve lesion

3.86   Answer: B

Serum amyloid (SAP) scan allows quantification of disease progression. Congo red staining shows apple-green appearance of amyloid deposits under polarised light. Beta-2 microglobin amyloid is found in dialysis-dependent patients.

3.87   Answer: A

Preservation of normal reflexes excludes significant upper or lower motor neurone involvement, and local muscle pathology is most likely.

3.88   Answer: C

Shoulder abduction is served by the deltoid muscle, which is subserved predominantly by C5 fibres carried by the axillary nerve.

3.89   Answer: B

For example, an isolated motor neuropathy or part of a mononeuritis multiplex secondary to rheumatoid arthritis. Supply biceps and brachioradialis muscles via musculoskeletal and radial nerves, respectively.

3.90 A 43-year-old labourer presents to the Emergency Department with low back pain. He is found to have weakness of hip flexion on the left side. What is the most likely explanation?

- ☑ A Disc prolapse and L2,3 nerve root compression
- ☐ B Disc prolapse and S1,2 nerve root compression
- ☐ C Dissecting abdominal aneurysm
- ☐ D Metastatic lumbar spine involvement
- ☐ E Paraneoplastic neuropathy

3.91 A 67-year-old man has experienced progressive difficulty with mobility, and is found to have significant weakness of left knee extension, associated with diminished knee jerk reflex on the left. What is the most likely explanation?

- ☐ A Generalised myositis secondary to statin therapy
- ☑ B L3,4 nerve root compression
- ☐ C Lead toxicity
- ☒ D Quadriceps wasting
- ☐ E Thoracic spine compression

3.92 A 42-year-old man attends the Emergency Department and is found to have weakness of pronation of the left forearm, and reduced power on testing wrist flexion on the same side. What is the most likely explanation for these findings?

- ☒ A Brachial plexus lesion
- ☑ B Injury to the median nerve at the elbow
- ☐ C Median nerve damage at the wrist
- ☐ D Radial nerve palsy
- ☐ E Ulnar nerve lesion at the elbow

3.93 A 23-year-old cyclist is rushed to the Emergency Department after being knocked off his bicycle by a motorist. He is found to have weakness of the small muscles of his right hand, which is held in a clawed posture. There is loss of sensation overlying the medial border of the right forearm and hand. What is the most likely cause?

- ☐ A Intracranial haemorrhage
- ☐ B Radial nerve compression in the upper limb
- ☐ C Stroke
- ☑ D T1 nerve root lesion
- ☒ E Ulnar nerve contusion at the elbow

3.90 Answer: A

Hip flexion usually mediated by iliopsoas muscle, supplied by nerve roots L1–L3.

3.91 Answer: B

Reduced power associated with diminished reflexes indicates a lower motor lesion. An alternative explanation is femoral nerve entrapment.

3.92 Answer: B

Causes include trauma, heavy metal poisoning and mononeuritis multiplex.

3.93 Answer: D

The features suggest a brachial plexus injury with features of T1 damage (Klumpke's paralysis). This can also be associated with ipsilateral Horner syndrome.

3.94 A 34-year-old woman attends the Emergency Department with sudden onset of speech impairment. On examination, she is found to have a severe expressive dysphasia. Which area of the brain is likely to be affected?

- ☑ **A** Left parietal lobe
- ☒ **B** Left temporal lobe
- ☐ **C** Occipital lobe
- ☐ **D** Right parietal lobe
- ☐ **E** Right temporal lobe

3.95 A 26-year-old man presents to the Emergency Department following an injury to his left leg. On examination he is found to have impaired sensation over the medial aspect of the dorsum of his left foot and lower leg. There is weakness of left ankle dorsiflexion and foot drop. Injury to which motor nerve is most likely to be responsible?

- ☑ **A** Common peroneal nerve
- ☐ **B** Femoral nerve
- ☐ **C** Lateral cutaneous nerve
- ☐ **D** Median popliteal nerve
- ☐ **E** Sacroiliac nerve

3.96 A 36-year-old man with diplopia is referred to the Ophthalmology Outpatient Department by his GP. On examination, the left eye looks down and out during forward gaze. Damage to which of the following nerves is most likely to be responsible?

- ☐ **A** Abducent nerve
- ☐ **B** Ciliary nerve
- ☐ **C** Cranial nerve II
- ☑ **D** Cranial nerve III
- ☐ **E** Trochlear nerve

3.94   Answer: A

Speech motor cortex is located in Broca's area of the dominant parietal lobe, whereas receptive dysphasia is more likely to result from a lesion affecting Wernicke's area in the dominant temporal lobe.

3.95   Answer: A

Most commonly, this nerve is damaged at the site where it wraps around the upper part of the fibula, just below the fibular head.

3.96   Answer: D

Oculomotor nerve, which supplies all the extraocular muscles except for lateral rectus (abducent nerve) and superior oblique (trochlear nerve).

3.97 A 45-year-old woman presents to the Emergency Department with impaired vision. She is found to have a left superior homonymous quadrantanopia. What is the most likely anatomical site of the lesion?

- A Right occipital lobe
- B Right optic nerve
- C Right optic tract
- D Right parietal lobe
- ☑ E Right temporal lobe

3.98 Which the following statements best describes the physiological role of gastrin?

- A Gastric distension inhibits its release
- B It is a high-molecular-weight glycopeptide
- C Its release is diminished in the presence of hypercalcaemia
- D Released from pancreatic β-islet cells
- ☑ E Stimulates intrinsic factor secretion

3.99 A number of different factors can influence the rate of gastric emptying. Which of the following is most likely to increase the rate of gastric emptying?

- A Amino acids in the duodenum
- B Emotional distress
- C Free fatty acids in the stomach
- ☑ D Gastrin
- E Secretin

3.100 Interactions between central nervous system neurotransmitters is believed to play an important role in epilepsy. Which of the following statements best describes γ-amino butyric acid (GABA) metabolism in the CNS?

- A GABA is a powerful stimulatory neurotransmitter
- B GABA is normally metabolised to glutamate
- ☑ C Gabapentin and vigabatrin potentiate the effects of GABA
- D Glutamate is an inhibitory neurotransmitter
- E Lamotrigine stimulates release of glutamate

3.97 Answer: E

The temporal lobe supplies fibres of the lower retina (upper visual field), whereas the parietal lobe supplies fibres of the upper retina (lower visual field).

3.98 Answer: E

Its release from G-cells in the gastric antrum is stimulated by hypercalcaemia, amino acids in the antrum, gastric distension and vagal stimulation. It also stimulates gastric acid and pepsin release.

3.99 Answer: D

Gastrin and distension of the stomach wall stimulate gastric emptying, whereas pain, headache, stress, fatty acids, secretin and low pH in the duodenum reduce gastric emptying.

3.100 Answer: C

Glutamate (stimulatory) is metabolised to GABA (inhibitory) by glutamic acid decarboxylase. Lamotrigine inhibits glutamate effects in the CNS. Note that gabapentin is a GABA pentamer.

3.101 Which of the following statements best describes the role of nitric oxide (NO) in human physiology?

☒ A cAMP mediates vascular relaxation responses to NO

☐ B NO increases platelet adhesiveness

☐ C Inducible NO synthase normally regulates vascular tone

☑ D Platelets generate and release NO in vivo

☐ E Serves an endocrine role in regulating vascular tone

3.102 A 45-year-old man is being treated for severe pneumonia and sepsis in the Intensive Care Unit. His blood pressure has been difficult to maintain despite adequate fluid administration and large quantities of intravenous noradrenaline. Which of the following agents is most likely to allow restoration of normal blood pressure?

☐ A Angiotensin I infusion

☐ B Endothelin antagonist

☐ C Interleukin 1

☑ D Nitric oxide synthase (NOS) inhibitor

☐ E NSAID

3.103 A number of potentially important inflammatory mediators have been studied in order to determine their role in human diseases. Which of the following statements is most correct with respect to interleukin 1 (IL-1)?

☐ A Alpha-subtype is formed predominantly by lymphocytes

☐ B Administration prevents fever in patients with sepsis

☑ C Beta subtype is increased after strenuous physical exercise

☒ D Oxidised LDL uptake inhibits vascular IL-1 expression

☐ E Stimulates release of vasoconstrictor molecules

3.104 Paracetamol has been shown to reduce fever, in addition to its analgesic properties. What is the most likely mechanism for this effect?

☐ A Bacteriostatic effects on Gram-positive organisms

☐ B Blockade of the TNFα receptor site

☐ C Cyclo-oxygenase (COX) inhibition

☑ D Decreased interleukin 1 formation

☐ E Enhanced nitric oxide release

3.101   Answer: D

Endothelium-derived NO is expressed constitutively by eNOS, and serves an autocrine/paracrine role in regulating vascular tone by stimulating vascular smooth muscle cGMP formation. It is rapidly broken down (hence no endocrine effects), inhibits leukocyte and platelet adhesion to endothelium.

3.102   Answer: D

A number of arginine analogues, eg L-N-monomethylarginine, inhibit NOS in vivo, and small studies have shown them to be effective in sepsis. None are licensed for treatment, but this supports the view that inducible NOS contributes to hypotension in sepsis.

3.103   Answer: C

Also sepsis, acute exacerbations of rheumatoid arthritis and other inflammatory states. Oxidised LDL stimulates endothelial IL-1 expression, which might contribute to plaque formation. IL-1 is formed predominantly by macrophages.

3.104   Answer: D

Hypothalamic effect to reset thermoregulation. Mechanism unclear, but IL-1 concentrations reduced. A number of studies have found inhibition of COX enzymes, but not consistent.

Clinical sciences answers

3.105 Which of the following statements most accurately describes the role of tumour necrosis factor (TNF)?

☐ A Causes powerful anti-inflammatory effects in vivo

☐ B Effective treatment for wide range of solid tumours

☐ C Inhibits monocyte and macrophage migration

☐ D TNFα inhibits monocyte production of interleukin 1

☑ E TNFβ synthesised by activated T lymphocytes

3.106 Central dopamine deficiency is believed to play an important role in the pathogenesis of Parkinson's disease. Which of the following statements is correct with regard to dopamine metabolism?

☐ A Dopa decarboxylase is found only in the CNS

☑ B Dopamine is metabolised to noradrenaline by dopamine hydroxylase

☐ C L-Dopa is formed by the action of dopa decarboxylase on tyrosine

☒ D Peripheral effects of dopa include vasoconstriction

☐ E Tyrosine is an essential dietary precursor of L-dopa

3.107 A number of factors are necessary for normal physiology, but some cannot be synthesised by human metabolism. Which of the following is an essential dietary amino acid?

☐ A Alanine

☒ B Cysteine

☐ C Glutamic acid

☑ D Phenylalanine

☐ E Tyrosine

3.108 A 51-year-old man is admitted to hospital with breathlessness, fever and tachycardia. A chest X-ray shows diffuse pulmonary consolidation throughout the right lower zones, and investigations show serum bicarbonate 14 mmol/l and lactate 7.2 mmol/l. Which of the following statements best explains his abnormal blood tests?

☐ A Decreased tissue oxygenation

☐ B Excess build-up of tissue carbon dioxide

☑ C Increased anaerobic glycolysis by peripheral tissues

☐ D Increased glycolysis

☐ E Reduced hepatic glycogenolysis

3.105 Answer: E

TNFα secreted by macrophages, eosinophils and natural killer (NK) cells. Anti-cancer effects of TNF disappointingly poor, and high level of serious adverse effects. TNF stimulates monocyte and macrophage activity (including IL-1 release). TNF and IL-1 have a synergistic pro-inflammatory effect, eg in rheumatoid arthritis.

3.106 Answer: B

Phenylalanine is an essential amino acid that is metabolised to tyrosine, which is in turn metabolised to dopa. Dopa is converted to dopamine by dopa decarboxylase; peripheral dopa decarboxylase inhibitors allow greater amounts of L-dopa to cross the blood–brain barrier in the treatment of parkinsonism.

3.107 Answer: D

Phenylalanine is an essential precursor to tyrosine, which is subsequently incorporated in the synthesis of dopa and thyroid hormones. The other amino acids listed can all be synthesised in vivo.

3.108 Answer: C

Normally, aerobic metabolism supplies energy via the glucose-6-phosphate and tricarboxylic acid (TCA) pathways. Anaerobic metabolism is increased when (i) oxygen availability is reduced, (ii) lactate utilisation is impaired (eg metformin), or (iii) both (eg sepsis). Glucose → Lactate + 2 H$^+$.

3.109 Factors that influence oxygen-binding capacity of haemoglobin play an important role in determining oxygen transport and delivery in the human circulation. Which of the following is most likely to be associated with high oxygen-binding affinity of haemoglobin?

- A Diabetes mellitus
- B High $PaCO_2$
- C High pH
- D High temperature
- E Raised 2,3-diphosphoglycerate (2,3-DPG)

3.110 Which of the following statements is correct with regard to normal oxygen carriage in a healthy individual breathing room air at rest?

- A 1 g haemoglobin carries 1.5 ml oxygen
- B 1 g haemoglobin carries 30 ml oxygen
- C 100 ml blood carries 0.1 ml oxygen
- D 100 ml plasma carries 10 ml oxygen
- E 100 ml plasma carries 100 ml oxygen

3.111 A 34-year-old woman has been attending the General Medical Outpatient Clinic for assessment of severe Raynaud's disease. You wish to check for the presence of cryoglobulins. How should the sample be handled?

- A Assay needs to be performed within 1 h of sample collection
- B Sample kept at 37 °C then cooled to −20 °C for separation
- C Separated immediately, then stored at −20 °C before assay
- D Transported and separated at 37 °C
- E Whole blood sample chilled to −20 °C immediately after collection

3.112 A 37-year-old woman is referred to the Outpatient Department for investigation of a skin rash overlying the bridge of her nose that is tender on palpation. She is found to have a white cell count of 12.2×10^9/l and raised C3 and C4 complement concentrations. What is the most likely diagnosis?

- A Glomerulonephritis
- B Infectious endocarditis
- C Streptococcal skin infection
- D Systemic lupus erythematosus (SLE)
- E Systemic sclerosis

3.109   Answer: C

Low temperature, reduced 2,3-DPG and low $PaCO_2$ are associated with high oxygen-binding affinity (eg stored blood) so that oxygen delivery to tissues may be impaired.

3.110   Answer: A

Haemoglobin is an efficient means of oxygen carriage, whereas comparatively smaller amounts are dissolved in plasma. Around 0.5 ml oxygen will be dissolved in 100 ml plasma.

3.111   Answer: D

Cryoglobulins precipitate at cool temperatures, around 4 °C, so that the sample must be kept at 37 °C before separation so that these are not lost from the supernatant.

3.112   Answer: C

Raised complement levels are a non-specific marker of inflammation. Low levels are seen in SLE, post-streptococcal glomerulonephritis, serum sickness and septicaemia, and can correlate with disease severity.

3.113 A 32-year-old woman attends the General Medical Outpatient Department for investigation of recurrent episodes of fever and abdominal pain associated with nausea and vomiting. Physical examination is normal. Each episode lasts for around 3–4 days, and have occurred three times in the past 8 months. Investigations show low levels of C3, but other complement components are normal. What is the most likely explanation?

- [ ] **A** Bacterial endocarditis
- [x] **B** Hereditary isolated C3 deficiency
- [x] **C** Recurrent pyelonephritis
- [ ] **D** Recurrent ureteric calculus formation
- [ ] **E** SLE

3.114 A 21-year-old man with a history of asthma is brought into the Emergency Department with wheeze and circulatory collapse around 1 h after being stung by a wasp. You suspect an anaphylactic reaction. What is the most appropriate initial management?

- [ ] **A** 5 ml of 1 in 10 000 adrenaline intravenously
- [x] **B** 0.5 ml of 1 in 1000 adrenaline intramuscularly
- [ ] **C** 100 mg of intravenous hydrocortisone
- [ ] **D** Intravenous chlorphenamine 4 mg
- [ ] **E** Intravenous saline at 500 ml/h

3.115 A young woman with well-controlled asthma is undergoing tests for suspected chronic urticaria. A skin-prick test shows the development of wheal and flare within 15 min, that gradually resolves within the next 45 min. What does this test indicate?

- [ ] **A** False positive due to inhaled corticosteroids
- [x] **B** Type I hypersensitivity
- [ ] **C** Type II hypersensitivity
- [ ] **D** Type III hypersensitivity
- [x] **E** Type IV hypersensitivity

3.113 Answer: C

Low C3 levels may occur with recurrent bacterial infections. Although infective endocarditis is a recognised cause, this is less likely in the absence of any other physical signs.

3.114 Answer: B

Potentially life-threatening condition; priority is to secure airway, support ventilation, and administer adrenaline to support circulation. Additional treatment includes antihistamine administration, and consideration of corticosteroid treatment (effects may be delayed for several hours).

3.115 Answer: B

The antigen reacts with pre-formed IgE bound to the surface of mast cells to cause mast cell degranulation and local release of vasoactive substances. Type I hypersensitivity is more common in patients with asthma, eczema and allergic rhinitis.

3.116 Which of the following conditions is an example of type III hypersensitivity?

- [ ] **A** Anaphylaxis after a bee sting
- [ ] **B** Graft-versus-host disease (GVHD)
- [x] **C** Methyldopa-induced haemolysis
- [ ] **D** Phenytoin-induced gum hypertrophy
- [ ] **E** Tuberculin skin reaction

3.117 A 47-year-old man has long-standing hepatitis C, acquired through previous intravenous drug use. During a follow-up appointment he is found to have lost a significant amount of weight over the past 6 months, and he has become jaundiced. Which of the following tumour markers most strongly suggests the development of hepatocellular carcinoma?

- [ ] **A** 5-Hydroxyindoleacetic acid
- [x] **B** Alpha-fetoprotein
- [ ] **C** Carcinoembryonic antigen
- [ ] **D** Human chorionic gonadotrophin
- [ ] **E** Vanillyl mandelic acid

3.118 Which of the following is most likely to account for a modestly elevated prostate-specific antigen concentration in an otherwise healthy 48-year-old man?

- [ ] **A** Ciprofloxacin treatment
- [x] **B** Digital rectal examination
- [ ] **C** Impaired renal function
- [ ] **D** Metastatic involvement of the prostate gland
- [ ] **E** Uncomplicated bacterial cystitis

3.119 A 46-year-old woman is undergoing investigation of recurrent headaches. Which of the following disorders is most likely to be responsible for the appearance of a monoclonal immunoglobulin band in the CSF?

- [x] **A** Lymphoma
- [x] **B** Multiple sclerosis
- [ ] **C** Sarcoidosis
- [ ] **D** SLE
- [ ] **E** Tuberculosis

3.116   Answer: C

Complement-dependent immune complex disease. This includes serum sickness, drug-induced haemolysis (also caused by penicillin), post-streptococcal glomerulonephritis, cryoglobulinaemia, SLE and rheumatoid arthritis.

3.117   Answer: B

Elevated concentrations are also seen in acute viral hepatitis, cirrhosis or with liver metastases. High maternal concentration can indicate twins or neural tube defect in the developing fetus.

3.118   Answer: B

Other causes include acute and chronic prostatitis and prostatic carcinoma. The prostate is rarely affected by metastases from elsewhere.

3.119   Answer: A

Multiple sclerosis, sarcoidosis and SLE are associated with raised CSF protein and oligoclonal bands, and TB is associated with high total protein concentration. Benign paraproteinaemia is another recognised cause of monoclonal CSF bands.

3.120   Which one of the following disorders is most likely to cause increased urinary calcium excretion?

- ☐ **A** Coeliac disease
- ☐ **B** Hyperthyroidism
- ☐ **C** Hypoparathyroidism
- ☒ **D** Vitamin D deficiency
- ☑ **E** Thiazide diuretic treatment

3.121   A 43-year-old hospital inpatient is noted to have very dark urine. Laboratory examination confirms the presence of urinary haemoglobin. What is the most likely underlying cause?

- ☐ **A** Crush injury
- ☑ **B** Haemolytic anaemia
- ☐ **C** Nephrotic syndrome
- ☐ **D** Polymyositis
- ☐ **E** Severe myositis secondary to statin therapy

3.122   Which pattern of inheritance best describes the genetic transmission of Huntington's disease?

- ☑ **A** Autosomal dominant with anticipation
- ☐ **B** Autosomal dominant with incomplete penetrance
- ☐ **C** Autosomal recessive
- ☐ **D** Spontaneous genetic mutation
- ☐ **E** X-linked recessive

3.123   Which of the following best describes the features associated with inheritance of neurofibromatosis?

- ☒ **A** Males affected more than females
- ☑ **B** Genetic testing by DNA analysis is available
- ☐ **C** Heterozygotes are phenotypically normal
- ☐ **D** Most cases arise from spontaneous genetic mutation
- ☐ **E** Skips generations

3.120   Answer: E

The others are recognised causes of reduced urinary calcium excretion. Thiazide diuretics lower urinary calcium clearance and can reduce the frequency of urinary calcium stone formation; they are a recognised cause of hypercalcaemia.

3.121   Answer: B

Haemoglobinuria can occur with severe haemolysis, eg transfusion reaction, paroxysmal nocturnal haemoglobinuria and burns injuries. Crush injuries and muscle damage result in myoglobinuria. Nephrotic syndrome is characterised by heavy proteinuria.

3.122   Answer: A

Both sexes affected equally. Complete penetration. Age at onset of disease becomes progressively earlier with successive generations (anticipation).

3.123   Answer: B

Typically inherited in an autosomal dominant pattern, therefore men and women equally affected, and manifests in every generation.

3.124 You are examining the family history of an index case in order to better understand the transmission of a particular disease. It appears that only men have been affected by the disease over the past three generations. What is the most likely inheritance pattern?

- [ ] **A** Autosomal dominant with incomplete expression
- [ ] **B** Autosomal recessive
- [ ] **C** Frequent single-gene mutations
- [x] **D** X-linked recessive
- [x] **E** X-linked dominant

3.125 Which one of the following disorders is characteristically inherited in an autosomal recessive manner?

- [ ] **A** Becker's muscular dystrophy
- [x] **B** Cystic fibrosis
- [ ] **C** Gardner syndrome
- [ ] **D** Glucose-6-phosphate dehydrogenase deficiency
- [ ] **E** Red–green colour blindness

3.126 Which of the following medications is most likely to cause bronchospasm in a patient with well-controlled asthma?

- [x] **A** Inhaled disodium cromoglicate
- [x] **B** Inhaled ipratropium bromide
- [ ] **C** Montelukast sodium
- [ ] **D** Oral salbutamol
- [ ] **E** Theophylline

3.124   Answer: D

X-linked recessive disorders are carried by phenotypically normal women. Men who inherit the abnormality on their single X chromosome express the disease; men who are phenotypically normal have inherited the normal X-chromosome. Women who express X-linked disorders indicates an X-linked dominant pattern of disease inheritance.

3.125   Answer: B

Gardner syndrome is inherited in an autosomal dominant manner, and the others are inherited in an X-linked manner.

3.126   Answer: A

Can prevent asthma, particularly in young patients, and is comparatively free of systemic adverse effects. However, particulate size is bigger than aerosolised medications and it can irritate the respiratory tract causing cough and bronchospasm.

4. DERMATOLOGY

4.1   A 41-year-old man with severe psoriasis is referred to the Dermatology Clinic. He has had extensive treatment with vitamin A analogues, coal tar-based therapies and UV light with little effect. You decide to treat him with an anti-TNF. Which one of the following represents the main cell type which produces TNF?

☐ **A**   B lymphocytes

☑ **B**   Macrophages

☐ **C**   Mast cells

☐ **D**   Neutrophils

☐ **E**   T lymphocytes

4.2   A 45-year-old woman presents to the plastic surgeons for reconstructive surgery because she thinks the bridge of her nose is collapsing. She is also suffering from nasal congestion and shortness of breath. Blood tests reveal a raised creatinine. Which one of the following blood tests is likely to help reveal the underlying condition?

☐ **A**   Anti-nuclear antibody (ANA)

☐ **B**   Anti smooth muscle antibodies

☑ **C**   c-ANCA

☑ **D**   p-ANCA

☐ **E**   Rheumatoid factor

4.3   A 74-year-old man is brought to the hospital by ambulance, accompanied by his daughter. He has been confined to bed and she is worried as he has a very large sacral pressure sore with extensive slough and macerated skin in the surrounding area. Which of the following is the correct dressing type for him?

☑ **A**   Calcium alginate

☐ **B**   Cotton dressing

☐ **C**   Hydrocolloid dressing

☐ **D**   Saline soaks

☐ **E**   Silver-based dressing

4.1 Answer: B

Macrophages are the main cell type that produces TNF.

4.2 Answer: C

The presentation suggests Wegener's granulomatosis.

4.3 Answer: A

Trials have shown calcium alginate to be superior to hydrocolloid.

4.4 A 43-year-old single male dancer comes to the clinic. He is concerned as he has multiple purple-red scaly patches, mainly on his legs. He has also suffered from oral candidiasis over the past month. Which of the following is the most appropriate next step?

- [ ] **A** HHV-8 testing
- [x] **B** HIV testing
- [ ] **C** Human herpesvirus 6 (HHV-6) testing
- [ ] **D** Papillomavirus testing
- [ ] **E** Topical steroid therapy

4.5 A 55-year-old man with a history of hypertension, mild left ventricular failure and chronic stable angina comes to the Dermatology Clinic complaining of alopecia. Which of the following is the most likely cause?

- [x] **A** Diltiazem
- [ ] **B** Furosemide
- [ ] **C** Nifedipine
- [x] **D** Ramipril
- [ ] **E** Simvastatin

4.6 A 60-year-old woman comes to the clinic complaining of a rash that is characterised by tense blisters, particularly affecting the flexural surfaces of her arms and legs. They heal without significant scarring. She never gets any lesions in her mouth. Which of the following is the most likely diagnosis?

- [ ] **A** Erythema multiforme
- [ ] **B** Flexural eczema
- [x] **C** Pemphigoid
- [x] **D** Pemphigus
- [ ] **E** Stephens–Johnson syndrome

4.4 Answer: B

These patches may be due to Kaposi's sarcoma, an AIDS-defining illness.

4.5 Answer: D

Ramipril and β-blockers are recognised causes of alopecia in some patients.

4.6 Answer: C

Pemphigoid characteristically spares mucous membranes.

4.7 A 24-year-old man comes to the clinic, concerned because he has a number of small, flesh-coloured, domed papules around the corona of his glans penis. He admits to having had unprotected sex on a number of occasions. Which of the following is the most likely diagnosis?

- ☐ **A** Condylomata acuminata
- ☐ **B** Gonorrhoea
- ☒ **C** Herpes simplex infection
- ☐ **D** Molluscum contagiosum
- ✓ **E** Pearly penile papules

4.8 A 75-year-old Jamaican woman attends the clinic. She has been with the same partner for 55 years. She has a large number of painless subcutaneous nodules over her shins which have been developing for years. Some of these have ulcerated to leave a well-defined edge and plenty of slough. VDRL and TPHA are both positive. Which of the following is the most likely diagnosis?

- ☐ **A** HIV
- ☐ **B** Pinta
- ☐ **C** Sarcoidosis
- ☒ **D** Syphilis
- ✓ **E** Yaws

4.9 A 32-year-old woman presents to the clinic with lesions on the anterior aspects of both legs. She complains that they are unsightly and prevent her from wearing a skirt. On examination she has bilateral non-pitting oedema with non-symmetrical papules and plaques on both legs. Her GP is currently treating her for anxiety. She has lost 4 kg in weight over the past 3 months. Which of the following is the most likely diagnosis?

- ☐ **A** Erythema multiforme
- ☐ **B** Erythema nodosum
- ☐ **C** Necrobiosis lipoidica
- ✓ **D** Pretibial myxoedema
- ☐ **E** Psoriasis

4.7   Answer: E

Pearly penile papules are not sexually transimitted.

4.8   Answer: E

Yaws is a relatively common condition in people of West Indian origin.

4.9   Answer: D

The rash is typical of pretibial myxoedema, and she has symptoms of thyrotoxicosis.

4.10   A 29-year-old woman complains of an intensely itchy, bullous rash over her scalp, buttocks and elbows. She has a past history of intermittent diarrhoea, diagnosed by the GP as irritable bowel. Which of the following is the most likely diagnosis?

☑ **A**   Dermatitis herpetiformis

☐ **B**   Eczema

☐ **C**   Pemphigoid

☐ **D**   Pemphigus

☐ **E**   Psoriasis

4.11   A 32-year-old woman is referred to the Dermatology Clinic due to development of unusual freckles over her face over the past few weeks. The patient denies any significant sun exposure and is taking no regular medications apart from the oral contraceptive pill. On examination there are raised pigmented papules over the cheeks, chin and forehead. Which of the following offers the most likely explanation?

☐ **A**   Acne vulgaris

☐ **B**   Addison's disease

☑ **C**   Chloasma

☐ **D**   Melanoma

☒ **E**   Vitiligo

4.12   You see a 45-year-old woman in the Hypertension Clinic and note a number of discrete areas of hypopigmentation on her hands and forearms. Which of the following is the most likely explanation for this appearance?

☐ **A**   Addison's disease

☐ **B**   Diabetes mellitus

☐ **C**   Neurofibromatosis

☐ **D**   Post-scarring hypopigmentation

☑ **E**   Vitiligo

4.10 Answer: A

The pattern of the rash and the diarrhoea raises the possibility of dermatitis herpetiformis and coeliac disease.

4.11 Answer: C

Usually symmetrical, more common in women and associated with the oral contraceptive pill and pregnancy. Benign condition.

4.12 Answer: E

Common site, also involves face and genitalia. Probable autoimmune aetiology, and can be associated with other autoimmune diseases. No satisfactory treatment, although repigmentation can occur spontaneously.

4.13 You are asked to review a 31-year-old man in the Medical Outpatient Department, and you note from his records that he has previously been diagnosed with Peutz–Jeghers syndrome. Which one of these statements is correct regarding this diagnosis?

- [ ] **A** *BRCA1* is the responsible gene
- [ ] **B** Inherited in X-linked manner
- [ ] **C** Often occurs as part of a multiple endocrine neoplasia syndrome
- [x] **D** Pigmentation of the lips is due to melanin deposition
- [x] **E** There is a substantially increased risk of colonic carcinoma

4.14 A 47-year-old woman had been referred to the Dermatology Outpatient Department for investigation of a widespread rash. Skin biopsy shows features of vasculitis with necrosis, particularly affecting the arterioles. What is the most likely diagnosis?

- [ ] **A** Allergic vasculitis
- [ ] **B** Henoch–Schönlein purpura
- [x] **C** Polyarteritis nodosa
- [ ] **D** SLE
- [ ] **E** Urticarial vasculitis

4.15 You are asked to review a 28-year-old woman who reports easy bruising after comparatively minor trauma. Which of the following features most strongly suggests a diagnosis of Ehlers–Danlos syndrome?

- [ ] **A** Delayed recoil of skin after stretching
- [x] **B** Hyperextensible joints
- [ ] **C** Keloid scarring after trauma
- [ ] **D** Poor dentition
- [ ] **E** Skin hyperextensible over lower limbs only

4.16 You review a 28-year-old man in the Outpatient Department who is very tall and has hyperextensible skin with delayed elastic recoil, which is most pronounced around his face and eyes. His past history includes two previous hospital admissions for investigation of suspected gastrointestinal bleeding. Which of the following best explains these features?

- [ ] **A** Ehlers–Danlos syndrome
- [ ] **B** Kleinfelter syndrome
- [ ] **C** Marfan syndrome
- [x] **D** Pseudoxanthoma elasticum
- [ ] **E** Zollinger–Ellison syndrome

4.13   Answer: D

Inherited in autosomal dominant manner due to the *LKB1* gene. Gastrointestinal polyposis, not associated with malignant transformation.

4.14   Answer: C

Classic and microscopic polyarteritis nodosa cause necrotising arteritis; the other listed disorders tend to cause necrotising venulitis.

4.15   Answer: B

Skin generally hyperextensible, with normal elastic recoil. After injury, scars tend to be thin and paper-like.

4.16   Answer: D

Skin features are usually most notable around the neck, and the condition is associated with gastrointestinal bleeding, and myocardial infarction at a young age.

4.17 You are examining a 73-year-old man admitted to the Acute Medical Admissions Unit earlier in the day, and note the appearance of multiple raised plaques overlying his back. These vary in colour from pale to dark-brown, and are flat with irregular margins. What is the most likely explanation for these skin abnormalities?

- [ ] **A** Adenocarcinoma
- [✓] **B** Basal cell papilloma
- [✗] **C** Keratoacanthoma
- [ ] **D** Melanocytic naevi
- [ ] **E** Neurofibroma

4.18 A 62-year-old man is referred to the Dermatology Outpatient Department for assessment of a blistering rash overlying both of his shins. The legs appear modestly erythematous with overlying scratch marks, and there are large fluid-filled bullae. What is the most likely diagnosis?

- [ ] **A** Bacterial cellulitis
- [✓] **B** Bullous pemphigoid
- [ ] **C** Chronic lymphoedema
- [ ] **D** Pemphigus vulgaris
- [ ] **E** Porphyria

4.19 A 38-year-old woman is being investigated for iron deficiency anaemia, and is noted to have multiple small blisters overlying both forearms, associated with overlying scratch marks. Which of the following features is most strongly suggestive of dermatitis herpetiformis?

- [ ] **A** Family history of the condition
- [✓] **B** Papillary IgA deposition seen by immunofluorescence of unaffected skin
- [ ] **C** Recent herpes simplex infection of her lower lip
- [ ] **D** Regional lymphadenopathy
- [ ] **E** Skin biopsy confirms blisters are intra-epidermal

4.17   Answer: B

Also known as seborrhoeic warts, these are common in elderly patients and entirely benign.

4.18   Answer: B

Typically the legs are very itchy. Treatment is with high-dose corticosteroids, and steroid-sparing agents (eg azathioprine) may be required.

4.19   Answer: B

IgA deposition also seen along the basement membrane. Rare blistering disorder with intensely itchy rash treated with dapsone.

4.20 A 35-year-old woman is referred to the Dermatology Outpatient Department for assessment of excess hair growth. She has become increasingly distressed by excessive hair growth, particularly over her face and forearms. Which of the following is most likely to be responsible?

- ☐ **A** Diabetes mellitus
- ☐ **B** Hyperthyroidism
- ☐ **C** Oral contraceptive pill use
- ☐ **D** Peripheral neuropathy
- ☑ **E** Phenytoin treatment

4.21 A 28-year-old man with type 1 diabetes complains of a rash overlying his lower limbs during a routine clinic appointment. He is noted to have a number of dark-purple lesions overlying both shins, which are tender on palpation. What is the most likely explanation?

- ☐ **A** Lipoatrophy
- ☐ **B** Necrobiosis lipoidica
- ☐ **C** Pyoderma gangrenosum
- ☑ **D** Sarcoidosis
- ☐ **E** Urticarial vasculitis

4.22 A 17-year-old girl is referred to the Dermatology Clinic for assessment of severe acne vulgaris affecting her face, shoulders and back. She is asking if isotretinoin could be given. Which of the following statements is most accurate with regard to retinoid treatment?

- ☐ **A** Around 35% of patients respond to treatment
- ☐ **B** Euphoria is a characteristic adverse effect
- ☐ **C** It lessens the likelihood of conception
- ☑ **D** It should normally only be prescribed by dermatology specialists
- ☐ **E** Patients should avoid pregnancy until treatment is stopped

4.23 Which of the following is best recognised as a feature of Stevens–Johnson syndrome?

- ☒ **A** Cutaneous target lesions
- ☑ **B** Necrotic genital ulcers
- ☐ **C** Preceding streptococcal infection in most patients
- ☐ **D** Sparing of the mucous membranes
- ☐ **E** Underlying tuberculosis in 30% of patients

4.20 Answer: E

Other effects include facial coarseness, acne vulgaris and gum hyperplasia. As a result, it is rarely used as first-line treatment in young patients with epilepsy.

4.21 Answer: D

Inflammation affects the dermis and subcutaneous layers (panniculitis), and is usually tender. The lesions vary in size and have the appearance of slightly raised bruises.

4.22 Answer: D

Retinoids are highly effective, with a 90% response rate and two-thirds cure rate. They are teratogenic and patients should avoid conception during and up to 2 years after stopping acitretin treatment. They can impair liver biochemical tests and are associated with myalgia and depression.

4.23 Answer: B

Often associated with mucosal involvement but, unlike erythema multiforme, there are few cutaneous target lesions. Most cases are drug-induced, eg sulphonamides, NSAIDs and the oral contraceptive pill.

4.24 You are reviewing a 55-year-old woman in the Outpatient Department when you notice that she has patchy areas of depigmentation on her hands and abdomen. You suspect that this appearance is due to vitiligo. Which one of these statements is most accurate regarding this condition?

- [ ] **A** It is post-inflammatory in most patients
- [✓] **B** Repigmentation can occur spontaneously
- [ ] **C** Skin involvement is most noticeable in white people
- [ ] **D** Topical corticosteroids are effective in most patients
- [ ] **E** Usually associated with high anti-melatonin antibody titre

4.25 A 45-year-old woman is noted to have dry, erythematous skin on the volar surfaces of both wrists. A diagnosis of atopic dermatitis is suspected. Which of the following features is most consistent with this diagnosis?

- [ ] **A** Hepatomegaly
- [✓] **B** Intensive itch
- [ ] **C** Local lymphadenitis
- [ ] **D** Nodules overlying the distal interphalangeal joints
- [ ] **E** Small vesicles with clear fluid

4.26 Which of the following statements most correctly describes the role of tacrolimus in treating skin disease?

- [✓] **A** Herpes simplex infection is a recognised complication of topical treatment
- [✗] **B** Inhibits eosinophil activity
- [ ] **C** It is ineffective in acne rosacea
- [ ] **D** It is a preferred first-line agent for atopic dermatitis
- [ ] **E** Oral treatment is reserved for psoriasis with joint involvement

4.24 Answer: B

Effects are most pronounced in Afro-Caribbean patients and those with tanned skin. The margins often appear hyperpigmented, but there is no evidence that this is the case. Patients should be advised to protect themselves against sunburn.

4.25 Answer: B

Affects 1–6% of adults. Distribution may be more atypical than in childhood, eg non-flexural sites, and family history of atopy less strong than in childhood atopic dermatitis.

4.26 Answer: A

Topical treatment is reserved for severe atopic dermatitis, and appears effective also for rosacea, psoriasis and other skin disorders. It inhibits T-cell activation and cytokine release, and systemic absorption can cause renal impairment.

4.27 A 41-year-old woman is reviewed in the Dermatology Outpatient Department with easy bruising. She has had long-standing rheumatoid arthritis, which is quiescent at present. Which of the following features is most likely a complication of repeated use of high-dose corticosteroid treatment?

- [ ] **A** Abdominal white striae
- [ ] **B** Acne
- [ ] **C** Gum hyperplasia
- [ ] **D** Hirsutism
- [x] **E** Paper-thin skin

4.28 Which one of these aspects of lifestyle advice would be most effective in controlling the extent of psoriasis in a 42-year-old woman with extensive plaques over her buttocks and lower limbs?

- [ ] **A** Lose weight
- [ ] **B** Moderate alcohol intake
- [ ] **C** Reduce salt intake
- [x] **D** Stop smoking cigarettes
- [ ] **E** Take more regular aerobic exercise

4.29 Which one of the following skin disorders is most likely to be worsened by exposure to strong sunlight?

- [ ] **A** Acne vulgaris
- [ ] **B** Eczema
- [ ] **C** Pityriasis versicolor
- [ ] **D** Psoriasis
- [x] **E** Rosacea

4.30 A 29-year-old woman presents to the Dermatology Clinic with a 2–4-week history of intermittent abdominal pain associated with a transient blanching erythematous rash overlying face, neck and trunk. She has noted a number of distinct wheals over her chest wall, but these have settled. What is the most likely diagnosis?

- [ ] **A** Acute intermittent porphyria
- [x] **B** Angioedema
- [ ] **C** Atopic dermatitis
- [ ] **D** Atypical migraine
- [ ] **E** Recurrent anaphylaxis

4.27   Answer: E

Although the others are recognised features, they are less specific. Of note, white striae are 'inactive', whilst purple–red striae are 'active'.

4.28   Answer: D

Cigarette smoking confers a threefold increased risk in women with psoriasis, and smoking cessation allows better recovery in both men and women.

4.29   Answer: E

Although this may be less important in most cases than was previously believed. Sunlight may worsen the other conditions, but is generally thought beneficial in eczema and psoriasis.

4.30   Answer: B

Acute angioedema (< 6 weeks) is common, affecting up to one third of adults at some point. Can be associated with skin, abdominal and respiratory symptoms.

4.31 A 56-year-old man presents with a 4-month history of rash overlying his trunk and upper and lower limbs. A skin biopsy is reported to show a leukocytoclastic vasculitis pattern. What is the most likely underlying cause?

☑ **A** Adverse drug reaction
☒ **B** Cryoglobulinaemia
☐ **C** Discoid lupus erythematosus
☐ **D** Polyarteritis nodosum
☐ **E** Wegener's granulomatosis

4.32 A 43-year-old man presented to the Dermatology Outpatient Department for assessment of multiple red–yellow papules which had developed over his lower limbs over the past 3 months. The appearance of the lesions is strongly suggestive of eruptive xanthomata. What underlying metabolic disturbance is most likely to be associated with these findings?

☐ **A** High LDL cholesterol
☑ **B** High serum triglycerides
☐ **C** High VLDL particle fraction
☐ **D** Low HDL cholesterol
☐ **E** Low lipoprotein-a concentrations

4.33 A 19-year-old woman develops a painful rash at the left angle of her mouth, associated with a cluster of small fluid-filled vesicles. The laboratory reports that a Tzanck test is positive. What is the most likely diagnosis?

☐ **A** Chickenpox
☐ **B** Dermatitis herpetiformis
☒ **C** Erysipelas
☑ **D** Herpes simplex virus (HSV)
☐ **E** Measles

4.31 Answer: A

Can occur as an adverse effect of any one of a large range of different drugs. Also a characteristic finding in urticarial vasculitis.

4.32 Answer: B

Sudden crops of red–yellow papules with erythematous halos, usually over buttocks or extensor surfaces of the limbs. Lesions contain lipids and lymphocytic infiltrate. Increased risk of pancreatitis.

4.33 Answer: D

The Tzanck test is a direct smear test for herpesvirus, but cannot distinguish varicella zoster virus (VZV) from HSV. Localisation of the lesions to one site, with peri-oral distribution, makes HSV more likely.

4.34 During pre-operative assessment before hip replacement surgery, a 79-year-old woman is noted to have thickening and disfiguration of a number of her toenails, and fungal infection is suspected. What is the most rapid means of confirming the diagnosis?

- ☐ **A** Fungal blood cultures
- ☐ **B** Fungal culture of toe scrapings
- ☐ **C** Plain X-ray of the foot and toes
- ☑ **D** Potassium hydroxide test
- ☒ **E** Wood's light

4.35 A 36-year-old woman with long-standing diabetes presented with plaques over both shins. She was found to have a 12-cm, yellow, atrophic, centrally scarred plaque over each shin, associated with surrounding swelling. What is the most likely diagnosis?

- ☐ **A** Dermatomyositis
- ☐ **B** Diabetic lipoatrophy
- ☑ **C** Necrobiosis lipoidica
- ☐ **D** Polymyositis
- ☐ **E** Sarcoidosis

4.36 A 64-year-old woman is under investigation in the General Medical Outpatient Department for fatigue and lethargy. On examination, you find that all her fingernails appear concave and brittle. What is the most likely cause?

- ☐ **A** Calcium deficiency
- ☑ **B** Iron deficiency
- ☐ **C** Iron poisoning
- ☐ **D** Trauma
- ☐ **E** Vitamin B_{12} deficiency

4.37 What is the most likely cause of angular cheilitis in a 56-year-old woman who is also found to have a bright-red tongue?

- ☒ **A** Folate deficiency
- ☑ **B** Iron deficiency
- ☐ **C** Rifampicin treatment
- ☐ **D** Streptococcal infection
- ☐ **E** Vitamin B_{12} deficiency

4.34 Answer: D

Nail sample is placed on a slide with potassium hydroxide and gently heated to dissolve the skin and nail cells, leaving the fungal cells, which may be visualised on light microscopy. Fungal culture can take 3–6 weeks.

4.35 Answer: C

Occurs predominantly (but not exclusively) in patients with diabetes. Threefold greater prevalence in women. Spontaneous remission occurs in a quarter of patients, and scarring is common.

4.36 Answer: B

Other recognised causes of koilonychia include trauma (unlikely to affect all nails) and lead poisoning, and it is associated with recurrent pleural effusions in yellow nail syndrome.

4.37 Answer: B

Classically, this leads to a cherry-red tongue appearance. Of note, rifampicin is associated with pink discoloration of body fluids and secretions, rather than organ discoloration.

4.38 A 43-year-old man is noted to have a painless white plaque along the left lateral border of his tongue. It is firmly adherent to the tongue, with a fine overlying pattern of striation visible on close inspection. What is the likeliest diagnosis?

- A Candidiasis
- B Leukoplakia
- ☑ C Lichen planus
- D Phosphorus burn
- E Streptococcal stomatitis

4.39 A 42-year-old man has recently been discharged from hospital after presenting with features of alcohol withdrawal and abdominal pain. He had been commenced on a number of new medications. He now re-attends the Emergency Department with fever symptoms. On examination, there is a new diffuse erythematous rash over his trunk and limbs, and investigations show white cell count $9.7 \times 10^9/l$ and eosinophils $0.8 \times 10^9/l$. Which of the following drugs is most likely to have caused his rash?

- A Diazepam
- B Metronidazole
- ☑ C Phenytoin
- D Quinine
- E Thiamine

4.40 A 34-year-old man is referred to the General Medicine Outpatient Clinic for investigation of urticarial symptoms. He has had a number of attacks over the past 3 months, characterised by swelling of the lips and tongue associated with a non-specific generalised rash. During the episodes, he experiences severe colicky abdominal pain for around 6–8 hours. Which of the following investigations might be most helpful?

- A Antibody to house dust mite antigen
- B Eosinophil count
- ☑ C C1-esterase inhibitor
- D IgE
- E Urinary porphyrins

4.38 Answer: C

This is a common condition. It is usually painless (unlike stomatitis) and firmly adherent to the tongue (unlike candidiasis). Phosphorus burns are often painless but associated with ulceration and sloughing. Wickham's striae are pathognomonic for lichen planus. Leukoplakia is a diagnosis of exclusion.

4.39 Answer: C

The diffuse distribution and raised eosinophil count suggest a hypersensitivity rash; other causes include a broad range of drugs, especially penicillins, salicylates and antihistamines. Note that phenytoin can also cause an SLE-like syndrome, erythema multiforme and fixed drug eruptions.

4.40 Answer: C

C1-esterase inhibitor deficiency is a rare condition that predisposes to urticarial reactions with prominent respiratory and gastrointestinal features. As with chronic urticaria, trigger factors are varied, including aspirin, NSAIDs, codeine, food additives, exercise and trauma.

5. ENDOCRINOLOGY

5.1 A 24-year-old woman presents with tachycardia, sweating, anxiety and weight loss. On examination there is no sign of thyroid enlargement, she has a resting tachycardia of 98/min. Her TSH is < 0.01 mIU/l. There is depressed uptake on thyroid scintigraphy. Which of the following is the most likely diagnosis?

- ☐ A Graves' disease
- ☐ B Hashimoto's thyroiditis
- ☒ C Riedel's thyroiditis
- ☐ D Sick euthyroid syndrome
- ☑ E Struma ovarii

5.2 A 29-year-old woman presents with anxiety, sweating and weight loss in the 20th week of her pregnancy. Her TSH is suppressed at < 0.01 mIU/l and she is thyroid autoantibody positive. Which of the following is the most appropriate management?

- ☐ A Carbimazole
- ☐ B Carbimazole and thyroxine (block replace)
- ☐ C Diazepam
- ☐ D Propanolol
- ☑ E Propylthiouracil

5.3 A man who is managed with thyroxine replacement for hypothyroidism comes to the clinic. He complains of tiredness and bony aches. He is known to have chronic renal failure. Blood results of note include: creatinine 227 µmol/l, calcium 2.08 mmol/l, ⬇ 1,25-dihydroxycholecalciferol 10 ng/l and parathyroid hormone ⬆(PTH) 16 pmol/l. Which of the following represents the most appropriate way to manage him?

- ☑ A Alphacalcidol
- ☐ B Cinacalcet
- ☐ C Ergocalciferol
- ☐ D Parathyroidectomy
- ☐ E Sevelamer

5.1 Answer: E

The clinical and biochemical features suggest primary hyperthyroidism, which is usually associated with increased uptake on thyroid scintigraphy. Reduced uptake suggests thyroid hormone from another source eg paraneoplastic sydrome or ingestion of thyroid hormone (thyrotoxicosis factitia).

5.2 Answer: E

Propylthiouracil is thought to be safer in pregnancy.

5.3 Answer: A

The elevated PTH and low calcium indicate secondary hyperparathyroidism which is common in chronic renal failure and may progress to tertiary hyperparathyroidism in some patients.

5.4 A 45-year-old man with long-standing type 1 diabetes is managed with a glargine basal-bolus regime because of frequent hypoglycaemia. He has also suffered from three syncopal attacks over the past 6 months. His lying BP is 155/100 mmHg, and his standing BP is 108/70 mmHg. Currently he takes ramipril and bendroflumethiazide. Which of the following is the most appropriate treatment for him?

- A   Start fludrocortisone
- B   Start hydrocortisone
- C   Recommend compression stockings
- ☑ D   Stop his bendroflumethiazide
- E   Stop his ramipril

5.5 A 66-year-old man with recently diagnosed type 2 diabetes comes to the Emergency Department after a myocardial infarction. His BMI is 32 kg/m² and his BP is 140/85 mmHg; cardiovascular and respiratory examination is unremarkable. Blood testing reveals an HbA1c of 8.8% (it was 9.1% at diagnosis) and a raised creatinine of 240 µmol/l. Which of the following is the most appropriate way to manage his blood glucose?

- A   Exenatide
- ☒ B   Gliclazide
- ☑ C   Insulin
- D   Metformin
- E   Rosiglitazone

5.6 A 66-year-old man with type 2 diabetes suffers an inferior myocardial infarction. His HbA1c on admission is 7.2% and he takes metformin for blood sugar control. On examination, his BP is 142/72 mmHg and he is not in cardiac failure. His creatinine is 132 µmol/l. Which of the following is the most appropriate way to manage his blood glucose?

- A   Add exenatide
- B   Add gliclazide
- C   Add rosiglitazone
- ☑ D   Continue his metformin
- E   Transition him to basal-bolus insulin

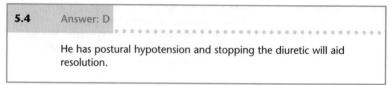

5.4 Answer: D

He has postural hypotension and stopping the diuretic will aid resolution.

5.5 Answer: C

There is either no experience in renal failure with the other agents or they are not suitable.

5.6 Answer: D

Early clinical trials suggested that insulin may improve outcome if given to all MI patients. However, this has been refuted by more recent studies (eg DIGAMI-2). He is relatively well controlled and can continue his metformin.

5.7 A 32-year-old woman presents with symptoms of weight loss, palpitations and anxiety. Her periods stopped 3 months ago. She has done a number of pregnancy tests which have all been negative. On examination she has an obvious left-sided thyroid nodule. Her TSH is < 0.01 mIU/l and a thyroid uptake scan reveals it to be a solitary nodule associated with increased activity. Which of the following is the most appropriate treatment?

- ☒ **A** Carbimazole
- ☐ **B** Lugol's iodine
- ☐ **C** Propylthiouracil
- ☑ **D** Radioiodine
- ☐ **E** Subtotal thyroidectomy

5.8 A 70-year-old woman is admitted with decreased consciousness. Apparently she has been unwell for a few days. On examination she is pyrexial at 37.9 °C and you can barely wake her from sleep. Her glucose is measured at 44.2 mmol/l, her creatinine is 240 µmol/l and her bicarbonate is 22 mmol/l. Which of the following is true of her underlying condition?

- ☐ **A** Bicarbonate is an important component of therapy
- ☐ **B** Mortality is less than 5%
- ☐ **C** She will be ketotic
- ☑ **D** The condition is a presenting feature in a significant number of patients with type 2 diabetes
- ☐ **E** There is likely to be no residual insulin production

5.9 A 68-year-old man who has ischaemic heart disease and chronic atrial fibrillation presents with acute gout affecting his right great toe. Blood testing reveals a raised uric acid, he is known to have chronic renal failure, and a recent creatinine was 185 µmol/l. Which of the following is the most appropriate treatment?

- ☐ **A** Allopurinol
- ☑ **B** Colchicine
- ☐ **C** Ibuprofen
- ☐ **D** Prednisolone
- ☐ **E** Rasburicase

5.7 Answer: D

Radioiodine avoids any possible complications associated with surgery.

5.8 Answer: D

This patient has hyperosmolar non-ketotic (HONK) syndrome with some residual insulin production, and is not ketotic.

5.9 Answer: B

Rasburcase is the most effective means of lowering total body urate burden, but may only be administered parenterally and is licensed only for tumour lysis syndrome.

5.10 A 49-year-old man is diagnosed with haemochromatosis. Which of the following conditions is *not* normally associated with haemochromatosis?

- [ ] **A** Chondrocalcinosis
- [ ] **B** Cirrhosis
- [✓] **C** Diabetes insipidus
- [ ] **D** Diabetes mellitus
- [ ] **E** Erectile dysfunction

5.11 A 60-year-old man presents to the Dyslipidaemia Clinic. His total cholesterol is 4.9 mmol/l, with an HDL of 0.7 mmol/l and raised triglycerides at 3.9 mmol/l. Which one of the following is likely to impact most on his HDL cholesterol?

- [ ] **A** Atorvastatin 10 mg
- [✗] **B** Colestyramine
- [ ] **C** Ezetimibe
- [✓] **D** Nicotinic acid
- [ ] **E** Simvastatin 40 mg

5.12 A 34-year-old man is referred to the Hypertension Clinic. He is currently managed with ramipril 10 mg and amlodipine 10 mg, but his BP is still elevated at 154/105 mmHg. There are no other abnormal findings on examination. His potassium is 3.1 mmol/l. Which of the following is the most likely diagnosis?

- [✓] **A** Conn syndrome
- [ ] **B** Cushing syndrome
- [ ] **C** Essential hypertension
- [ ] **D** Phaeochromocytoma
- [ ] **E** Polycystic kidney disease

5.10   Answer: C

Anterior pituitary-driven disorders are more common.

5.11   Answer: D

Nicotinic acid is likely to have most effect in increasing his HDL cholesterol; although it is associated with a high incidence of adverse effects eg 'flushing headache'.

5.12   Answer: A

Persistent hypokalaemia and hypertension despite ACE inhibition suggests Conn syndrome.

5.13   A 19-year-old woman comes to the clinic. She is obese and has
problems with both acne and hirsutism. She has not had a period
for the past 4 months and denies sexual intercourse. Her BP is
elevated at 152/92 mmHg. Which of the following is the most likely
diagnosis?

- ☐ **A** Congenital adrenal hyperplasia (CAH)
- ☐ **B** Hypothyroidism
- ☑ **C** Polycystic ovarian syndrome (PCOS)
- ☐ **D** Pregnancy
- ☐ **E** Prolactinoma

5.14   A 26-year-old woman comes to the clinic. She has been diagnosed
with PCOS and now wants to discuss starting a family as she has
recently married. She only has a period on average once every
3 months. On examination her BP is 144/82 mmHg and her BMI is
32 kg/m². Which of the following is the most appropriate initial plan
to restore her periods?

- ☑ **A** Get her to lose weight
- ☐ **B** Start her on clomifene
- ☐ **C** Start her on Dianette
- ☐ **D** Start her on metformin
- ☐ **E** Start her on rosiglitazone

5.15   A 64-year-old woman presents with a second Colles' fracture. You
arrange to check her bone mineral density (BMD) and her T-score is
−3.5. Which of the following is the most appropriate therapy for
her?

- ☐ **A** Alendronate
- ☐ **B** Calcium
- ☐ **C** Calcium and vitamin D
- ☑ **D** PTH analogue
- ☒ **E** Zolendronate

5.13   Answer: C

The obesity, acne and hirsutism is relatively typical of polycystic ovarian syndrome.

5.14   Answer: A

If she can lose weight, then that is the most appropriate initial treatment for her. Metformin, rosiglitazone and clomifene all induce ovulation.

5.15   Answer: D

Her BMD falls into the critically low range, so anabolic therapy with a PTH analogue is the most appropriate treatment.

5.16 You are asked to interpret thyroid function test results from a 42-year-old woman who has been attending the Medical Outpatient Department with weight loss. These show thyroid-stimulating hormone (TSH) undetectable and free T$_4$ 18 pmol/l. What is the most likely underlying diagnosis?

- [ ] **A** Early primary hypothyroidism
- [ ] **B** Graves' disease
- [x] **C** Primary hyperthyroidism
- [ ] **D** Subclinical hyperthyroidism
- [x] **E** T$_3$ thyrotoxicosis

5.17 A previously healthy 42-year-old man is referred to the Medical Outpatient Department with a 3-month history of weight loss and persistent sinus tachycardia. Thyroid function tests show TSH 2.4 mIU/l, free T$_4$ 25 pmol/l and free T$_3$ 6.2 pmol/l. What is the most likely underlying diagnosis?

- [ ] **A** Primary hyperthyroidism
- [x] **B** Secondary hyperthyroidism
- [x] **C** Sick euthyroid syndrome
- [ ] **D** Subclinical hypothyroidism
- [ ] **E** Viral thyroiditis

5.18 A 51-year-old woman is being investigated for obesity and hypertension in the Medical Outpatient Department. Investigations indicate hypothyroidism, and antibody tests are positive for anti-thyroid peroxidase (anti-TPO), positive for anti-thyroglobulin and negative for anti-TSH receptor. What is the most likely underlying diagnosis?

- [x] **A** Autoimmune hypothyroidism
- [x] **B** Hashimoto's thyroiditis
- [ ] **C** Graves' disease
- [ ] **D** Pituitary failure
- [ ] **E** SLE

5.16   Answer: E

Comprises 5% of hyperthyroidism. T_4 is often normal, whereas free T_3 concentrations are abnormally high. Complete suppression of TSH can, less commonly, be associated with primary hyperthyroidism where free T_4 is in the upper part of the normal reference range.

5.17   Answer: B

In the setting of primary hyperthyroidism, TSH would be completely suppressed. Detectable levels strongly suggest secondary hyperthyroidism (excess pituitary TSH secretion) or, in rare cases, tertiary hyperthyroidism (excess hypothalamic TRF secretion).

5.18   Answer: A

Not definitive, but anti-TSH receptor antibodies are more usually positive in Graves' disease, whereas the others are less commonly so.

5.19 A 47-year-old woman is noted to have a non-tender thyroid nodule during a routine physical examination. Which of the following statements best describes the role of fine-needle aspiration cytology (FNAC)?

A Around 20–30% specificity

B Infection occurs after the procedure in 5–10% of patients

C Outdated modality now being replaced by MRI scanning

☑ D Overall diagnostic accuracy more than 90%

E Virtually 100% sensitivity

5.20 You review a 30-year-old man in the Endocrinology Outpatient Department who has recenly been diagnosed with Graves' ophthalmopathy. Which of these statements is correct regarding this condition?

☑ A Corneal ulceration is a recognised complication

B Most patients have biochemical hyperthyroidism

C Only 5–10% ever develope extra-ocular features of Graves' disease

☒ D Smoking cessation can worsen progression

E Targeted radiotherapy is useful in most patients

5.21 Which of the following is most commonly found in patients with Hashimoto's thyroiditis?

A Anti-TSH receptor antibodies inhibiting thyroid release

☑ B Extensive thyroid gland infiltration by plasma cells

C Early fibrosis and scarring of the thyroid gland

D Pretibial swelling and skin thickening

E Proptosis

5.22 Which of the following treatments is most likely to be useful in the management of non-toxic multinodular goitre?

A Carbimazole

B Non-selective β-blockers

C Radioiodine

☑ D Surgery

E Thyroxine

5.19   Answer: D

Values vary between centres and operators, but sensitivity and specificity are both around 90% too, and false-negative rate is around 5%.

5.20   Answer: A

Due to non-closure of the eyelid and corneal dryness. Specific treatment is usually not required for Graves' ophthalmopathy in most cases, other than to ensure corneal lubrication. Corticosteroids and radiotherapy may be effective in severe cases complicated by optic nerve compression.

5.21   Answer: B

Typically associated also with anti-TPO and anti-thyroglobulin antibodies and, less commonly, anti-TSH receptor antibodies (unlike those in Graves' disease, these tend to be stimulatory).

5.22   Answer: D

Surgery is most often indicated because of tracheal compression or cosmetic appearance. Radioiodine may also be useful in some cases.

5.23   A 51-year-old woman is found to have bitemporal hemianopia and is being investigated for a suspected pituitary tumour. Which of the following investigations provides optimal views to determine whether the pituitary gland is enlarged?

- ☐ **A** Contrast-enhanced CT brain
- ☐ **B** Functional positron emission tomography (PET)scan
- ☐ **C** Plain skull X-ray
- ☑ **D** T1-weighted MRI scan
- ☐ **E** Transcranial Doppler ultrasound

5.24   Which of the following tests would most reliably detect a deficiency of the growth hormone (GH) axis in a 19-year-old man?

- ☐ **A** ACTH stimulation test
- ☐ **B** Arginine test
- ☒ **C** Glucagon test
- ☑ **D** Insulin tolerance test
- ☐ **E** Thyroid-releasing hormone (TRH) administration test

5.25   You see a patient in the Outpatient Department with blood pressure 102/64 mmHg who is found to have: sodium 132 mmol/l and potassium 5.1 mmol/l. You suspect a diagnosis of hypopituitarism. Which of the following would be the most appropriate next step in the patient's management?

- ☐ **A** CT brain
- ☒ **B** Glucagon test
- ☑ **C** Insulin tolerance test
- ☐ **D** MRI brain scan
- ☐ **E** Short Synacthen test

5.23 Answer: D

T1-weighted MRI shows brain tissue as white, and pituitary adenomata typically are of lower signal intensity than surrounding tissue. Contrast-enhancement may help distinguish the nature of larger tumours.

5.24 Answer: D

Insulin is administered to provoke a stress response, with subsequent release of growth hormone and ACTH. Glucagon also stimulates growth hormone release, but less directly. Arginine stimulates growth hormone secretion, and may be used as a second-line test.

5.25 Answer: C

Hypoglycaemia stimulates ACTH and GH release. Glucagon gives a similar, although less potent, stimulus. Short Synacthen test provides information about the glucocorticoid axis only, and not the growth hormone axis.

5.26 A 52-year-old man attends the Endocrinology Outpatient Department for review of his hypopituitarism. He is currently taking prednisolone 4 mg in the mornings and 2 mg in the evenings. What is the most reliable test to ensure that his glucocorticoid treatment is not excessive?

- A ACTH concentrations in serum
- B Blood pressure
- C Dipstick urinalysis for glucose
- D Random plasma glucose
- ☑ E Urinary free cortisol measurements

5.27 A 16-year-old boy attends the Endocrinology Clinic for the first time, having previously attended a specialist paediatric unit for review of his growth hormone deficiency. Which of the following statements most accurately describes the effect of growth hormone treatment in this condition?

- A Hypercholesterolaemia is a recognised feature
- B Impaired quality of life is a recognised adverse effect of treatment
- ☑ C May become unnecessary in around 50% of patients in whom deficiency resolves
- D Tends to cause obesity in most patients
- E Treatment is generally unnecessary in adults

5.28 Which of the following factors is most likely to cause an increase in prolactin levels?

- ☑ A Breast stimulation
- B Cranial irradiation
- C Hyperthyroidism
- D L-Dopa
- E Obstructive jaundice

5.26   Answer: E

Aiming to keep these within the normal daily limits, so as to avoid development of diabetes, hypertension and reduced bone mineral density.

5.27   Answer: C

Therefore, retesting should be considered. Associated with improved quality of life, exercise capacity, increased lean body mass and reduced fat mass and serum cholesterol.

5.28   Answer: A

Other causes include dopamine antagonists (antipsychotics and anti-emetics), opiates, primary hypothyroidism (TSH stimulates prolactin release) and renal failure (accumulation).

5.29 Which of the following is most likely to be a feature associated with acromegaly?

- A Histology shows adenocarcinoma in 15–20%
- B Local invasion is common
- C Most cases are diagnosed at 18–30 years of age
- D Pituitary adenoma is found in fewer than 30% of cases
- E Threefold increased prevalence in women

5.30 A 46-year-old man is referred to the Medical Outpatient Department for advice on the management of his hypertension and diabetes. On examination, he is noted to have a plethoric face, hirsutism, thin skin, multiple bruises and active striae across the abdominal wall. What is the most likely underlying cause?

- A ACTH-dependent pituitary adenoma
- B Adrenal carcinoma
- C Alcoholism
- D Depression
- E Ectopic ACTH syndrome

5.31 A 44-year-old woman is undergoing investigations for an underlying cause of obesity. Thyroid function tests and 24-h urinary free cortisol and overnight dexamethasone tests are all normal. Which one of these statements is correct?

- A 24-h urinary free cortisol test has 5–10% false-negative rate
- B Cushing syndrome has been excluded
- C Low-dose dexamethasone suppression test may provide additional information
- D Midnight cortisol measurement has low sensitivity but is highly specific
- E Overnight dexamethasone suppression test is more sensitive in obese patients

5.29   Answer: B

Most cases are diagnosed aged 40–60 years. Carcinoma is rare, and pituitary adenoma is found in > 99% of cases. Equal gender prevalence.

5.30   Answer: A

Alcoholism and severe depression account for around 1% of all cases of Cushing syndrome, whereas ACTH-dependent pituitary adenoma is found in around two-thirds of patients.

5.31   Answer: C

Overnight suppression test has a false-negative rate of 2% (similar rate to low-dose dexamethasone suppression test) but this is higher in obese patients. Midnight cortisol has virtually a 0% false-negative rate, ie highly sensitive.

5.32 Which one of the following drugs is most likely to stimulate prolactin release?

☐ A Bromocriptine

☐ B Cabergoline

☐ C L-Dopa

☑ D Metoclopramide

☐ E Ropinirole

5.33 A 30-year-old woman is referred to the Medical Outpatient Department for investigation of excessive thirst and polydipsia. A fluid deprivation test is performed and shows a urine osmolality of 280 mOsm/kg. After administration of desmopressin, urine osmolality is 920 mOsm/kg. What is the most likely underlying diagnosis?

☑ A Cranial diabetes insipidus (DI)

☐ B Nephrogenic diabetes insipidus

☐ C Psychogenic polydipsia

☐ D Syndrome of inappropriate ADH secretion

☐ E Sample contamination giving an erroneous result

5.34 Which of the following features is most strongly suggestive of the syndrome of inappropriate ADH secretion?

☒ A Headache

☒ B Hyponatraemia with raised plasma osmolality

☐ C Hypovolaemia

☐ D Impaired renal function

☑ E Normal urine osmolality despite abnormally low serum osmolality

5.32 Answer: D

Dopamine antagonist. The others have dopamine agonist effects, which suppress prolactin release.

5.33 Answer: A

Low urine osmolality due to lack of ADH effect, indicative of diabetes insipidus; restoration by ADH indicates cranial cause, lack of response to ADH would indicate nephrogenic DI (insensitivity to ADH). After fluid deprivation, osmolality is high in psychogenic polydipsia.

5.34 Answer: E

Normal osmolality is inappropriate; it would be expected to be low.

5.35 A 72-year-old man with known diabetic nephropathy presents to hospital with a history of diarrhoea and vomiting over the last 3 days. He reports he is not passing much urine. His temperature is 38.7 °C, and laboratory investigations show glucose 26 mmol/l, sodium 137 mmol/l, potassium 7.0 mmol/l, urea 18.2 mmol/l, creatinine 320 μmol/l and C-reactive protein (CRP) 150 mg/l. What is the most appropriate immediate treatment?

- ☑ **A** Calcium gluconate
- ☐ **B** Co-amoxiclav
- ☐ **C** Insulin and dextrose infusion
- ☒ **D** Intravenous hydration
- ☐ **E** Urethral catheter insertion and monitoring of urine output

5.36 An obese 55-year-old man presents with a 6-week history of thirst and polyuria. His fasting glucose is 7.6 mmol/l. Which of the following is the best initial treatment?

- ☐ **A** Advise that results are satisfactory and offer reassurance
- ☑ **B** Institute lifestyle modification to lose weight and increase fitness
- ☐ **C** Start glipizide
- ☒ **D** Start metformin
- ☐ **E** Start rosiglitazone

5.37 A 24-year-old woman is referred to the Diabetic Clinic by her GP, who has diagnosed diabetes on the basis of glycosuria and a 6-month history of polyuria and polydipsia. Her weight has been stable for the past year. There is a strong family history of diabetes. A glucose tolerance test is positive, with a post-prandial glucose of 12.6 mmol/l. Which of the following diagnoses is most likely?

- ☐ **A** Latent autoimmune diabetes of adulthood (LADA)
- ☑ **B** Monogenic diabetes (MODY)
- ☐ **C** Secondary diabetes
- ☐ **D** Type 1 diabetes
- ☐ **E** Type 2 diabetes

5.35 Answer: A

The immediate risk is arrhythmia secondary to hyperkalaemia.
Thereafter, dextrose infusion and insulin should be used to shift
potassium into tissues to reduce circulating potassium
concentrations, in addition to controlling circulating glucose
concentrations.

5.36 Answer: B

A fasting glucose > 7 mmol/l confirms diabetes mellitus. Advice
regarding diet, weight loss and exercise is appropriate first-line
treatment and, if this is insufficient, then oral hypoglycaemics could
be introduced.

5.37 Answer: B

The lack of weight loss despite prolonged osmotic symptoms makes
type 1 DM less likely. Normal BMI without hypertension or
hyperlipidaemia makes type 2 less likely. Family history makes MODY
more likely than LADA.

5.38　An 18-year-old man with known type 1 diabetes presents to the Emergency Department with general malaise. Dipstick urinalysis is strongly positive for ketones, and an arterial blood gas confirms a metabolic acidosis. You suspect diabetic ketoacidosis (DKA). Which one of the following findings would be *least* likely to occur, and might suggest an alternative diagnosis?

- [ ] **A**　CRP 50 IU/l
- [ ] **B**　Leukocyte count 16.2 × 10⁹/l
- [ ] **C**　Serum glucose 36 mmol/l
- [✓] **D**　Serum sodium 162 mmol/l
- [ ] **E**　Urea 13.8 mmol/l

5.39　A 34-year-old man is referred to the Endocrinology Clinic for investigation of gynaecomastia. Which of the following investigations would be most appropriate in his initial management?

- [ ] **A**　24-h urinary cortisol
- [ ] **B**　Chest X-ray
- [ ] **C**　Mammography
- [✓] **D**　Serum testosterone
- [ ] **E**　Testicular ultrasound

5.40　A 65-year-old man is found to have serum calcium of 2.72 mmol/l and albumin 34 g/l. Further investigation shows chest X-ray is normal and serum parathyroid hormone is 0.7 IU/l. What is the most likely diagnosis?

- [ ] **A**　Dietary vitamin D excess
- [✓] **B**　Primary hyperparathyroidism
- [ ] **C**　Medullary thyroid carcinoma
- [ ] **D**　Small-cell lung carcinoma
- [ ] **E**　Squamous cell lung carcinoma

5.41　A 34-year-old woman is found to have serum calcium 2.64 mmol/l and phosphate 0.3 mmol/l. Which of the following statements regarding the aetiology of hypercalcaemia is correct?

- [ ] **A**　Hyperthyroidism is the commonest cause in young adults
- [ ] **B**　It is less common in patients taking calcium-channel blockers
- [✓] **C**　It is a recognised feature of vitamin A toxicity
- [ ] **D**　Milk-alkali syndrome has become increasingly common recently
- [ ] **E**　Sarcoidosis is a recognised cause due to delayed calcium excretion

5.38   Answer: D

It is unusual to see hypernatraemia in DKA; it is normally more suggestive of hyperosmotic, non-ketotic syndrome (HONK).

5.39   Answer: D

Other tests include liver biochemistry, serum oestradiol, luteinising hormone (LH) and follicle-stimulating hormone (FSH), prolactin, human chorionic gonadotrophin (hCG) and sex-hormone binding globulin (SHBG).

5.40   Answer: B

Hypercalcaemia suppresses parathyroid hormone (PTH) release, which should be undetectable. Hypercalcaemia is often seen in squamous cell carcinoma, breast and renal carcinoma and is thought to be due to PTH-related peptide.

5.41   Answer: C

Hypercalcaemia in sarcoidosis is thought due to production of active 1,25-D3 by granulomata. Common causes include hyperparathyroidism and malignancy. Rarer causes include hyperthyroidism, phaeochromocytoma, Addison's disease and thiazide use.

5.42 Which of the following is a recognised adverse effect of chronic hypercalcaemia?

- [ ] **A** Asthma
- [ ] **B** Fatty liver infiltration
- [X] **C** Osteoarthritis
- [✓] **D** Peptic ulcer disease
- [ ] **E** Varicose veins

5.43 A 29-year-old woman is being investigated for muscle cramps and fatigue in the General Medical Outpatient Clinic. Investigations show modest elevation of PTH and calcium concentrations, and normal creatinine phosphokinase. What is the most likely underlying diagnosis?

- [X] **A** Diffuse parathyroid hyperplasia
- [✓] **B** Functional parathyroid adenoma
- [ ] **C** Hyperthyroidism
- [ ] **D** Multiple myeloma
- [ ] **E** Multiple parathyroid adenomata

5.44 Which of the following is most likely to cause raised circulating serum calcium concentrations?

- [ ] **A** Chronic renal failure
- [ ] **B** Malabsorption
- [ ] **C** Rhabdomyolysis
- [✓] **D** Tertiary hyperparathyroidism
- [ ] **E** Tumour lysis syndrome

5.45 A 71-year-old woman has recently sustained a fractured left femoral head after a minor fall. Dual-enery X-ray absorptiometry (DEXA) scanning shows a femoral neck bone density T-score of –2.8. What does this mean?

- [ ] **A** 2.8% of the population have lower bone density
- [✓] **B** Bisphosphonates should be considered
- [ ] **C** Less than normal but treatment not required
- [ ] **D** Lifestyle modification is ineffective beyond 60 years of age
- [ ] **E** Ten-year fracture risk is 2.8%

5.42 Answer: D

Due to excess gastrin production. Other features include myopathy, constipation, nephrolithiasis and nephrogenic diabetes insipidus.

5.43 Answer: B

The absence of PTH suppression in the presence of raised serum calcium is strongly suggestive of primary hyperparathyroidism. The vast majority of cases arise from a solitary functional nodule; less commonly due to multiple adenomata or diffuse hyperplasia.

5.44 Answer: D

A feature of primary and tertiary hyperparathyroidism (autonomous PTH production regardless of serum calcium), whereas calcium is often slightly low or normal in secondary hyperparathyroidism. The other listed options are all recognised causes of hypocalcaemia.

5.45 Answer: B

This means 2.8 standard deviations lower than gender-matched population mean. Bisphosphonate therapy can reduce the risk of subsequent fracture by up to 50%.

5.46 Which of the following conditions is most likely to account for a serum magnesium concentration of 1.7 mmol/l?

☐ **A** Acute pancreatitis

☐ **B** Bartter syndrome

☑ **C** Chronic renal impairment

☐ **D** Diarrhoea

☒ **E** Thiazide diuretics

5.47 A 24-year-old man attends the Endocrinology Outpatient Department for a routine follow-up appointment for alkaptonuria. Which of these is the most common feature of the condition?

☐ **A** Gastrointestinal obstruction

☐ **B** Haematuria

☐ **C** Liver disease

☑ **D** Nephrolithiasis

☐ **E** Psoriatic arthropathy

5.48 A 20-year-old man is admitted to hospital with colicky abdominal and flank pain, and a CT scan shows calculus partially obstructing the distal left ureters. He has had two previous hospital admissions for ureteric calculi. Which of the following conditions is most likely to predispose to nephrolithiasis?

☐ **A** Diabetes insipidus

☒ **B** Homocystinuria

☐ **C** Ketoacidosis

☐ **D** Lactic acidosis

☑ **E** Oxalosis

5.49 A 53-year-old woman presents with sudden onset of pain in the first metatarsophalangeal joint in her left foot. The pain is severe and she is unable to weight-bear. On examination, the joint is swollen and red with limited mobility, and temperature is 37.1 °C. Serum calcium is 2.26 mmol/l, albumin 42 g/l and urate 0.26 mmol/l. What is the most likely diagnosis?

☑ **A** Acute gout

☐ **B** Atheroembolism

☐ **C** Osteoarthritis

☒ **D** Septic arthritis

☐ **E** Subluxation

5.46   Answer: C

Uncommon, but usually associated with excess administration of conventional intravenous fluids such as normal saline or 5% dextrose. The other listed causes are recognised causes of hypomagnesaemia.

5.47   Answer: D

Rare disorder with autosomal recessive inheritance, deficiency of the enzyme homogentisic acid oxidase. Homogentisate polymers, alkapton, accumulate in urine (darkens on standing) and cartilage (osteoarthritis). Rarer features include ocular involvement and aortic valve incompetence.

5.48   Answer: E

Metabolic abnormality causing overproduction of oxalate. Features include bone disease, recurrent nephrolithiasis and premature cardiovascular disease.

5.49   Answer: A

The site and characteristics are strongly suggestive. There is no correlation between serum urate and risk of gout; risk is dependent on total body urate, which varies from 0.5–1.0 g in healthy individuals to 10–30 g in patients with hypertension or heart failure.

5.50 An 18-year-old man is being investigated in the Medical Outpatient Department for abnormal liver function tests. Which of the following most strongly suggests an underlying diagnosis of Wilson's disease?

- ☐ **A** Decreased urinary copper excretion
- ☐ **B** Dilatation of the biliary tree on ultrasound scan
- ☑ **C** Hypoparathyroidism
- ☐ **D** Increased serum caeruloplasmin
- ☐ **E** Scattered corneal microdeposits

5.51 A 46-year-old man is referred to the Medical Outpatient Clinic for investigation of hepatomegaly. You note that he appears to have excessive skin pigmentation. Which of these most strongly suggests haemochromatosis?

- ☐ **A** ESR 38 mm/h
- ☐ **B** Haematocrit 0.58
- ☐ **C** Hb 16.1 g/dl
- ☐ **D** Serum ferritin 560 µg/l
- ☑ **E** Transferrin saturation 76%

5.52 A 55-year-old woman is found to have serum transferrin 66% and serum ferritin 620 µg/l. You suspect a possible diagnosis of haemochromatosis. Which of the following is most likely to be responsible?

- ☑ **A** Alcohol excess
- ☐ **B** COPD
- ☐ **C** Excessive iron intake
- ☐ **D** Living at high altitude
- ☐ **E** Long-standing smoking

5.53 A 45-year-old woman is admitted to hospital with generalised abdominal pain. Physical examination is normal. Her urine is found to turn dark-red on standing. What is the most likely explanation for these features?

- ☑ **A** Acute intermittent porphyria
- ☐ **B** Acute interstitial nephritis
- ☐ **C** Alkaptonuria
- ☐ **D** Porphyria cutanea tarda
- ☐ **E** Rifampicin overdose

5.50 Answer: C

Other features include cirrhosis and chronic hepatitis, haemolysis, tremor, chorea, seizures, arthropathy and Kayser–Fleischer corneal rings. Diagnosis is usually based on decreased serum caeruloplasmin and increased urinary copper excretion, and copper deposition can be demonstrated on liver biopsy.

5.51 Answer: E

Features also include raised ferritin (this is less specific) and liver iron concentrations > 180 μmol/g on biopsy specimens. There is increased prevalence of diabetes mellitus, hypogonadism and cardiomyopathy.

5.52 Answer: A

Other causes of secondary haemochromatosis include liver disease, parenteral iron overload (eg in patients with chronic renal disease), and ineffective erythropoiesis (eg β-thalassaemia).

5.53 Answer: A

Unlike porphyria cutanea tarda, there is no skin involvement or photosensitivity. Rifampicin causes pink-red discoloration of body fluids and urine, whereas urine in alkaptonuria turns black on standing.

5.54 A 56-year-old man is given radio-labelled iodine treatment for hyperthyroidism associated with a diffuse multinodular goitre. Which of these is most frequently recognised as a feature of this treatment?

- ☐ **A** Doses up to 800 MBq do not cause extracorporeal radiation emission
- ☐ **B** Most patients require repeated administration
- ☐ **C** Risk of cancer is increased by around 1% per year
- ☑ **D** Should be avoided in pregnant women
- ☐ **E** There is predominantly α-particle emission

5.55 A 54-year-old woman is referred to the Hypertension Clinic because she has failed to respond to combination of three antihypertensive agents. Blood pressure is 168/98 mmHg in her right arm, and initial investigations show: sodium 146 mmol/l, potassium 3.0 mmol/l and bicarbonate 32 mmol/l. What is the most likely diagnosis?

- ☐ **A** Addison's disease
- ☑ **B** Conn syndrome
- ☐ **C** Cushing's disease
- ☐ **D** Phaeochromocytoma
- ☐ **E** Renal artery stenosis

5.56 A 60-year-old man is found to have resistant hypertension, and investigations show hypokalaemic alkalosis. Two weeks after commencing spironolactone therapy his blood pressure is found to have decreased from 182/95 mmHg to 156/82 mmHg and his metabolic disturbance has resolved. What is the most likely underlying cause of his hypertension?

- ☐ **A** Adrenal carcinoma
- ☑ **B** Benign adenoma in adrenal cortex
- ☐ **C** Diffuse hyperplasia of the adrenal medulla
- ☐ **D** Phaeochromocytoma
- ☐ **E** Severe essential hypertension

5.54 Answer: D

Causes emission of α-particles predominantly (poor penetration and range) and, to a lesser extent, gamma rays (higher penetration); 10–15% require further radioiodine. Women of childbearing age should avoid pregnancy for at least 4 months.

5.55 Answer: B

Typically, patients have hypertension resistant to conventional therapy and the syndrome is thought to be present in 2–10% of all hypertensive patients. Good blood pressure and electrolyte response to spironolactone. Cushing's could cause the same abnormalities, but would be expected to manifest other clinical features.

5.56 Answer: B

Scenario strongly suggestive of hyperaldosteronism. Single functional adrenocortical adenoma (Conn syndrome) accounts for 75% of cases.

5.57 A 24-year-old man is referred to the Medical Outpatient Department for assessment of anorexia and weight loss over the past 6 months. On examination, he is found to have a 22-mmHg difference between seated and standing systolic blood pressure readings. Investigations show: sodium 132 mmol/l, potassium 4.7 mmol/l and ESR 28 mm/h. What is the most likely diagnosis?

- ☑ **A** Addison's disease
- ☐ **B** Conn syndrome
- ☐ **C** Diabetes insipidus
- ☐ **D** Diabetes mellitus
- ☐ **E** Tuberculosis

5.58 A 43-year-old woman is found to have adrenal insufficiency in the context of a number of other autoimmune disorders. Which of the following features most strongly suggests autoimmune polyglandular syndrome type 1 (APS-1)?

- ☐ **A** Autosomal dominant familial pattern
- ☐ **B** Diabetes insipidus
- ☑ **C** Hypoparathyroidism
- ☐ **D** Primary gonadal failure
- ☐ **E** Vitiligo

5.59 A 32-year-old woman is referred to the local Hypertension Clinic for investigation of high blood pressure. Recordings have been highly variable, ranging from 148/86 mmHg to 182/106 mmHg with no obvious diurnal pattern. Which of the following is the most appropriate initial test in screening for underlying phaeochromocytoma?

- ☑ **A** 24-h urinary free catecholamine measurement
- ☐ **B** 24-h urinary metanephrine measurement
- ☐ **C** Clonidine suppression test
- ☐ **D** 123I-labelled MIBG scan
- ☐ **E** Plasma catecholamines

5.57   Answer: A

Other features include pigmentation (generalised or in creases), arthralgia, symptoms resembling hypoglycaemia, and investigations also show modestly elevated urea and calcium and eosinophilia.

5.58   Answer: C

Not seen in APS-2. The features of APS-1 are chronic candidiasis, adrenal insufficiency, hypoparathyroidism, primary hypogonadism and hypothyroidism, and (rarely) hypopituitarism and diabetes insipidus.

5.59   Answer: A

Should be performed at least twice because of variability in readings. Free catecholamine assay is more sensitive than metabolites (metanephrine and vanillyl mandelic acid (VMA)). Suppression tests are reserved for cases where diagnosis is questionable, and MIBG scans are used for localisation rather than diagnosis.

5.60 A 46-year-old man presents with a 1-year history of intermittent headaches and dizziness. Blood pressure is found to be 144/92 mmHg seated, and 126/84 mmHg standing. 24-h cardiac monitoring shows pulse rate varying between 92/min and 132/min in sinus rhythm. What is the most likely underlying diagnosis?

- A Addison's disease
- B Adrenal carcinoma
- C Generalised anxiety disorder
- D Hyperthyroidism
- ☑ E Phaeochromocytoma

5.61 A 23-year-old woman is referred to the Endocrinology Department for assessment of amenorrhoea for the past 4 months. Her weight has decreased from 72 kg to 58 kg over the past 6 months. What is the most likely cause of her amenorrhoea?

- ☑ A Excessive exercise
- B Gastric carcinoma
- C Pregnancy
- D Premature ovarian failure
- E Turner syndrome

5.62 You are asked for advice regarding hormone replacement therapy (HRT) in a 61-year-old woman with symptoms of hot flushes. Which statement most correctly describes the role of HRT?

- A Can lower systemic blood pressure
- B Improves overall survival
- C Increases overall cardiovascular risk
- ☑ D Reduces symptoms of vaginal dryness
- E Should be considered in all women aged 45 years or more

5.63 A 61-year-old man attends the Diabetic Outpatient Department for routine follow-up. He mentions that he has been impotent for some time, and is interested in possible treatment. Which of these statements best characterises the role of sildenafil in this situation?

- A Ineffective in patients with type 2 diabetes
- B Normally taken orally 12 h before intercourse attempted
- ☑ C Sudden cardiac death is a recognised adverse effect
- D Therapeutic effects enhanced by nitrate co-administration
- ☒ E Therapeutic effects mediated by enhanced cyclic AMP

5.60 Answer: E

Hypertension and postural hypotension are characteristic features, the latter due to functional stiffening of the blood vessels. Diagnosis should be confirmed by at least two 24-h urinary catecholamine assays.

5.61 Answer: A

Although weight loss alone would be sufficient; may suggest anorexia. Pregnancy should be excluded; however, weight loss makes this less likely. Turner syndrome and Kallman syndrome cause primary amenorrhoea.

5.62 Answer: D

HRT offers effective symptomatic relief for hot flushes and other post-menopausal symptoms. There is a reduction in cardiovascular disease risk and improvement in bone mineral density, offset by an increased risk of hepatobiliary disease and thromboembolism.

5.63 Answer: C

Mostly in patients with pre-existing heart disease. Potentially hazardous interaction with nitrate therapy, causing hypotension. Treatment is given as a single 50–100-mg dose 1 h before intercourse.

5.64 Which of the following factors most strongly indicates the need for surgical intervention in primary hyperparathyroidism?

- ☑ **A** Chronic renal impairment
- ☐ **B** Impaired liver function
- ☒ **C** Patient < 50 years age
- ☐ **D** Serum calcium 2.60 mmol/l or above
- ☐ **E** Single episode of ureteric colic

5.65 A 43-year-old woman is referred to the Endocrinology Outpatient Department for assessment of a number of metabolic abnormalities. Calcium is 2.45 mmol/l, phosphate is 0.2 mmol/l, bicarbonate 12 mmol/l and dipstick urinalysis shows ketones + and glucose +++. What is the most likely underlying diagnosis?

- ☒ **A** Bartter syndrome
- ☐ **B** Diabetic ketoacidosis
- ☑ **C** Fanconi syndrome
- ☐ **D** Felty syndrome
- ☐ **E** Lactic acidosis

5.66 A 51-year-old man with long-standing diabetes is referred to the Medical Outpatient Department for investigation of his right foot. He had fallen 4 weeks earlier, and X-rays of the foot and ankle at that time showed no fractures. On examination, the left foot feels warmer than the right, and peripheral pulses are intact. A repeat X-ray is normal, and bone scintigraphy shows increased uptake overlying the left foot. What is the most likely diagnosis?

- ☐ **A** Avascular necrosis
- ☑ **B** Charcot neuroarthropathy
- ☐ **C** Osteomyelitis
- ☒ **D** Reflex sympathetic dystrophy
- ☐ **E** Stress fracture

5.64 Answer: A

Other criteria are serum calcium > 3.00 mmol/l, urinary calcium excretion of > 10 mmol/day, nephrocalcinosis, recurrent ureteric calculi and evidence of bone disease. Less strict criteria are young age, patient preference and single episode of calculus disease.

5.65 Answer: C

Characteristic renal wasting of glucose, bicarbonate, phosphate and amino acids due to tubular defect, often leading to osteomalacia.

5.66 Answer: B

Diabetes is the commonest cause of this disorder. Peripheral pulses are often intact, whereas there is usually evidence of a sensory neuropathy. It may be precipitated by minor trauma.

5.67 A 43-year-old man presents to the Emergency Department with a 12-h history of loin and back pain, fever and rigors. Examination shows temperature 39.4 °C. Investigations show: sodium 134 mmol/l, potassium 5.4 mmol/l, urea 25 mmol/l, creatinine 164 µmol/l, bicarbonate 12 mmol/l, serum osmolality 332 mOsm/kg. What is the most likely diagnosis?

- [ ] **A** Alcoholic hepatitis
- [✓] **B** Diabetic ketoacidosis
- [ ] **C** Lactic acidosis
- [ ] **D** Methanol ingestion
- [✗] **E** Pancreatitis

5.68 A 45-year-old man has had well-controlled diabetes for 27 years. What finding would be most likely on physical examination?

- [✓] **A** Background diabetic retinopathy
- [ ] **B** Hepatomegaly
- [ ] **C** Hypertension
- [ ] **D** Lipoatrophy
- [ ] **E** Peripheral sensorimotor neuropathy

5.69 A 28-year-old man is admitted to the High Dependency Unit via the Emergency Department with diabetic ketoacidosis. Which one of these statements is most accurate with respect to his initial management?

- [ ] **A** Hydration should provide 1.5 l in the first 24 h
- [ ] **B** Hyponatraemia should be corrected rapidly
- [✗] **C** Potassium supplements should be withheld in the first hour
- [ ] **D** Resuscitation should be with saline only
- [✓] **E** Urine output should be monitored at least hourly in the first 24 h

5.67 Answer: B

Osmolality is very high. Estimated by [(Na⁺ + K⁺) × 2 + urea + glucose], therefore glucose is probably 27 mmol/l.

5.68 Answer: A

Background (non-proliferative) retinopathy is dependent on the duration of diabetes, and is present in around 80% of patients who have had diabetes for 20 years or more.

5.69 Answer: E

The mainstay of treatment is fluid replacement, insulin administration and careful monitoring of fluid balance and electrolyte status.

5.70   A 34-year-old man is admitted via the Emergency Department
following a collapse and reduced conscious level. He has had long-
standing diabetes, which has been well controlled with insulin. On
arrival in the Emergency Department, a BM glucose reading was
1.0 mmol/l and his conscious level responded rapidly to
administration of intravenous glucose. What test will be most
helpful in establishing the underlying cause of his hypoglycaemia?

☑ A HbA1c

☒ B Post-prandial glucose

☒ C Serum insulin concentration

☐ D Short Synacthen test

☐ E Urinary C-peptide excretion

5.71   A 30-year-old woman is referred to the Endocrinology Department
for investigation of weight loss despite a healthy appetite. Thyroid
function tests show free T_4 = 36 pmol/l and TSH is undetectable.
Which of the following signs is most likely to be present on
examination?

☐ A Atrial fibrillation

☐ B Bitemporal hemianopia

☐ C Exophthalmos

☑ D Lid lag

☐ E Pretibial myxoedema

5.72   A 55-year-old woman attending the Hypertension Clinic is found to
have elevated 24-h urinary catecholamine excretion on two
successive tests, suggesting a diagnosis of phaeochromocytoma.
Which of the following statements is most accurate regarding this
condition?

☐ A Around one third are malignant

☐ B Family history is common

☑ C More than 85% are solitary adrenal medullary tumours

☐ D Radio-labelled iodine is a recognised treatment

☐ E Surgical resection normalises blood pressure in > 95% of patients

5.70 Answer: A

The most common explanation for hypoglycaemia is overly-aggressive insulin therapy, which will be reflected by a low HbA1c concentration. In some cases Addison's disease should be considered as an alternative diagnosis.

5.71 Answer: D

This is a feature of hyperthyroid states, as is tachycardia. Atrial fibrillation is a less consistent complication, and exophthalmos and pretibial skin changes are features of Graves' disease regardless of thyroid state.

5.72 Answer: C

Around 10–15% are diffuse, bilateral or extramedullary. Between 8% and 12% are malignant. Radioiodine-labelled metaiodobenzylguanidine (MIBG) can help localise functionally active tumour. Surgical correction alleviates symptoms and can make hypertension easier to control with conventional therapy; in only a small proportion of patients can treatment be completely withdrawn.

5.73 A 56-year-old man with diabetes since childhood is referred to the General Medical Outpatient Department for assessment. Over the past 6 weeks he has been complaining of increased sweating and abdominal bloating. He also describes blurred vision on rising from bed in the mornings associated with dizziness. What is the best explanation for his symptoms?

- A Addison's disease
- B Autonomic neuropathy ☑
- C Nocturnal hypoglycaemia
- D Postural hypotension
- E Thyrotoxicosis

5.74 A 34-year-old woman is 24 weeks pregnant. She is referred for further assessment because her weight gain has been much greater than anticipated. In addition, her husband is concerned that she has become harder to rouse from sleep in the mornings and she has been rather confused after waking. What is the most likely diagnosis?

- A Alcoholism
- B Gestational diabetes ☒
- C Glucagonoma
- D Hepatic failure
- E Insulinoma ☑

5.75 Which of the following is most likely to be associated with increased insulin sensitivity?

- A Acromegaly
- B Phaechromocytoma
- C Polycystic ovarian syndrome
- D Smoking cessation
- E Weight loss ☑

5.73   Answer: B

Blurred vision and dizziness are suggestive of postural hypotension; additional features of excessive sweating and abdominal bloating suggest a more generalised autonomic impairment. Other features include gustatory sweating, gastroparesis, vomiting and diarrhoea.

5.74   Answer: E

Uncommon cause of hypoglycaemia, typically associated with weight gain. Can be demonstrated by prolonged fasting, up to 72 h. Other causes of hypoglycaemia include soft-tissue sarcomas that secrete insulin-like growth factor, liver disease and alcoholism.

5.75   Answer: E

This has been shown to completely normalise insulin sensitivity in obese patients with impaired glucose tolerance. Smoking cessation would be expected to increase sensitivity, but this has not been demonstrated so convincingly. The other listed condtions are associated with increased insulin resistance.

6. GASTROENTEROLOGY

6.1 A 58-year-old publican who smokes 20 cigarettes per day complains of increasing nausea and epigastric pain which radiates through to his back. He has lost 5 kg in weight over the past 4 months. His BMI is 19 kg/m² and he has epigastric tenderness on palpation. His Hb is 10.5 g/dl, with a macrocytosis; other bloods are normal and upper gastrointestinal (GI) endoscopy reveals mild oesophagitis. What is the best next investigation?

- ☑ **A** CT abdomen
- ☐ **B** Endoscopic retrograde cholangiopancreatography (ERCP)
- ☐ **C** pH monitoring
- ☐ **D** Repeat endoscopy after acid suppression
- ☐ **E** Sigmoidoscopy

6.2 A 52-year-old woman presents with anorexia, joint pains, diarrhoea and intermittent fevers. She has lost 5 kg in weight over the past 6 months and feels tired out. There is a history of hypertension, for which she takes indapamide, but nil else of note. Her BMI is 17.5 kg/m², BP is 132/72 mmHg, and there is palpable inguinal lymphadenopathy. She is anaemic (Hb 10.0 g/dl), with an albumin of 22 g/l. Small-bowel biopsy shows expanded villi with PAS-positive macrophages. Which of the following is the most likely diagnosis?

- ☐ **A** Coeliac disease
- ☐ **B** Bacterial overgrowth syndrome
- ☐ **C** Intestinal lymphoma
- ☐ **D** Tropical sprue
- ☑ **E** Whipple's disease

6.1   Answer: A

Two very important differentials are chronic pancreatitis and pancreatic carcinoma.

6.2   Answer: E

The small-bowel biopsy picture is characteristic of Whipple's disease.

6.3 A 54-year-old man is referred with symptoms of chronic liver disease. His GP has referred him to try and elucidate an underlying diagnosis. He also has a history of chondrocalcinosis of both knees and impaired glucose tolerance. Medication of note includes Viagra, which he takes for erectile dysfunction. He has a chronically raised ALT which is around the 150 IU/l mark and a decreased albumin of around 29 g/l; his Hb is normal. He claims not to drink any alcohol as he is a taxi driver. His BMI is 27 kg/m². Which of the following is the most likely diagnosis?

- A Alcoholic cirrhosis
- B Chronic active hepatitis
- ☑ C Haemochromatosis
- D Steatohepatitis
- E Wilson's disease

6.4 A 42-year-old woman with a history of chronic alcohol abuse presents to the clinic with increasing abdominal swelling. On examination there are signs of chronic liver disease, jaundice, ascites and spider naevi. She has a macrocytic anaemia and a raised CA-125 of 65 units/ml. Which of the following is the most likely cause of her raised CA-125?

- A Ascites
- ☑ B Cirrhosis
- C Colon cancer
- D Hepatocellular carcinoma
- E Ovarian cancer

6.5 A 32-year-old man is referred to the clinic by his GP, who suspects irritable bowel syndrome. He has intermittent bouts of diarrhoea, problems with bloating, and flatulence. He has been feeling increasingly tired over the past few months. He is pale and has a BMI of 21 kg/m². Bloods reveal mild anaemia and small-bowel biopsy shows partial villus atrophy and increased lymphocytes. What is the most appropriate treatment?

- A Ciprofloxacin
- ☑ B Gluten-free diet
- C Lactose-free diet
- D Metronidazole
- E Prednisolone

6.3 Answer: C

Clinically, the constellation of chondrocalcinosis, cirrhosis and impaired glucose tolerance raises haemochromatosis as a possibility.

6.4 Answer: B

A CA-125 level in this range can be due to cirrhosis; if ovarian carcinoma was suspected, the CA-125 could well be very much more elevated.

6.5 Answer: B

Coeliac disease can be missed in this age group. The anaemia and small-bowel picture are typical of this underlying diagnosis.

6.6   A 40-year-old man comes to the clinic with symptoms of indigestion over the past 18 months. He is very worried because his father died of oesophageal carcinoma. His blood tests are normal, endoscopy reveals *Helicobacter pylori* gastritis, and he is treated with eradication therapy. What can you advise with respect to his risk of gastric carcinoma? Select one option.

☑ **A** He can be reassured that his risk of gastric carcinoma has been significantly reduced

☐ **B** He is at risk of gastric lymphoma

☐ **C** He should restrict alcohol to less than 10 units/week

☐ **D** He should re-take eradication therapy every 2 years

☐ **E** The risk will definitely be increased

6.7   A 40-year-old pub owner comes to the clinic with worsening shortness of breath, made better by lying flat. He is an alcoholic with significant signs of liver disease, including marked ascites. He has bilateral pleural effusions, is tachycardic with a pulse of 100/min, and his BP is 95/60 mmHg. He is hypoxic and hypocapnic on arterial blood gas (ABG) testing (PaO$_2$ 7.6 kPa, PaCO$_2$ 3.6 kPa). Which of the following is the most likely diagnosis?

☐ **A** Cardiac failure

☐ **B** COPD

☑ **C** Hepatopulmonary syndrome

☐ **D** Pulmonary embolus

☐ **E** Pulmonary fibrosis

6.8   A 28-year-old man who has type 1 diabetes presents to the clinic with tiredness and lethargy. He doesn't admit to any particular bowel upset. He has a family history of autoimmune diseases, with other members of the family known to suffer from vitiligo and hypothyroidism. On examination he looks thin (BMI 18 kg/m^2). Bloods reveal a macrocytic anaemia (Hb 9.9 g/dl, MCV 114 fl). His albumin is low at 30 g/l. Which of the following is the most likely diagnosis?

☐ **A** Bacterial overgrowth

☑ **B** Coeliac disease

☐ **C** Crohn's disease

☐ **D** Hypothyroidism

☒ **E** Pernicious anaemia

6.6   Answer: A

H. pylori is associated with increased risk of both gastric carcinoma and gastric maltoma. Eradication therapy is associated with a significant reduction in these risks.

6.7   Answer: C

Pulmonary embolus is very unlikely here as these patients are auto-anticoagulated. Hepatopulmonary syndrome occurs due to arteriovenous shunting, is progressive and life-threatening. Liver transplant is the only effective treatment.

6.8   Answer: B

Occult coeliac disease is surprisingly common in this group, and is suggested by the low albumin and the macrocytic anaemia (folate deficiency).

6.9 A 61-year-old man presents with unexplained lethargy and fatigue. He has lost a few kg in weight over the past few months. His BMI is 19 kg/m²; physical examination including per rectal (PR) is unremarkable. His bloods reveal an Hb of 9.4 g/dl with an MCV of 75 fl. Upper GI endoscopy is normal and flexible sigmoidoscopy reveals mild diverticular disease. Which of the following would you consider the most likely underlying diagnosis?

- [ ] **A** Angiodysplasia
- [ ] **B** Crohn's disease
- [ ] **C** Diverticulosis
- [✓] **D** Right-sided colonic carcinoma
- [ ] **E** Small-bowel lymphoma

6.10 A 62-year-old woman with atrial fibrillation comes to the Emergency Department. She is anticoagulated with warfarin and her most recent INR was 2.1. She complains of sudden onset of central abdominal pain. On examination she is in great pain and her abdomen is very tender, with absent bowel sounds. She is hypotensive, with a BP of 100/60 mmHg, and tachycardic (105/min, irregular). Which of the following diagnoses would you consider highest on your list?

- [ ] **A** Acute pancreatitis
- [ ] **B** Colonic perforation
- [✓] **C** Ischaemic bowel
- [ ] **D** Retroperitoneal bleed
- [ ] **E** Ruptured aortic aneurysm

6.11 A 61-year-old man presents with a long history of dysphagia, first to liquids, then to solids, then to either intermittently. This has been going on for months. He has no other past history of note, but has had to be moved from his job as a labourer in the local warehouse to a desk-based one due to fatigue. On examination he has a purple-red rash on his face and his BMI is 31 kg/m². Blood testing is unremarkable apart from positive anti-nuclear antibodies. Which of the following is the most likely diagnosis?

- [ ] **A** Achalasia
- [✓] **B** Dermatomyositis
- [ ] **C** Oesophageal carcinoma
- [ ] **D** Oesophageal reflux
- [ ] **E** SLE

6.9 Answer: D

The lack of significant GI symptoms, combined with weight loss and anaemia is suggestive of a possible right-sided colonic tumour.

6.10 Answer: C

Although she is anticoagulated, this doesn't exclude the possibility of an arterial embolus leading to acute ischaemic bowel. Early diagnosis is essential, to allow for limited resection if possible.

6.11 Answer: B

Dermatomyositis can present with oesophageal symptoms because of dysmotility. The rash and generalised weakness fit well with the diagnosis.

6.12   A 40-year-old alcoholic is admitted with sudden-onset severe epigastric pain and vomiting. You suspect that the underlying diagnosis is acute pancreatitis. Bloods include: Hb 12.1 g/dl, white cell count (WCC) 13.3 × 10⁹/l, platelets 190 × 10⁹/l, sodium 140 mmol/l, potassium 4.4 mmol/l, creatinine 139 µmol/l, urea 17.1 mmol/l, amylase 1210 IU/l, albumin 28 g/l, PaO₂ 7.8 kPa, ALT 182 IU/l. Which one of the following blood results is associated with a worse prognosis?

☐ **A**   ALT 182 IU/l

☐ **B**   Amylase 1210 IU/l

☐ **C**   Creatinine 139 µmol/l

☑ **D**   PaO₂ 7.8 kPa

☐ **E**   WCC 13.3 × 10⁹/l

6.13   A 36-year-old woman with long-standing Crohn's disease comes to the clinic. She is worried because she is on oral mesalazine but still has diarrhoea and rectal bleeding and has required three courses of prednisolone this year. She has active disease, as indicated by an Hb of 10.4 g/dl and an ESR of 47 mm/h. Colonoscopy reveals Crohn's skip lesions but with much more active distal disease, in keeping with her symptoms. Which of the following is the most appropriate way to manage her?

☐ **A**   Give her a further course of oral steroids

☒ **B**   Give her intravenous infliximab

☐ **C**   Give her rectal budesonide

☑ **D**   Give her rectal mesalazine

☐ **E**   Increase her oral mesalazine

6.14   A 28-year-old woman who is 29 weeks pregnant comes to the Gastroenterology Clinic. She has Crohn's disease but it has been quiescent for 18 months and she stopped her medication (sulfasalazine) before getting pregnant. She now has severe diarrhoea and abdominal pain. Her abdomen is consistent with a 30-week pregnancy, so is difficult to assess further. Her ESR is elevated at 50 mm/h, and she is mildly anaemic with an Hb of 10.7 g/dl. Which one of the following will you give her to manage her Crohn's?

☐ **A**   Infliximab

☐ **B**   Methotrexate

☐ **C**   Metronidazole

☑ **D**   Prednisolone

☐ **E**   Sulfasalazine

6.12 Answer: D

The Glasgow pancreatitis scoring system scores severity on: age > 55 years, WCC > 15 × 10⁹/l, urea > 16 mmol/l, glucose > 10 mmol/l and PaO_2 < 8.0 kPa.

6.13 Answer: D

The most appropriate next step would be rectal mesalazine, which has been shown in clinical trials to be more effective than rectal steroids in controlling symptoms of distal Crohn's disease.

6.14 Answer: D

Corticosteroids have the most experience with respect to use in pregnancy and are probably the safest option of those given.

6.15 A 28-year-old man who had a renal transplant 2 years ago has just returned from a family holiday to Morocco with watery diarrhoea. He takes extensive immunosupressive treatment. On examination he has a 20-mmHg postural drop in BP and is pyrexial (38.5 °C). His creatinine has risen to 185 µmol/l (142 µmol/l pre-holiday) and oocysts are seen in his stool. How will you manage him?

- ☒ A Ciprofloxacin
- ☐ B Loperamide
- ☐ C Metronidazole
- ☑ D Nitazoxanide
- ☐ E Supportive management only

6.16 A 34-year-old woman attends the Gastroenterology Clinic for investigation of intermittent crampy abdominal pain. On examination, you note that she has oral ulceration, glossitis and angular stomatitis. Which of the following diagnoses is most likely to cause these physical findings?

- ☑ A Coeliac disease
- ☐ B Erythema multiforme
- ☐ C Peutz–Jeghers syndrome
- ☐ D Porphyria
- ☐ E Ulcerative colitis

6.17 A 65-year-old man attends his GP complaining of 'food sticking in his throat'. Which of the following is correct regarding oesophageal dysphagia?

- ☐ A Bolus transit time is usually not affected
- ☐ B Characteristically there is difficulty initiating swallowing
- ☐ C Dysphagia for solids is usually due to altered oesophageal motility
- ☑ D Functional dysphagia can be intermittent and non-progressive
- ☐ E Stricture (benign or malignant) is an uncommon cause

6.15 Answer: D

Nitazoxanide blocks the ability of the parasites to generate energy by blocking the pyruvate ferridoxin reaction. *Cryptosporidium* might not need to be treated in all patients but, given the immunosupression and increased creatinine, treatment seems prudent here.

6.16 Answer: A

Coeliac disease is also associated with dermatitis herpetiformis. Erythema multiforme gives target-like rash with mucosal blistering and ulceration. Peutz–Jeghers syndrome involves mucosal freckling and intestinal polyposis. Oral ulceration can be a feature of Crohn's disease, but not ulcerative colitis.

6.17 Answer: D

Bolus transit time is reduced, or completely impeded. Dysphagia for solids is most commonly due to a structural lesion, most commonly a stricture. Oropharyngeal dysphagia more typically causes difficulty initiating swallowing and may be associated with nasopharyngeal regurgitation.

6.18 A 37-year-old woman attends the Emergency Department after sudden onset of moderately severe central chest pain associated with nausea and sweating. Physical examination is normal, and serial ECGs show sinus rhythm and normal morphology. Oesophageal spasm is thought the most likely explanation for her symptoms. Which of the following statements related to oesophageal spasm is correct?

- A 10% of patients with recurrent non-cardiac chest pain have oesophageal dysfunction
- ☑ B Can be provoked by food ingestion
- C It is a recognised cause of globus
- D Pain can be relieved by sublingual GTN
- E Rarely associated with gastro-oesophageal reflux

6.19 You review a 56-year-old woman in the Medical Outpatient Department following recent inpatient investigation of dyspepsia. At that time she had been commenced on regular therapy with omeprazole 20 mg bd. Which of the following is a characteristic adverse effect of proton pump inhibitor therapy?

- A Constipation
- ☒ B Headache
- ☑ C Salmonellosis
- D Viral gastroenteritis
- E Visual disturbance

6.20 A 56-year-old woman is investigated for symptoms of progressive dysphagia, and is diagnosed with benign oesophageal stricture. Which of the following conditions is most likely to have caused this disorder?

- ☒ A Accidental ingestion of bleach 6 years before
- B Achalasia
- C Barrett's oesophagus
- ☑ D Long-standing gastro-oesophageal reflux
- E Prolonged nasogastric tube insertion 1 year earlier

6.18 Answer: B

Can be provoked by food ingestion or reflux, but no obvious precipitant in most cases. Up to 50% of patients with recurrent non-cardiac chest pain have oesophageal dysfunction. Globus (lump in the throat sensation) occurs at the laryngeal level.

6.19 Answer: C

Reduced stomach acid defences predispose to gastroenteritis, particularly that caused by *Salmonella* and other bacteria. Diarrhoea is a characteristic adverse effect, particularly in patients treated with lansoprazole. Administration of lansoprazole 30 mg daily suppresses gastric acid production by 50–75% overall, whereas administration of omeprazole 40 mg daily suppresses acid production by 75–100%.

6.20 Answer: D

So-called peptic stricture is the most common cause. Other recognised causes include corrosive ingestion, prolonged nasogastric tube insertion and radiotherapy.

6.21   A 32-year-old woman attends the Gastroenterology Outpatient Department for investigation of retrosternal pain after swallowing, which is worst after solid foods. Which of the following conditions is most likely to account for her symptoms?

☒ A   Achalasia

☑ B   Herpes simplex oesophagitis

☐ C   Mallory–Weiss syndrome

☐ D   Oesophageal pouch

☐ E   Plummer–Vinson syndrome

6.22   You are asked to review a 38-year-old man who has regularly been attending the Infectious Diseases Unit for the past 4 years. He has been complaining of progressively worsening odynophagia over the past 5 weeks. Which of the following conditions is most likely to account for his symptoms?

☐ A   Benign oesophageal stricture

☐ B   Gastro-oesophageal reflux

☑ C   Herpes simplex oesophagitis

☐ D   Oesophageal lymphoma

☐ E   Oesophageal perforation

6.23   You are asked to review a 62-year-old man in the Medical Outpatient Department. For the past 7 weeks, he has complained of progressive difficulty swallowing. He has lost around 15 kg weight in the past year. Which of the following factors is most strongly associated with underlying oesophageal carcinoma?

☐ A   Abstinence from alcohol

☑ B   Achalasia

☐ C   High dietary intake of root vegetables

☐ D   History of intermittent febrile illness

☐ E   Hypertension

6.21   Answer: B

Oesophagitis can cause severe pain on swallowing, whereas the other conditions listed are typically painless.

6.22   Answer: C

Oesophagitis is particularly common in immunocompromised patients, eg HIV-positive, corticosteroid users, and can be due to *Candida*, HSV, CMV.

6.23   Answer: B

Other risk factors are tobacco use, heavy alcohol intake, Plummer–Vinson syndrome, coeliac disease and long-standing gastro-oesophageal reflux. Diets high in cereal and *N*-nitroso compounds appear to increase risk.

6.24 You are asked to review a male patient in your Gastroenterology Outpatient Clinic for consideration of an upper GI endoscopy. He has been complaining of progressive dysphagia for 4 months, associated with intermittent dyspepsia. Which of the following factors is most likely to increase the risk of underlying oesophageal carcinoma?

- A 5-kg weight loss in past 4 months
- B Age 60–70 years
- C Dysphagia for liquids only
- D History of intermittent dysphagia
- E Strong family history of oesophageal carcinoma

6.25 An elderly female patient is referred to the Medical Outpatient Department for investigation of progressive weight loss and dysphagia over the past 6 months. Which of the following investigations is most appropriate for initial investigation of her symptoms?

- A Abdominal ultrasound scan
- B Barium swallow
- C Cervical lymph node biopsy
- D CT scan thorax
- E Plain chest X-ray

6.26 One of the nursing staff on your ward has been experiencing intermittent dyspepsia. She has read some information on the internet about *H. pylori* infection, and wondered how to test for this. Which of the following is the most sensitive test for detecting gastrointestinal infection with *H. pylori*?

- A Blood culture and sensitivities
- B ^{13}C-urea breath test
- C IgG antibody titres
- D IgM antibody titres
- E Stool culture

6.24   Answer: B

Weight loss is common in dysphagia, typically associated with increased appetite with benign strictures, and anorexia with carcinoma.

6.25   Answer: B

Alternatively, endoscopy is a useful first investigation that allows biopsy, but extraluminal tumour (eg lymphoma) can be overlooked. CT or endoscopic ultrasound is useful for assessing the extent of spread and lymph node involvement.

6.26   Answer: B

Sensitivity 98%, specificity 95%. Stool cultures have 90% sensitivity and 95% specificity, and IgG titres have 85% sensitivity. Breath testing can be used to confirm eradication after treatment.

6.27   A 64-year-old lifelong smoker presents with a 3-month history of weight loss and progressive dysphagia. He is found to weigh 46 kg and an irregular, hard liver edge is palpable. Which of the following is the most likely explanation for his symptoms?

- **A**   Adenocarcinoma of the upper oesophagus
- **B**   Adenocarcinoma of the lower third of the oesophagus
- **C**   Metastatic thyroid carcinoma
- **D**   Oesophageal lymphoma
- **E**   Squamous carcinoma of the lower third of the oesophagus

6.28   A 51-year-old man presents with a 2-month history of 14-kg weight loss and fatigue. Upper GI endoscopy is reported as normal. He is seen in the clinic and reports progressive dysphagia for solids over the past 4 weeks. Which of the following investigations would be most helpful next?

- **A**   Barium swallow
- **B**   Coeliac antibody screening
- **C**   CT scan of thorax
- **D**   Iron studies
- **E**   Plain chest X-ray

6.29   A 34-year-old patient presents with epigastric pain radiating to the back, associated with haematemesis. Endoscopy reveals a 2 × 2 cm peptic ulcer and he is commenced on omeprazole 40 mg daily. Which of the following statements regarding its mechanism of action is correct?

- **A**   Blocks H^+ release from G-cells
- **B**   Enhances HCO_3^- release from G-cells
- **C**   Increases chief cell secretions
- **D**   Inhibits H^+ release from parietal cells
- **E**   Potentiates the effects of gastrin

6.27 Answer: B

These account for around 45% of all oesophageal malignancies. Squamous carcinoma of the middle part of the oesophagus accounts for around 40%. Lymphoma is less common and can be more diffuse and submucosal.

6.28 Answer: C

Endoscopy can miss important diagnoses: extrinsic compressive tumours and submucosal intrinsic oesophageal lesions (eg lymphoma). Obstruction can be demonstrated in some cases by barium swallow, but CT is more detailed and the investigation of choice, or endoscopic ultrasound.

6.29 Answer: D

Parietal cells are responsible for H^+ and intrinsic factor secretion, chief cells secrete pepsinogen, while G-cells secrete gastrin (which stimulates parietal cell H^+ secretion).

6.30 A 52-year-old man is admitted to hospital after suspected haematemesis. Which of the following statements most accurately describes this condition?

☐ **A** 20–30% of patients require surgery to stop blood loss

☐ **B** 75% of patients have had a similar admission in the past 12 months

☐ **C** Bleeding resolves spontaneously in 30–40% within 48 h

☐ **D** Early endoscopy is recommended for all patients

☑ **E** Shock suggests a significant volume blood loss

6.31 A GP telephones you for advice. One of his patients has been found to have a positive faecal occult blood (FOB) stool test during a general health check. The patient is a 42-year-old banker who does not report any specific abdominal symptoms. Which of the following represents the best course of initial action?

☐ **A** Admit for urgent inpatient investigation

☐ **B** Arrange outpatient barium enema

☐ **C** Arrange outpatient colonoscopy

☑ **D** Repeat further stool FOB test

☐ **E** Request mesenteric angiography

6.32 Which of the following statements is correct with regard to gastrin?

☐ **A** Causes gastric pH to increase

☐ **B** Concentrations fall significantly during proton pump inhibitor (PPI) treatment

☐ **C** Inhibits parietal cell secretion

☒ **D** Mainly located in the gastric cardia

☑ **E** Stimulates gastric mucosa growth

6.33 Which of the following statements best describes the role of motilin?

☐ **A** Causes smooth muscle relaxation

☑ **B** Circulating levels increase during erythromycin treatment

☐ **C** Decreases the rate of gastric emptying

☒ **D** Relaxes the lower oesophageal sphincter

☐ **E** Secreted only by pancreatic β cells

6.30 Answer: E

Bleeding resolves spontaneously in around 90% within 48 h, and the use of urgent endoscopy is best directed towards those requiring endoscopic treatment, or where the diagnosis will alter immediate patient management. Shocked patients should receive blood transfusion early.

6.31 Answer: D

Despite the fact that there is a high false-positive rate for FOB tests, they now form part of the bowel cancer screening programme. In this case there is unlikely to be significant underlying pathology.

6.32 Answer: E

Gastrin located mainly in the fundus, stimulates acid secretion by parietal cells, hence pH falls. Gastrin concentrations are not altered directly by PPI treatment.

6.33 Answer: B

Motilin stimulates gastric emptying and small-bowel propulsion. It is secreted from the whole GI tract and metabolised by the liver. Erythromycin is an enzyme inhibitor that increases motilin levels (GI adverse effect of the drug).

6.34 A number of peptides are involved in regulation of gut motility. Which of the following statements best describes their role in normal gastrointestinal physiology?

- [ ] **A** Cholecystokinin inhibits gut motility
- [x] **B** Ghrelin enhances gastric emptying and appetite
- [ ] **C** Glucagon-like peptide 1 (GLP-1) inhibits insulin secretion
- [ ] **D** Motilin stimulates colonic propulsion
- [ ] **E** Vasoactive intestinal polypeptide (VIP) inhibits small-bowel secretion

6.35 A 35-year-old woman is referred to the Gastroenterology Outpatient Department for investigation of intermittent abdominal pain and bloating over the past 6 months. On direct questioning, she reveals that her stools have been pale and more difficult to flush away than usual. Which of the following is the most likely explanation?

- [ ] **A** Achalasia of the oesophagus
- [x] **B** Coeliac disease
- [ ] **C** Crohn's disease
- [ ] **D** Meckel's diverticulum
- [x] **E** Ulcerative colitis

6.36 A 44-year-old woman has long-standing coeliac disease, and is referred to the General Medical Outpatient Department for investigation of anaemia. Her results show Hb 9.8 g/dl and MCV 97 fl. Which of the following initial investigations would be most helpful in determining her subsequent management?

- [x] **A** Blood film microscopy
- [ ] **B** Dipstick urinalysis
- [ ] **C** ESR and serum calcium
- [ ] **D** Faecal occult blood test
- [ ] **E** Serum urea and electrolytes

6.34   Answer: B

Ghrelin antagonists are being examined as potential adjuncts to aid weight loss. Cholecystokinin stimulates colonic motility, GLP-1 stimulates insulin release and VIP increases intestinal secretion.

6.35   Answer: B

The history of steatorrhoea strongly suggests small-bowel malabsorption. This can be a feature of Crohn's disease, but is less likely in the absence of any other constitutional features.

6.36   Answer: A

This will help distinguish a normocytic anaemia from a dimorphic anaemia caused by mixed folate and iron deficiency.

6.37   A 52-year-old woman presents to the Outpatient Department with a
5-month history of passing pale stools that smell offensive and are
difficult to flush away. Which of the following statements best
describes confirmation of fat malabsorption?

☑ **A**   Breath $^{14}CO_2$ after labelled-fat administration can be used to indicate
the extent of fat malabsorption

☐ **B**   Faecal fat > 8 g per day is diagnostic

☒ **C**   Impaired triglyceride absorption indicates pancreatic dysfunction

☐ **D**   Stool densiometry is a valuable diagnostic test

☐ **E**   Vitamin B_{12} deficiency often co-exists with fat malabsorption

6.38   You are reviewing a middle-aged woman in the Medical Outpatient
Department who is undergoing investigation of iron deficiency
anaemia. Gastroscopy and colonoscopy investigations are normal.
Which of the following factors would most strongly suggest a
diagnosis of coeliac disease?

☐ **A**   Co-existent folate deficiency

☑ **B**   IgA endomysial antibodies

☐ **C**   Poor haemoglobin response to iron therapy

☐ **D**   Positive anti-reticulin antibody

☐ **E**   Thickened small-bowel mucosal folds on barium follow-through

6.39   A 48-year-old woman has recently been attending the
Gastroenterology Department and is diagnosed with coeliac disease.
During a further attendance she asks for your opinion on a
blistering rash that has erupted around both elbows and her left
forearm. Which of the following is the most likely diagnosis?

☐ **A**   Acne rosacea

☑ **B**   Dermatitis herpetiformis

☐ **C**   Erythema ab igne

☐ **D**   Fixed drug eruption

☐ **E**   Herpes simplex dermatitis

6.37   Answer: A

Diagnosis can be confirmed by faecal fat > 6 g/day during a standard 100 g/day diet. Impaired triglyceride absorption is a feature of pancreatic and small-bowel pathology. Often associated with malabsorption of fat-soluble vitamins (A, D, E and K).

6.38   Answer: B

The other stems are recognised features, but only this test is sensitive and specific for coeliac disease. Up to 20% of patients are IgA-deficient; this should be measured simultaneously to avoid false-negative tests.

6.39   Answer: B

This is an unusual non-infective condition, associated with similar jejunal morphology to coeliac disease and malabsorption, although typically less severe.

6.40 A 50-year-old man is admitted to the General Medical Ward for investigations for weight loss and malabsorption. You note an erythematous rash with multiple small vesicles, and suspect dermatitis herpetiformis. Which of the following represents the best immediate management of this patient?

- A Calorie-controlled diet
- B Dapsone therapy
- C Gluten-free diet
- D Oral co-amoxiclav
- E Topical hydrocortisone

6.41 You see a 42-year-old woman in the Medical Outpatient Department. Her GP performed a full blood count and found Hb 9.2 g/dl and MCV 126 fl. Which of the following is the most likely explanation for these findings?

- A Excess alcohol intake
- B Hepatic steatosis
- C Hypothyroidism
- D Intestinal bacterial overgrowth
- E Ulcerative colitis

6.42 Which of the following diagnostic tests is the most useful for establishing a diagnosis of intestinal bacterial overgrowth?

- A ^{14}C-glycocholate breath test
- B Blood cultures
- C Hydrogen breath test
- D Intubation and aspiration of intestinal fluid
- E Stool culture

6.43 A 40-year-old woman has recently undergone massive intestinal resection for extensive Crohn's disease, resulting in ileostomy formation. Her Crohn's disease is now quiescent, and you are preparing to discharge her home. Which of the following is a frequently recognised long-term complication?

- A Constipation
- B Hypercalcaemia
- C Osteoporosis
- D Peptic ulcer disease
- E Urinary calculi

6.40 Answer: C

Both malabsorption and rash in dermatitis herpetiformis will improve. Dapsone is at least partly effective against the skin rash, but will not improve absorption.

6.41 Answer: D

The findings suggest folate or vitamin B_{12} deficiency, rather than a simple macrocytosis. Vitamin B_{12} is normally absorbed in the terminal ileum. Reduced absorption due to overgrowth can be established by performing a Schilling test before and after antibiotic treatment.

6.42 Answer: C

This has largely replaced the ^{14}C-glycocholate breath test and gut aspiration, and depends on liberation of hydrogen from lactulose by intestinal bacteria.

6.43 Answer: E

Reduced bile salt absorption stimulates increased bile turnover and more frequent gallstone formation. Reduced fat and vitamin absorption is important. Bile salts entering the colon stimulate oxalate absorption, increasing the risk of urinary calculi.

6.44 A 58-year-old man is undergoing radiotherapy for metastatic bowel cancer. Shortly after his irradiation course, he develops nausea, abdominal pain and diarrhoea. Which of the following statements is correct in relation to radiation enteritis?

- ☐ **A** Bleeding risk increases due to peptic ulcer disease
- ☐ **B** Corticosteroids should be avoided
- ☐ **C** Early surgery is indicated in most patients
- ☑ **D** Malabsorption can occur due to bacterial overgrowth
- ☐ **E** Risk is unrelated to dose of radiation

6.45 A 22-year-old medical student has recently returned from her 'elective', and is complaining of persistent diarrhoea and steatorrhoea, abdominal bloating and weight loss. Which of the following diagnoses is the most likely cause of her symptoms?

- ☐ **A** Coeliac disease
- ☐ **B** Crohn's colitis
- ☑ **C** Giardiasis
- ☐ **D** Hyperthyroidism
- ☒ **E** Tropical sprue

6.46 A 58-year-old woman presents to hospital with sudden onset of central abdominal pain and vomiting. Her pulse is irregular, blood pressure 102/68 mmHg and abdomen tender, with absent bowel sounds. Which of the following diagnoses requires most urgent consideration?

- ☐ **A** Aortic aneurysm rupture
- ☑ **B** Intestinal ischaemia
- ☐ **C** Myocardial infarction
- ☐ **D** Perforated duodenal ulcer
- ☐ **E** Severe gastroenteritis

6.44   Answer: D

Enteritis is associated with ulceration and ischaemia, which heal by scarring and formation of telangiectasia (which increase bleeding risk). Partial obstruction is common, and surgery should be reserved for cases of suspected perforation or complete obstruction.

6.45   Answer: C

Infection with *Giardia intestinalis* is the commonest parasitic infection in travellers returning to the UK. Tropical sprue presents with a similar malabsorptive syndrome, usually after viral gastroenteritis.

6.46   Answer: B

Acute small-bowel ischaemia is most commonly caused by thromboembolic occlusion of the superior mesenteric artery, eg in atrial fibrillation. Mortality is high, and early surgical resection of ischaemic bowel is indicated.

6.47 A 52-year-old woman is referred to the Gastroenterology Outpatient Clinic for investigation of abdominal pain and recurrent episodes of profuse watery diarrhoea. On examination she is found to have facial telangiectasia. Which of the following diagnoses is most likely to account for her symptoms?

- A Churg–Strauss syndrome
- B Crohn's disease
- ☑ C Functional enterochromaffin cell malignancy
- D Hereditary haemorrhagic telangiectasia
- E Scleroderma

6.48 A 29-year-old man attends the Gastroenterology Outpatient Clinic for follow-up. There is a strong family history of intestinal polyposis, thought due to Peutz–Jeghers syndrome. Which of these statements is correct regarding this condition?

- A Endoscopy and X-ray follow-up should be undertaken every 5 years
- B Extensive polyposis is best treated by small-bowel resection
- C Genetic testing is not yet available
- D It is inherited in an X-linked recessive manner
- ☑ E Malignant transformation of polyps is a recognised complication

6.49 A 40-year-old woman is under regular review in the Gastroenterology Outpatient Clinic for ulcerative colitis. Which of the following best describes the familial basis of inflammatory bowel disease?

- A 3-fold increased prevalence amongst women versus men
- ☑ B 10-fold increased risk in first-degree relatives
- C Heritability is greater in ulcerative colitis than Crohn's disease
- D Incidence is falling due to effective patient counselling
- E Inherited in autosomal dominant manner with incomplete expression

6.50 Which of the following is *not* recognised as an effective treatment for patients with inflammatory bowel disease?

- A 6-Mercaptopurine
- B Balsalazide
- C Hydrocortisone
- ☑ D Ibuprofen
- E *Lactobacillus* spp.

6.47 Answer: C

The features are consistent with carcinoid syndrome, which occurs in 5% of patients with carcinoid tumour, usually when there are liver metastases. Other features include tricuspid incompetence and pulmonary stenosis.

6.48 Answer: E

The Peutz–Jeghers gene (*LKB1*) is inherited in an autosomal dominant manner. Follow-up should be at least every 2 years in view of the risk of malignancy.

6.49 Answer: B

The incidence of ulcerative colitis is stable, while that of Crohn's is rising. Genetic factors, some related to human leukocyte antigen (HLA), appear to be important, but environmental factors are also of great importance.

6.50 Answer: D

NSAIDs may increase the frequency of relapse in inflammatory bowel disease, and are associated with the development of lymphocytic colitis. The role of probiotics in IBD is not fully established, but they appear effective for pouchitis in Crohn's disease.

6.51 Which of the following statements is correct regarding the extra-gastrointestinal features of inflammatory bowel disease (IBD)?

- ☐ **A** Ankylosing spondylitis occurs in 20% of patients with ulcerative colitis
- ☐ **B** Cholelithiasis is common in ulcerative colitis
- ☒ **C** Erythema nodosum is more common in ulcerative colitis than in Crohn's
- ☑ **D** Ocular complications occur in around 10% of IBD patients
- ☐ **E** Ureteric calculi complicate ulcerative colitis but not Crohn's disease

6.52 A middle-aged woman is undergoing outpatient investigation of diarrhoea, weight loss and abdominal pain. Which of the following barium enema findings would most strongly suggest a diagnosis of ulcerative colitis?

- ☒ **A** Cobblestone appearance on barium enema
- ☐ **B** Deep mucosal ulceration
- ☑ **C** Loss of normal colonic features and superficial ulceration
- ☐ **D** Narrowing and stricturing around the terminal ileum
- ☐ **E** Obscuration of the psoas muscle outline

6.53 A 38-year-old man attends the Gastroenterology Outpatient Clinic for review. He has had inflammatory bowel disease for 6 years, and is currently asymptomatic. Which of the following investigations is most useful in assessing disease activity?

- ☑ **A** ESR
- ☐ **B** IgA
- ☐ **C** Iron studies
- ☐ **D** p-ANCA
- ☐ **E** Serum calcium

6.54 Which of the following interventions is *least* likely to be of value in the management of Crohn's disease?

- ☑ **A** Acetaminophen
- ☒ **B** Codeine phosphate
- ☐ **C** Rectal hydrocortisone
- ☐ **D** Smoking cessation
- ☐ **E** Sulfasalazine

6.51   Answer: D

Including uveitis, episcleritis and conjunctivitis. Erythema nodosum and pyoderma gangrenosum, gallstones and ureteric stones are more common in Crohn's disease than in ulcerative colitis.

6.52   Answer: C

Cobblestone appearance, with deep ulceration and stricturing is indicative of Crohn's disease. Loss of the psoas shadow on an adequately penetrated abdominal film suggests retroperitoneal fluid, and can be seen in acute flare-ups of colitis or proctitis.

6.53   Answer: A

Other markers of acute inflammation include raised C-reactive protein, platelet count and ferritin concentrations.

6.54   Answer: A

Codeine can help reduce stool frequency; smoking cessation reduces the frequency of relapses.

6.55 A 29-year-old man has had ulcerative colitis for the past 3 years, usually maintained on balsalazide. He has been admitted with a severe attack, having had two recent hospital admissions for high-dose corticosteroid treatment. Which of the following factors would most strongly indicate the need to consider surgical intervention?

- A Allergy to sulfasalazine
- B Excessive corticosteroid requirement
- ☑ C Failure of medical therapy to control sepsis
- D Number of previous hospital admissions
- E Patient preference

6.56 A 27-year-old man has a 2-year history of ulcerative colitis. Over the past 5 days, he has experienced tenesmus and diarrhoea with blood and mucus. His GP had commenced him on oral sulfasalazine 2 days ago, but the frequency of his diarrhoea has worsened and he refers the patient to you for advice. Which of the following would be the most appropriate initial step in his management?

- A Add oral azathioprine and rectal budesonide
- B Commence intravenous hydrocortisone
- C Commence oral prednisolone
- ☑ D Commence rectal hydrocortisone
- ☑ E Substitute rectal mesalazine

6.57 A 54-year-old woman attends her GP requesting laxative treatment for constipation. She is taking a number of medications. Which of the following is most likely to be responsible for her symptoms?

- A Digoxin
- ☑ B Diltiazem
- ☑ C Furosemide
- D Lansoprazole
- E Simvastatin

6.55 Answer: C

Other factors are active gastrointestinal haemorrhage, perforation or toxic bowel dilatation. Excess corticosteroid requirements, frequent admissions and patient choice are important considerations in chronic management.

6.56 Answer: D

Appropriate for proctitis and left-sided proctocolitis. If the patient fails to respond or there are moderate to severe symptoms, then oral prednisolone would be appropriate before considering other treatments.

6.57 Answer: B

Other possible causes include other calcium-channel blockers, opiates and drugs with anticholinergic properties, eg amitriptyline. Lansoprazole is an important cause of diarrhoea.

6.58 Which of the following metabolic disturbances is most likely to cause constipation?

☑ **A** Hypercalcaemia

☐ **B** Hyperglycaemia

☐ **C** Hyperkalaemia

☐ **D** Hyperthyroidism

☐ **E** Hyponatraemia

6.59 A 51-year-old woman complains of long-standing constipation. She is taking no regular medications, and is otherwise in good health. You decide to prescribe treatment for symptomatic relief. Which of the following statements is most accurate regarding the mechanism of action of laxative treatments?

☐ **A** Bisacodyl is a bulking agent

☒ **B** Ispaghula husk is a stimulant laxative

☑ **C** Magnesium sulphate is an osmotic laxative

☐ **D** Methylcellulose is an osmotic laxative

☐ **E** Senna suppositories are effective for slow-transit constipation

6.60 A 49-year-old man has regularly been taking over-the-counter laxative preparations for constipation. Which of the following is the most commonly recognised adverse effect of treatment?

☑ **A** Diarrhoea

☐ **B** Dry mouth

☐ **C** Hyperkalaemia

☐ **D** Postural hypotension

☐ **E** Toxic megacolon

6.61 A 65-year-old woman is admitted via the Emergency Department with abdominal pain, fever and constipation. On examination, there is tenderness overlying the left iliac fossa. Which of the following should be considered the most likely diagnosis?

☑ **A** Acute diverticulitis

☐ **B** Acute proctocolitis

☐ **C** Crohn's colitis

☐ **D** Diverticular disease of the descending colon

☐ **E** Ulcerative colitis

6.58 Answer: A

Other possible causes include: hypothyroidism, hypokalaemia, porphyria, diabetes mellitus, spinal cord lesions and parkinsonism.

6.59 Answer: C

Other osmotic laxatives include lactulose. Stimulant laxatives include bisacodyl and senna, and bulking agents include methylcellulose and ispaghula husk. Bisacodyl and glycerol can be given rectally.

6.60 Answer: A

Long-term use of stimulant laxatives can cause colonic atonia.

6.61 Answer: A

Diverticulosis affects around half of people over 50 years of age, and is asymptomatic. Constipation is a common feature, unlike colitis, where diarrhoea often predominates.

6.62 A 52-year-old woman is being investigated for chronic abdominal pain, and her GP arranged for a plain abdominal X-ray. The report indicates the presence of multiple gaseous cysts, suggesting the diagnosis of pneumatosis cystoides intestinalis. Which of the following is a recognised treatment of this condition?

- [ ] **A** Cephalosporin
- [x] **B** Oxygen administration
- [ ] **C** Prednisolone
- [ ] **D** Segmental colonic resection
- [ ] **E** Transabdominal ultrasonography

6.63 A 45-year-old man undergoes barium enema for investigation of altered bowel habit and is found to have multiple colonic polyps. Which of the following statements most strongly indicates a risk of malignancy?

- [ ] **A** Histology shows mild dysplasia
- [x] **B** Multiple rather than a single polyp
- [ ] **C** Pedunculated polyp rather than flat
- [x] **D** Squamous metaplasia
- [ ] **E** Tubular architecture on microscopy

6.64 A 48-year-old man with long-standing Crohn's disease presents to the Gastroenterology Outpatient Clinic for investigation of chronic watery diarrhoea. ESR is 18 mm/h, C-reactive protein is < 10 g/dl and clinical examination is normal. Which of the following is the most likely explanation for his symptoms?

- [ ] **A** Crohn's colitis
- [ ] **B** Laxative abuse
- [x] **C** Malabsorption of bile salts
- [ ] **D** Psychogenic polydipsia
- [ ] **E** Terminal ileal inflammation

6.62 Answer: B

Treatment is often unnecessary. Oxygen can help disperse the cysts, which have a high nitrogen content.

6.63 Answer: D

Multiple versus single polyp is, to a lesser extent, associated with increased risk, along with severe dysplasia, sessile or flat polyp shape, villous architecture and large polyps > 1.5 cm.

6.64 Answer: C

Often underdiagnosed, caused by ileal disease in coeliac disease, cystic fibrosis and post-infective gastroenteritis. Bile salts in the colon cause water secretion and increase oxylate absorption and ureteric calculi can occur.

6.65 A 42-year-old woman attends the Medical Outpatient Department. She has recently undergone sigmoidoscopy and barium enema investigations of altered bowel habit, which are both normal. You suspect a diagnosis of irritable bowel syndrome (IBS). Which of the following is a recognised diagnostic criterion?

- [ ] A Abdominal bloating
- [x] B Abdominal pain for 12 consecutive weeks in the past year
- [x] C Abdominal pain relieved by defecation
- [ ] D Altered stool frequency
- [ ] E Change in form or appearance of stool

6.66 A 52-year-old woman presents with progressive jaundice over a 3–4-month period. Which of the following antibody tests would best confirm a diagnosis of primary biliary cirrhosis?

- [ ] A Anti-basement membrane antibody
- [ ] B Anti-kidney microsomal antibody
- [x] C Anti-mitochondrial antibody
- [ ] D Anti-nuclear antibody
- [ ] E Anti-nuclear cytoplasmic antibodies (ANCA)

6.67 A 52-year-old man presents with nausea and anorexia for the past 5 weeks. He has recently returned from a holiday in Paris. Investigations show bilirubin 55 µmol/l, ALT 256 IU/l, ALP 98 IU/l and GGT 62 IU/l. Which of the following statements is correct in relation to further management?

- [ ] A Abdominal ultrasound is the most appropriate next step
- [ ] B Anti-hepatitis A virus (HAV) IgG antibodies confirm acute hepatitis A infection
- [ ] C Corticosteroids are indicated in proved cases of hepatitis A infection
- [x] D Hepatitis A can be prevented by immunoglobulin administration
- [ ] E Post-hepatitis A syndrome is due to recurrent viral infection

6.65   Answer: B

Alternatively, at least two of C, D or E are required for diagnosis (Rome II criteria). Other features often include bloating, urgency, straining, sensation of incomplete defecation and passage of mucus.

6.66   Answer: C

Positive in over 95% of patients. Anti-nuclear and anti-smooth muscle antibody titres are typically raised in autoimmune chronic active hepatitis.

6.67   Answer: D

Hepatitis A can be controlled by good hygiene. Infection can also be prevented when travelling to endemic areas by live inactivated HAV vaccine. Post-hepatitis A syndrome can cause debility for several months after infection, and is a functional disorder.

6.68   A 36-year-old doctor is referred to the Liver Unit with a 6-week history of jaundice. You are arranging a number of investigations, including screening for hepatitis B infection. Which of the following tests would be most helpful for confirming acute hepatitis B infection?

- [ ] **A**   Anti-HBc IgG antibody positive
- [ ] **B**   Anti-HBs IgM antibody positive
- [ ] **C**   Anti-mitochondrial antibody positive
- [ ] **D**   HBcAg positive
- [x] **E**   HBsAg positive

6.69   A 22-year-old woman is transferred to the Liver Unit from the local Medical Assessment Unit. She had been admitted 2 days earlier, having alleged to have taken a paracetamol overdose. Investigations show that her liver function has been deteriorating, with ALT 25 500 IU/l and bilirubin 134 μmol/l. Which of the following most strongly suggests a need for liver transplantation?

- [ ] **A**   Age less than 30 years
- [x] **B**   Arterial pH 7.2
- [ ] **C**   Grade II encephalopathy
- [ ] **D**   Prothrombin time 58 s
- [ ] **E**   Serum creatinine 180 μmol/l

6.70   A 90-kg woman attends the Medical Outpatient Clinic for assessment of deranged liver biochemistry detected on a routine test, which shows bilirubin 14 μmol/l, ALT 124 IU/l, ALP 76 IU/l and GGT 64 IU/l. She denies alcohol intake and is taking no regular medications. Hepatitis viral serological tests are negative. Which is the most likely explanation for these findings?

- [ ] **A**   Chronic autoimmune hepatitis
- [x] **B**   Non-alcoholic steatohepatitis
- [ ] **C**   Primary biliary cirrhosis
- [ ] **D**   Recurrent gallstones
- [ ] **E**   Undisclosed paracetamol use

6.68 Answer: E

Also HBV DNA, suggesting active viral replication. HBsAg appears from about 6–12 months after infection, then disappears (persistence indicates chronic infection). Anti-HBc IgM appears early, and persists after HBsAg has disappeared. Anti-HBc IgG indicates past infection. Anti-HBs antibodies appear late and indicate immunity.

6.69 Answer: B

King's criteria are pH < 7.3 despite resuscitation, or serum creatinine > 300 μmol/l and prothrombin time > 100 s and grade III–IV encephalopathy.

6.70 Answer: B

Other possible causes should be considered, including chronic autoimmune hepatitis (less likely), Wilson's disease and haemochromatosis. Non-alcoholic steatohepatitis is associated with fatty infiltration and inflammation of the liver, more common in patients with diabetes or obesity.

6.71 Which of the following disorders is most likely to cause cirrhosis without a preceding hepatitis?

- [ ] **A** Alcoholism
- [ ] **B** Autoimmune hepatitis
- [ ] **C** Paracetamol overdose
- [x] **D** Primary biliary cirrhosis
- [ ] **E** Wilson's disease

6.72 A 56-year-old woman with alcohol-induced cirrhosis is regularly admitted to the Liver Unit. On this occasion, she is admitted after an episode of haematemesis, and has heart rate 98/min and blood pressure 96/54 mmHg. She is transfused 2 units of packed red cells and given fluid resuscitation. Which of the following is the most appropriate initial step in her management?

- [ ] **A** Administration of oral propranolol
- [ ] **B** Infusion of somatostatin
- [x] **C** Intravenous administration of terlipressin
- [ ] **D** Intravenous omeprazole
- [x] **E** Urgent upper GI endoscopy

6.73 A 65-year-old patient is found to be jaundiced. His investigations show bilirubin 78 μmol/l, ALT 86 IU/l, ALP 176 IU/l and albumin 39 g/l. He is taking a number of different medications. Which of these is most likely to account for his jaundice?

- [ ] **A** Alpha-methyldopa
- [x] **B** Atorvastatin
- [ ] **C** Methotrexate
- [x] **D** Nifedipine
- [x] **E** Rifampicin

6.71 Answer: D

In most other cases, cirrhosis is a late consequence of liver inflammation. Paracetamol overdose is notable for its ability to cause hepatitis but not cirrhosis. Hepatic fibrosis is a recognised adverse effect of methotrexate.

6.72 Answer: E

This will allow bleeding varices to be sclerosed or banded, and identify other potential sources of upper GI blood loss, eg peptic ulcer. Propranolol, somatostatin and terlipressin reduce bleeding risk (terlipressin improves survival).

6.73 Answer: D

Can cause cholestasis and hepatitis. The others may cause hepatitis (α-methyldopa is antibody-mediated). Other causes of cholestasis are co-amoxiclav, erythromycin and chlorpromazine.

6.74 A 38-year-old man is admitted via the Emergency Department with a short history of abdominal pain and vomiting. Which of the following would most strongly suggest a diagnosis of acute pancreatitis?

☒ **A** Epigastric pain radiating to the back

☐ **B** Haemoglobin concentration 9.6 g/dl

☐ **C** Serum amylase 192 IU/l (normal range 60–80 IU/l)

☑ **D** Serum calcium 1.94 mmol/l

☐ **E** Serum triglycerides 1.8 mmol/l

6.75 A 23-year-old man has been admitted with a recurrent episode of acute pancreatitis. Liver ultrasonography is normal, and he denies excess alcohol intake. Which of the following is most likely to increase the risk of a further episode?

☑ **A** Corticosteroid treatment

☐ **B** Hypercholesterolaemia

☐ **C** Hyperglycaemia

☐ **D** Hypocalcaemia

☐ **E** Thiazide diuretic use

6.74   Answer: D

Amylase may be elevated in peptic ulcer perforation, biliary peritonitis, intestinal ischaemia and renal impairment. Pain characteristically radiates to the back in posterior duodenal ulceration.

6.75   Answer: A

Other provoking factors include alcohol, gallstones, viral infection, hypertriglyceridaemia and hypercalcaemia.

7. HAEMATOLOGY and ONCOLOGY

7.1   A 70-year-old woman comes to the clinic complaining of extensive bruising on both arms. She had an MI 2 years ago and takes ramipril, amlodipine, aspirin, atorvastatin and atenolol. On examination she is apyrexial, her BP is 140/80 mmHg, pulse 75/min and regular. There is no lymphadenopathy or hepatosplenomegaly and she has extensive bruising on both forearms. The platelet count is normal, as is the Hb; the prothrombin time (PT) is 16.2 s and the activated partial thromboplastin time (APTT) is 33.1 s. Which of the following is the most likely diagnosis?

- ☑ **A** Aspirin-related ecchymoses
- ☐ **B** Disseminated intravascular coagulation (DIC)
- ☐ **C** Idiopathic thrombocytopenic purpura (ITP)
- ☐ **D** Thrombotic thrombocytopenic purpura (TTP)
- ☐ **E** Traumatic bruising

7.2   A 45-year-old woman presents to the clinic with chronic myeloid leukaemia (CML). You decide that she is a suitable candidate for imatinib therapy. Which one of the following correctly describes the mode of action of imatinib?

- ☐ **A** Inhibitor of epidermal-derived growth factor
- ☐ **B** Inhibitor of MAP kinase
- ☐ **C** Inhibitor of serine kinase
- ☑ **D** Inhibitor of tyrosine kinase
- ☐ **E** Inhibitor of VEGF

7.3   A 21-year-old woman presents to the Haematology Clinic with jaundice and pallor. She has recently suffered from an upper respiratory tract infection. She tells you that her father had an elective splenectomy. On examination her temperature is 37.4 °C, she is pale and has jaundiced sclerae. She has splenomegaly; the blood film reveals anaemia (Hb 9.8 g/dl) and uniform spherocytes. Which of the following is the best way to confirm the diagnosis?

- ☐ **A** Cold agglutinins
- ☐ **B** Coombs' test
- ☐ **C** Haemoglobin electrophoresis
- ☐ **D** *Mycoplasma* serology
- ☑ **E** Osmotic fragility testing

7.1   Answer: A

Inhibition of platelet aggregation leads to increased propensity for bruising. No specific intervention is required.

7.2   Answer: D

Imatinib is specific for tyrosine kinases coded for by the *abl* proto-oncogene, c-kit and tyrosine kinase activity related to the platelet-derived growth factor receptor.

7.3   Answer: E

The suspected diagnosis is hereditary spherocytosis, with a haemolytic crisis after respiratory tract infection.

7.4 A 72-year-old man who attended the GP some months ago because of a rash on his shins comes to the clinic complaining of a lump at the base of his neck and cold, blue fingertips. On further questioning he admits to having had sweats at night over the past few months. On examination he has supraclavicular lymphadenopathy and acrocyanosis. While awaiting follow-up tests he suffers a lower respiratory tract infection and is given a macrolide. Investigations reveal anaemia (Hb 10.1 g/dl), a raised WCC of 19.2 × 10⁹/l and a platelet count of 408 × 10⁹/l. He also has an elevated lacate dehydrogenase (LDH). Which of the following is the most likely diagnosis?

   ☐ **A** Bronchial carcinoma

   ☐ **B** Drug-induced haemolysis

   ☒ **C** Gastric carcinoma

   ☐ **D** Hodgkin's lymphoma

   ☑ **E** Non-Hodgkin's lymphoma

7.5 A woman who is 74 years old attends the pre-clerking clinic for right total knee replacement. She has a history of hypertension but is otherwise completely well. Investigations reveal an Hb of 12.0 g/dl, a WCC of 20.0 × 10⁹/l with lymphocytes of 19 × 10⁹/l, platelets of 149 × 10⁹/l. Her ECG shows an old inferior infarct, and her chest X-ray shows left ventricular hypertropy but nil else of note. Which of the following represents the most appropriate plan with respect to her surgery?

   ☐ **A** Cancel her surgery

   ☑ **B** Go ahead with surgery and refer to Haematology post-op

   ☐ **C** Start alemtuzumab

   ☐ **D** Start chlorambucil

   ☐ **E** Start fludarabine

7.6 A 68-year-old man comes to the clinic with extreme tiredness and dull abdominal pain which is making it difficult for him to eat. His wife is very worried about him and has come to the surgery with him. He has a very enlarged spleen and an abnormal full blood count (FBC): Hb 8.4 g/dl, WCC 29.3 × 10⁹/l, platelets 654 × 10⁹/l. What other finding is most likely on examination?

   ☐ **A** Ascites

   ☐ **B** Hepatomegaly

   ☐ **C** Inguinal lymph nodes

   ☐ **D** Lymphoedema

   ☑ **E** Petechiae/ecchymoses

7.4 Answer: E

Mild anaemia, raised white count, LDH and cold agglutinins, coupled with the propensity for lower respiratory tract infection fits with non-Hodgkin's lymphoma.

7.5 Answer: B

She has chronic lymphocytic leukaemia (CLL), which is often asymptomatic for a considerable period of time. Symptoms, severe anaemia or a rapid increase in the white count dictate commencement of chemotherapy.

7.6 Answer: E

While hepatomegaly does commonly occur with lymphoproliferative disorders, it is a more variable finding than petechiae or ecchymoses, which occur due to disordered platelet function.

7.7 A 22-year-old smoker of 3–5 cigarettes per day presents to the clinic with recurrent haemoptysis that has got worse over the past 18 months. He has been treated for three episodes of pneumonia over the past 2 years. On examination he looks thin and you suspect he might have left upper lobe collapse. This is confirmed on chest X-ray; bloods are normal. Which of the following is the most likely diagnosis?

- ☑ **A** Bronchial carcinoid
- ☐ **B** Bronchial carcinoma
- ☒ **C** Bronchiectasis
- ☐ **D** Inhaled foreign body
- ☐ **E** Left upper lobe pneumonia

7.8 An 80-year-old man with metastatic prostatic carcinoma is admitted to a hospice for pain control. He is taking MST, paracetamol and Oramorph for breakthrough pain. He has continuing pain but doesn't want to take more morphine because of drowsiness and confusion. What would you advise with respect to pain control?

- ☑ **A** Keep MST stable, reduce Oramorph and add a non-steroidal
- ☐ **B** Reduce his MST and add a non-steroidal
- ☐ **C** Stop the MST and start a non-steroidal
- ☐ **D** Transfer him to fentanyl patches
- ☐ **E** Stop the MST and titrate the Oramorph to his pain

7.9 A 60-year-old woman with a 35-year history of rheumatoid arthritis comes to the clinic. She has taken a number of second-line agents, including sulfasalazine and, most recently, methotrexate, but these were all stopped due to lack of effect. Anaemia was noted 18 months ago and she was commenced on iron. She also takes naproxen and ranitidine. On examination there is evidence of active rheumatoid and splenomegaly. FBC: Hb 8.0 g/dl, WCC 3.9 × 10⁹/l, platelets 109 × 10⁹/l. She also has a raised alkaline phosphatase of 180 IU/l. Which of the following is the most likely diagnosis?

- ☐ **A** Anaemia of chronic disease
- ☑ **B** Felty syndrome
- ☐ **C** Folate deficiency
- ☐ **D** Iron deficiency anaemia
- ☒ **E** Methotrexate-related myelosupression

7.7   Answer: A

The relatively benign course of his disease, coupled with recurrent haemoptysis and left upper lobe collapse, suggests a carcinoid.

7.8   Answer: A

Multi-modal pain relief is crucial in this situation, and combining paracetamol, opiates and a non-steroidal is most appropriate here. He can only be transferred to fentanyl when his morphine dose is stable.

7.9   Answer: B

Anaemia with reduced white count and low platelets, coupled with splenomegaly is typical of Felty syndrome, seen against the background of active rheumatoid.

7.10 A 32-year-old man is about to undertake chemotherapy for acute lymphoblastic leukaemia. You are considering renoprotection for tumour lysis syndrome. Which one of the following agents would be most appropriate?

☐ **A** Allopurinol

☐ **B** Colchicine

☐ **C** Furosemide

☐ **D** Prednisolone

☑ **E** Rasburicase

7.11 A 32-year-old man has recently completed intensive chemotherapy for acute myeloid leukaemia. He is passing very large volumes of urine and is thirsty and drinking fluids all the time to keep up with it. Bloods reveal: Hb 10.2 g/dl, WCC 9.3 × 10⁹/l, platelets 160 × 10⁹/l, sodium 140 mmol/l, potassium 4.5 mmol/l, urea 18.3 mmol/l, creatinine 192 μmol/l, calcium 2.41 mmol/l, glucose 5.7 mmol/l. Which of the following is the most likely diagnosis?

☐ **A** Hypercalcaemia of malignancy

☐ **B** Leukaemia-related cranial diabetes insipidus

☑ **C** Post-chemotherapy nephrogenic diabetes insipidus

☐ **D** Psychogenic polydypsia

☒ **E** Tumour lysis syndrome

7.12 A 17-year-old girl with heavy periods comes to the clinic. She is known to have von Willebrand's disease type 1, and usually manages fine, but over the past few months the number of days that she bleeds have been longer and heavier. Her Hb is low at 11.0 g/dl, the PT is 14 s and the APTT is 37.5 s. Which of the following is the most appropriate treatment?

☑ **A** DDAVP

☐ **B** Factor VIII replacement

☐ **C** Factor IX replacement

☐ **D** Mefenamic acid

☒ **E** Tranexamic acid

7.10 Answer: E

Rasburicase catalyses oxidation of uric acid to produce allantoin, which is water-soluble and easily excreted. It is licensed for prophylaxis against and treatment of tumour lysis syndrome.

7.11 Answer: C

The calcium is mildly elevated and this is likely to relate to dehydration. A number of agents, including cyclophosphamide and methotrexate, can lead to the condition.

7.12 Answer: A

DDAVP promotes a 2- to 4-fold increase in von Willebrand factor, and a 3- to 6-fold rise in factor VIII. If symptoms are still no better, tranexamic acid can be substituted or added.

7.13 A 32-year-old woman suffers a very large post-partum haemorrhage after giving birth vaginally to her fourth child. She receives a 4-unit blood transfusion and returns home. Some 3 weeks later she goes to see the GP complaining of severe tiredness and a fever. Her temperature is 37.9 °C and she has mild hepatic tenderness. Which of the following is the most likely diagnosis?

- ☑ **A** Post-transfusion cytomegalovirus (CMV) infection
- ☐ **B** Post-transfusion hepatitis A infection
- ☐ **C** Post-transfusion hepatitis B infection
- ☐ **D** Post-transfusion hepatitis C infection
- ☐ **E** Post-transfusion hepatitis E infection

7.14 A 66-year-old man who is a 40 pack-year smoker attends the Oncology Clinic. He has had a chronic cough for the past 4 months and is now complaining of haemoptysis. He has a dull ache on the left side of the chest and his chest X-ray is suspicious of a hilar carcinoma. Which of the following is a contraindication for radical radiotherapy?

- ☐ **A** Adenocarcinoma
- ☐ **B** $FEV_1 < 60\%$
- ☐ **C** Hilar tumour
- ☑ **D** Malignant pleural effusion
- ☐ **E** Superior vena caval obstruction

7.15 A 21-year-old man had a splenectomy after a motorcycle accident 2 years ago. Since then he has suffered two episodes of pneumococcal infection (pneumonia and meningitis). His bloods are normal. What type of immunodeficiency is he suffering from?

- ☐ **A** Cell-mediated
- ☐ **B** Complement
- ☑ **C** Humoral
- ☐ **D** IgA
- ☐ **E** IgM

7.13 Answer: A

Post-transfusion CMV infection is known to occur after whole blood transfusion, with symptoms peaking some 3–4 weeks after the transfusion. The infection is self-limiting in immunocompetent patients; others need white cell-depleted blood.

7.14 Answer: D

Studies have illustrated that a malignant pleural effusion is associated with a much poorer prognosis in radical radiotherapy for bronchial carcinoma.

7.15 Answer: C

Pneumococcal antigens fall into the T1–2 antigen class, and splenectomy leaves the individual particularly susceptible to this type of infection.

7.16 An 18-year-old man attends his GP with symptoms of fatigue and lethargy. He has been a strict vegan for the past 2 years, and is concerned that he may have become anaemic. Investigations show: Hb 10.8 g/dl, MCV 118 fl, WCC 6.5 × 10^9/l, platelets 212 × 10^9/l. What is the most likely explanation for these findings?

- ☐ **A** Coeliac disease
- ☐ **B** Folate deficiency
- ☐ **C** Hypothyroidism
- ☐ **D** Iron deficiency
- ☑ **E** Vitamin B$_{12}$ deficiency

7.17 A 79-year-old man lives alone, and is referred to clinic for investigation of anaemia. Investigations show: Hb 10.4 g/dl, MCV 92 fl, WCC 4.5 × 10^9/l, platelets 212 × 10^9/l. What is the most likely explanation for these findings?

- ☐ **A** Bone marrow infiltration
- ☐ **B** Folate deficiency
- ☐ **C** Iron deficiency
- ☑ **D** Mixed iron and vitamin B$_{12}$ deficiency
- ☐ **E** Subclinical inflammatory bowel disease

7.18 You request a peripheral blood film on one of your patients with unexplained anaemia. Which of the following features would most strongly suggest an underlying diagnosis of iron deficiency?

- ☐ **A** Elliptocytes
- ☐ **B** Howell–Jolly bodies
- ☐ **C** Red cell inclusion bodies
- ☑ **D** Target cells
- ☐ **E** Tear-drop cells

7.16 Answer: E

Macrocytic anaemia in a young vegan strongly suggests vitamin B_{12} deficiency; supplements are recommended, along with calcium, vitamin D, iron and zinc. Note coeliac disease typically causes iron deficiency anaemia, and low MCV.

7.17 Answer: D

Normal MCV can also suggest anaemia of chronic disease, but lack of clinical history makes IBD unlikely.

7.18 Answer: D

Also seen in liver disease, post-splenectomy and haemoglobinopathies.

7.19 You are asked to review a 19-year-old woman in the Emergency Department. She has recently arrived in the UK from Cyprus, and presents with a short history of fever and productive cough. Investigations show: Hb 9.4 g/dl, MCV 58 fl, WCC 16.5 × 10⁹/l, platelets 342 × 10⁹/l, and a chest X-ray shows bilateral patchy infiltration. What is the most likely explanation for her anaemia?

- [ ] **A** Bone marrow suppression
- [ ] **B** Pulmonary haemorrhage
- [ ] **C** Splenomegaly
- [✓] **D** Thalassaemia trait
- [ ] **E** Wegener's granulomatosis

7.20 Which of the following statements is most accurate regarding the abnormal haemoglobin (HbS) found in patients with sickle cell disease compared to normal?

- [ ] **A** Binds oxygen more avidly
- [✗] **B** Has similar survival time to normal haemoglobin
- [ ] **C** It has no carbon dioxide-carrying capacity
- [ ] **D** More susceptible to infection by malarial parasites
- [✓] **E** Oxygen dissociation curve is shifted to the right

7.21 A 48-year-old man is attending the Medical Outpatient Department. His full blood count shows: Hb 10.0 g/dl, MCV 72 fl, WCC 5.1 × 10⁹/l, platelets 184 × 10⁹/l. You suspect iron deficiency anaemia. Which of the following findings would most strongly support this diagnosis?

- [ ] **A** High serum folate concentration
- [ ] **B** Low serum ferritin
- [ ] **C** Low serum iron concentration
- [✓] **D** Low serum transferrin saturation
- [✗] **E** Total iron-binding capacity (TIBC) is increased

7.19   Answer: D

Defect of β-chain manufacture, gives microcytic anaemia with very low MCV. The high WBC is due to underlying pneumonia.

7.20   Answer: E

Therefore, oxygen dissociates more readily to tissues, and anaemia can be well tolerated.

7.21   Answer: D

Serum iron can be reduced and serum ferritin increased in patients with inflammatory disorders. TIBC is generally increased. Transferrin saturation is more reliable than serum iron or TIBC alone.

7.22   A 51-year-old woman is found to have anaemia during a routine check-up recently. Which of the following additional tests would most strongly suggest haemolysis as an underlying explanation for her anaemia?

☐ **A**   Microcytic cells on blood film

☒ **B**   Mildly elevated bilirubin

☑ **C**   Red cell fragments on peripheral blood film

☐ **D**   Reticulocyte count of 1%

☐ **E**   Urine strongly positive for bilirubin

7.23   You are currently investigating a 43-year-old man in clinic for unexplained anaemia. Which of the following statements best describes the direct Coombs' test?

☑ **A**   Detects antibody on the patient's red cells

☐ **B**   Detects anti-RBC antibody in the patient's serum

☐ **C**   False-positive test often arises in sepsis

☐ **D**   Involves incubation of patient serum with test red cells

☐ **E**   Positive test indicates extravascular haemolysis

7.24   A 56-year-old woman is admitted to hospital with fever, confusion and renal impairment. Investigations show: Hb 9.6 g/dl, MCV 98 fl, WCC 8.5 × 10⁹/l, platelets 103 × 10⁹/l, and peripheral blood film shows red cell fragments and polychromasia. Which of the following is the most likely explanation for these features?

☐ **A**   Chronic alcohol excess

☐ **B**   Meningococcal septicaemia

☐ **C**   Penicillin-induced haemolytic anaemia

☑ **D**   TTP

☐ **E**   von Willebrand's disease

7.25   Which of the following mechanisms is most strongly linked to the pathophysiology of paroxysmal nocturnal haemoglobinuria (PNH)?

☑ **A**   Can be diagnosed by immunophenotyping

☒ **B**   Caused by excessive RBC transmembrane glycoprotein expression

☐ **C**   Involvement is specific to red blood cells only

☐ **D**   Erythrocytes prone to excess lysis only in vivo

☐ **E**   There is increased risk of acute lymphocytic leukaemia

7.22 Answer: C

Slightly elevated bilirubin and/or mild jaundice is a recognised feature, but often associated with other causes. Red cell fragments suggest microangiopathic haemolytic anaemia.

7.23 Answer: A

The indirect test detects antibodies in the patient's serum against a number of red cell surface antigens.

7.24 Answer: D

Similar to haemolytic uraemic syndrome (HUS) where renal failure and fever are the predominant features, whereas in TTP neurological features predominate. Due to excessive endothelium–platelet adhesiveness.

7.25 Answer: A

Deficiency of a transmembrane glycoprotein (RBCs, white cells and platelets) that is normally associated with factors that inhibit complement. Excess lysis ex vivo is the basis of Ham's test. Increased prevalence of acute myeloid leukaemia.

7.26 A 46-year-old woman who is taking a number of different medications is referred to the General Medical Outpatient Department for further assessment of raised white cell count. Her full blood count shows WCC 12.4 × 10⁹/l with 85% neutrophils. Which of the following medications is most likely to be responsible?

- ☐ A Chloramphenicol
- ☐ B Furosemide
- ☑ C Lithium
- ☐ D Propranolol
- ☒ E Topical betnovate ointment

7.27 During routine investigation of a 27-year-old man before elective orchidopexy, FBC investigation shows eosinophils 1.6 × 10⁹/l. Which of the following is the most likely explanation for this finding?

- ☑ A Asthma
- ☐ B Corticosteroid treatment
- ☐ C Eosinophilic leukaemia
- ☐ D Recreational drug use
- ☐ E Tropical eosinophilia

7.28 A 42-year-old man is admitted with abdominal pain thought to be due to acute haemorrhagic pancreatitis, and a blood sample is sent to the local transfusion service for 'Group and Save'. Which of the following best explains how the sample will be processed?

- ☐ A A unit of ABO and Rhesus-matched blood will be set aside
- ☑ B If antibody screening is negative, serum will be held and cross-matched later if blood is needed
- ☐ C Normally 2–3 units of matched whole blood are set aside
- ☐ D The sample will be held and examined only when blood is required
- ☐ E Two units of group O Rhesus-negative blood will be forwarded urgently

7.26 Answer: C

A number of non-inflammatory conditions are associated with neutrophilia. Drugs such as corticosteroids and lithium decrease peripheral margination of white blood cells (normally around 50% of the circulating pool).

7.27 Answer: A

Other common causes include hay fever and eczema. Less common causes include parasitic infection, Hodgkin's disease, sarcoidosis, polyarteritis nodosa and dermatitis herpetiformis.

7.28 Answer: B

Rapid cross-matching can be undertaken using spin cross-match. If atypical antibodies are detected, then compatible blood may need to be cross-matched and held.

7.29 A 62-year-old man is admitted with lassitude and fatigue due to severe anaemia, and is being transfused with 4 units of packed red cells. You are asked to review him because he has developed fever and tachycardia 30 min after commencing transfusion of the second unit. What is the most likely explanation?

- ☒ **A** ABO incompatibility
- ☐ **B** Hepatitis C
- ☐ **C** Immediate transfusion reaction
- ☐ **D** Iron overload
- ☑ **E** Leukocyte-based transfusion reaction

7.30 A 52-year-old woman has undergone hysterectomy, and has required transfusion with 3 units of packed red cells. Around 6 h after commencing the transfusion, she develops rigors, tachycardia and fever. Which of the following statements is correct regarding febrile transfusion reactions?

- ☒ **A** Aspirin is contraindicated due to the risk of Reye syndrome
- ☐ **B** Commonest in patients who have never had blood transfusion before
- ☑ **C** More common in multiparous than nulliparous women
- ☐ **D** More likely after transfusion of leukocyte-depleted blood
- ☐ **E** Most cases are due to viral infection

7.31 Which of the following is most likely to give rise to neutropenia in a previously healthy adult?

- ☐ **A** Acute gout
- ☐ **B** Bacterial skin infection
- ☒ **C** Oral prednisolone treatment
- ☑ **D** Respiratory viral illness
- ☐ **E** Vitamin B_{12} deficiency

7.32 You are asked to see a previously healthy 26-year-old woman in the Outpatient Department. She has been referred for investigation of easy bruising of her limbs after relatively minor trauma. Which of the following diagnoses is most likely?

- ☐ **A** Aplastic anaemia
- ☑ **B** Easy bruising syndrome
- ☐ **C** Hereditary haemorrhagic telangiectasia
- ☐ **D** Primary biliary cirrhosis
- ☒ **E** von Willebrand's disease

7.29 Answer: E

Non-haemolytic transfusion reaction, delayed haemolytic reaction or urticarial or anaphylactic reactions.

7.30 Answer: C

Due to development of leukocyte antibodies; also more common if previously transfused. Aspirin or paracetamol can reduce fever.

7.31 Answer: D

Viral illnesses in general, also severe bacterial infections, overwhelming sepsis, bone marrow suppression and autoimmune disease.

7.32 Answer: B

Benign disorder characterised by increased small-vessel fragility.

7.33 Which of the following statements best describes the pathophysiology of haemophilia A?

☑ **A** Around one third of cases are sporadic with no family history

☐ **B** Inheritance in an autosomal recessive manner

☐ **C** It is an autoimmune disorder

☐ **D** Low levels of von Willebrand factor

☒ **E** Low levels of factor IX

7.34 Which one of the following statements most accurately describes the mechanisms involved in von Willebrand's disease?

☐ **A** Abnormally high levels of vWF

☑ **B** Deficiency of factor VIII:C

☐ **C** Excessive platelet adhesiveness

☐ **D** Inheritance is X-linked recessive

☐ **E** Profound thrombocytopenia is a common feature

7.35 A 51-year-old man required transfusion of 10 units of packed red cells after a motorcycle accident and emergency orthopaedic surgery. A coagulation screen on arrival at hospital was normal, but now shows PT 15 s and APPT 54 s. Which of the following is most likely to be responsible for his abnormal coagulation?

☐ **A** Acute liver failure

☑ **B** Factor V and VIII deficiency

☐ **C** Immediate transfusion reaction

☐ **D** Thrombocytopenia

☐ **E** von Willebrand's disease

7.36 You are asked to review a 45-year-old woman who was referred to the Emergency DVT Clinic by her GP. She had noted swelling of her left calf that morning. Which of the following factors most strongly increases the risk of deep vein thrombosis?

☑ **A** Anti-β_2 glycoprotein 1 antibody

☐ **B** Excess prothrombin activity

☐ **C** Lupus anticoagulant

☐ **D** SLE

☐ **E** Total cholesterol > 10 mmol/l

7.33 Answer: A

Due to gene mutation, rather than non-paternity. Usually inherited in X-linked manner, and due to low levels of factor VIII:C.

7.34 Answer: B

Deficiency of vWF causes low factor VIII:C levels, endothelial dysfunction and impaired platelet function. Mild thrombocytopenia can occur. Usually, autosomal dominant inheritance pattern.

7.35 Answer: B

Factors V and VIII are depleted in stored blood and FFP or platelet transfusion should be considered after massive blood transfusion.

7.36 Answer: A

Lupus anticoagulant also contributes, but poses greatest risks when present in addition to antibody against β_2 glycoprotein 1 or anti-prothrombin antibody.

7.37 A 58-year-old woman has recently undergone right hemicolectomy for colonic carcinoma. She required 4 units of packed red cells to be transfused for correction of peri-operative blood loss. Several hours after transfusion, she became breathless and hypoxic, and you suspect a clinical diagnosis of transfusion-related acute lung injury (TRALI). Which one of the following is a characteristic feature of this condition?

    A Men are more commonly affected than women

    ☒ **B** Mortality is around 50–75%

    C Most commonly occurs after administration of pooled plasma products

    D Onset 18–24 h after transfusion was commenced

    ☑ **E** Pulmonary infiltrates are seen on plain chest X-ray

7.38 With respect to the ABO blood grouping system, which of the following statements is correct regarding a patient who is 'blood group A'?

    A Genotype must be 'AA'

    B Group A or group AB blood can safely be transfused

    C The group is inherited in an X-linked manner

    ☑ **D** They will have circulating anti-B antibodies

    E This accounts for 5–10% of the UK population

7.39 You review a 61-year-old woman with anaemia, and note her blood film report showing irregular red blood cells, target cells and the presence of Howell–Jolly bodies. Which of the following underlying diagnoses is most likely?

    A Acute myeloid leukaemia

    B Chronic lymphocytic leukaemia

    C Diabetes mellitus

    ☑ **D** Essential thrombocythaemia

    E Felty syndrome

7.37   Answer: E

Often mimics adult respiratory distress syndrome (ARDS) but outcome is generally better, with mortality around 10–15%. Multiparous women and previously transfused people are at greatest risk. Most common after blood transfusion; rare after pooled products.

7.38   Answer: D

In the UK, 45% are group A, 44% group O, 8% group B and 3% group AB. Genotype could be 'AA' or 'AO', and only group O or A can be transfused safely.

7.39   Answer: D

The appearance suggests splenic atrophy which is also seen in sickle cell disease, ulcerative colitis, coeliac disease and dermatitis herpetiformis.

7.40 A 48-year-old woman is referred for assessment of anaemia associated with mild jaundice. Which of the following features most strongly suggests haemolysis as an underlying cause?

- [ ] **A** High conjugated serum bilirubin
- [ ] **B** Positive urine bilirubin test
- [ ] **C** Raised serum haptoglobin concentrations
- [ ] **D** Red cell polymorphism
- [x] **E** Reticulocytosis

7.41 A 58-year-old lifelong smoker is referred for investigation of breathlessness, and a chest X-ray shows an abnormality in the left perihilar region. Other investigations show: sodium 134 mmol/l, potassium 3.4 mmol/l, urea 4.5 mmol/l, and serum and urine osmolalities of 258 mOsm/kg and 324 mOsm/kg, respectively. What is the most likely underlying diagnosis?

- [ ] **A** Adenocarcinoma of the lung
- [ ] **B** Adrenal carcinoma with metastases
- [ ] **C** Carcinoid
- [x] **D** Small-cell lung carcinoma
- [x] **E** Squamous cell lung carcinoma

7.42 A 35-year-old woman is being investigated for vague abdominal symptoms, and a CT scan reveals a small nodule in the head of pancreas. Which of the following most strongly suggests a diagnosis of insulinoma?

- [ ] **A** Fasting plasma glucose 2.8 mmol/l
- [ ] **B** Progressive weight loss
- [ ] **C** Recurrent blackouts after standing upright from a seated position
- [ ] **D** Random plasma glucose 2.5 mmol/l
- [x] **E** Sweating, tremor and personality change after a prolonged fast

7.40 Answer: E

High unconjugated serum bilirubin, high urinary urobilinogen and diminished serum haptoglobin concentrations are typical findings. Red cell fragments and abnormal morphology are also recognised features.

7.41 Answer: D

Associated with SIADH. May also be associated with ectopic adrenocorticotropic hormone (ACTH) secretion and Cushing syndrome.

7.42 Answer: E

Prolonged fasting will provoke the typical symptoms of hypoglycaemia, which can be confirmed by biochemical testing. Frequent snacks to prevent symptoms, and the effects of insulin on carbohydrate storage encourage weight gain.

7.43 A 58-year-old man is referred to the Outpatient Department for investigation of progressive weight loss and fatigue. He is a lifelong smoker, and there is marked clubbing of fingers and toes. Which of the following diagnoses is most likely to account for these findings?

- [ ] **A** Gastric carcinoma
- [ ] **B** Nasopharyngeal carcinoma
- [✓] **C** Non-small-cell lung carcinoma
- [ ] **D** Oesophageal adenocarcinoma
- [ ] **E** Squamous lung carcinoma

7.44 A 43-year-old man with established small-cell lung cancer is referred for investigation of progressive ataxia, unsteady gait and dysarthria. Examination shows bilateral impairment of coordination in both upper and lower limbs, but there is no nystagmus. What is the most likely explanation for these findings?

- [ ] **A** Eaton–Lambert syndrome
- [✗] **B** Midline cerebellar metastases
- [✓] **C** Non-infiltrative cerebellar degeneration
- [ ] **D** Polymyositis
- [ ] **E** Raised intracranial pressure

7.45 A 76-year-old man is admitted for palliative care. He has widespread metastases involving his thoracic spine, which is causing significant back pain. Routine investigations show Hb 17.4 g/dl, which is thought to be a paraneoplastic phenomenon. Which of the following disorders is *least* likely to be associated with erythrocytosis?

- [ ] **A** Cerebellar haemangioblastoma
- [ ] **B** Hepatoma
- [ ] **C** Renal cell carcinoma
- [✓] **D** Thyroid carcinoma
- [ ] **E** Wilms' tumour

7.43   Answer: C

Tobacco use probably increases the likelihood of all of these, but finger clubbing is more typically associated with this cancer than the others.

7.44   Answer: C

Paraneoplastic phenomenon thought to be antibody-mediated, relative lack of nystagmus, can also occur with other tumours (eg breast, thyroid). Eaton–Lambert and polymyositis are recognised complications, but lead to muscle weakness.

7.45   Answer: D

The others are associated with an increased risk of erythrocytosis, which can increase the likelihood of complications due to vascular occlusion.

7.46 You review a rather anxious 33-year-old woman in the General Medical Outpatient Department, who is seeking advice about genetic screening. Which of the following might most strongly suggest a need for breast cancer genetic screening tests?

- ☐ A History of oral contraceptive pill use for 16 years
- ☐ B Large breasts that are difficult to self-examine
- ☑ C One first-degree relative with male breast cancer
- ☐ D Second-degree relative with bilateral breast cancer
- ☐ E Two first-degree relatives diagnosed with breast cancer aged 70 years

7.47 Which one of the following statements is true regarding breast cancer screening programmes that use mammography?

- ☑ A Cancer is advanced or fungating at presentation in 75% of patients in developing countries that do not have screening programmes
- ☐ B Cost per life saved is around £5000 in the UK
- ☐ C Diagnostic yield is around 0.7% in the UK
- ☐ D Postal invitations for screening can breach patient confidentiality
- ☐ E Uptake for screening invitations is around 15–20% in Western societies

7.48 A 38-year-old pre-menopausal woman has recently been diagnosed with breast cancer. Which of the following statements is most accurate regarding hormonal treatment in this case?

- ☑ A Endometrial hyperplasia is a recognised adverse effect of tamoxifen
- ☐ B Fulvestrant blocks oestrogen receptors less effectively than tamoxifen
- ☐ C Letrozole is likely to be a useful adjunctive treatment in this patient
- ☒ D Response rate to tamoxifen is greater in oestrogen receptor-positive disease
- ☐ E Tamoxifen is an oestrogen antagonist

7.46 Answer: C

Potential for paternal inheritance. Other factors include a first-degree relative with bilateral breast cancer or onset < 40 years, two or more relatives diagnosed at < 60 years, or three or more relatives diagnosed at any age.

7.47 Answer: A

A number of factors contribute in addition to lack of mammographic screening, including poor education, lack of general surgical facilities and cultural factors. Diagnostic yield is less than 0.01% and is said to cost between £0.5 and 1.5 million per life saved.

7.48 Answer: A

Tamoxifen is a partial oestrogen receptor agonist, whereas fulvestrant is an oestrogen receptor antagonist used if tamoxifen is ineffective. Letrozole is an aromatase inhibitor used in post-menopausal women.

7.49   A 64-year-old man attends the Urology Outpatient Department with a progressive 6-month history of symptoms suggestive of prostatic hypertrophy. Which one of the following features would most strongly suggest prostate carcinoma, rather than benign hyperplasia?

- ☑ **A**   Hard enlarged prostate palpable on rectal examination
- ☐ **B**   History of low back pain
- ☐ **C**   Prostate-specific antigen (PSA) 5.2 µg/l
- ☐ **D**   Serum calcium 2.52 mmol/l
- ☐ **E**   Strong family history

7.50   You are asked to review the analgesia prescription of a 62-year-old man with metastatic lung carcinoma, who is complaining of chest wall and back pain. Which of the following statements best describes the effects of palliative analgesics in this patient?

- ☐ **A**   Agitation is a characteristic adverse effect of baclofen
- ☒ **B**   Amitriptyline is effective in 75% of patients with neuropathic pain
- ☑ **C**   Carbamazepine can reduce the effects of other existing treatments
- ☐ **D**   Dexamethasone is effective only for cerebral metastases
- ☐ **E**   High doses of ibuprofen should be avoided due to the risks of gastrointestinal haemorrhage

7.51   A 56-year-old woman is found to have Hb 98 g/l and MCV 72 fl. You suspect iron deficiency as the cause of her anaemia. Which of the following is most likely to have contributed to the development of this condition?

- ☐ **A**   Corticosteroid treatment
- ☒ **B**   Diverticulitis
- ☑ **C**   Omeprazole treatment
- ☐ **D**   Terminal ileitis secondary to inflammatory bowel disease
- ☐ **E**   Vitamin C tablets

7.49   Answer: A

Raised PSA > 4 µg/l is suggestive, but false positive results can occur.

7.50   Answer: C

Enzyme inducer, so other drugs are metabolised more readily, eg corticosteroids. Dexamethasone can be useful for visceral pain. Treatments for neuropathic pain are only effective in around 20% of patients.

7.51   Answer: C

Iron absorption occurs in the proximal small intestine, and is greatest for haem rather than non-haem iron, and enhanced in the ferrous (Fe^{2+}) state. Gastric acid and ascorbic acid prevent conversion to ferric iron (Fe^{3+}) and enhance gastrointestinal absorption.

7.52 You are asked for general advice regarding the potential benefits or harm of iron supplementation in pregnancy. Which of the following statements is most accurate?

- ☐ **A** Ferrous sulphate is teratogenic and should be avoided in the first trimester
- ☐ **B** High antenatal body mass index carries a 2- to 3-fold increased risk of post-partum iron deficiency
- ☑ **C** Iron deficiency is uncommon among pregnant women in Western societies
- ☐ **D** Post-partum iron deficiency can cause psychosis
- ☒ **E** Post-partum iron stores return to normal before haemoglobin is restored

7.53 Which of the following statements is correct regarding vitamin B_{12} absorption in humans?

- ☐ **A** Absorption is enhanced in the presence of vitamin B_{12} deficiency
- ☐ **B** Intrinsic factor is synthesised by the liver and secreted in bile
- ☑ **C** Intrinsic factor–vitamin B_{12} complexes bind to enterocyte receptors
- ☐ **D** Transcobalamin is found only in extracellular fluids
- ☐ **E** Vitamin B_{12} is synthesised de novo from cobalt and essential amino acids

7.54 A 61-year-old man is admitted in extremis after collapsing at home. He has been taking warfarin for atrial fibrillation, and describes a short history of melaena. His INR is found to be 8.5, and you suspect that he has had a large gastrointestinal haemorrhage. Which of the following would be the most appropriate means of reversing his anticoagulation?

- ☑ **A** Administration of clotting factor concentrates
- ☐ **B** Fresh frozen plasma
- ☐ **C** Intravenous vitamin K 1–2 mg
- ☐ **D** Intravenous vitamin K 10 mg
- ☐ **E** Pooled platelet administration

7.52	Answer: C

Post-partum anaemia impairs physical work capacity, contributes to cognitive and mood problems. Haemoglobin may appear normal, although iron stores are depleted. Iron requirements are high during pregnancy, but the incidence of iron deficiency anaemia remains uncommon in Western societies.

7.53	Answer: C

Intrinsic factor is a gastric glycoprotein; complexes bind to receptors before endocytosis. Vitamin B_{12} cannot be formed de novo in people. Transcobalamin (transport protein) is also found in the gut.

7.54	Answer: A

In life- or limb-threatening haemorrhage, the priority is rapid reversal of anticoagulation. Fresh frozen plasma (FFP) has comparatively low concentrations of factor IX, and is less good. Low-dose vitamin K should only be used for low-risk bleeding for reversal towards therapeutic anticoagulation.

7.55 A 56-year-old man with established chronic liver disease presents with a 12-h history of upper gastrointestinal bleeding. Which of the following factors would most strongly support administration of platelet concentrate?

- ☐ **A** Activated partial thromboplastin time 53 s
- ☐ **B** Bleeding time 13 s
- ☑ **C** Platelet count 18×10^9/l
- ☐ **D** Preceding aspirin therapy
- ☐ **E** Prothrombin ratio 2.4

7.56 A 57-year-old woman is due to undergo combination chemotherapy for breast carcinoma. Which of the following treatments is most likely to be effective in preventing neutropenic sepsis as a complication?

- ☐ **A** Corticosteroids
- ☐ **B** Factor VIII administration
- ☑ **C** Granulocyte colony-stimulating factor
- ☐ **D** Granulocyte transfusion
- ☐ **E** Treatment administered in a quiet ward side-room

7.57 A 60-year-old man is diagnosed with non-Hodgkin's lymphoma, and is due to undergo autologous stem cell transplantation (ASCT). Which of the following statements best describes the role of ASCT in this patient?

- ☐ **A** Disease relapse is comparatively rare
- ☑ **B** Rituximab reduces the risk of disease recurrence
- ☐ **C** Shorter courses of chemotherapy are needed but morbidity is higher
- ☐ **D** Stem cells are transfused from a matched donor first-degree relative
- ☐ **E** Transplant rejection is a common limitation of this technique

7.55 Answer: C

Platelet administration should be considered if count is very low, eg $< 10 \times 10^9/l$, or at levels $< 25 \times 10^9/l$ if the patient is actively bleeding.

7.56 Answer: C

Granulocyte CSF and granulocyte–macrophage CSF administration enhances circulating neutrophil counts and reduces the prevalence and severity of neutropenic sepsis. Granulocyte transfusion has been studied, but the potential benefits remain unproven.

7.57 Answer: B

Stem cells are harvested from the patient and used to repopulate the haemopoietic system after high-dose chemotherapy. The risk of relapse is lower for allogenic transplantation, but rejection is a problem. Rituximab is a monoclonal antibody to CD20.

7.58 A 58-year-old woman undergoes renal biopsy for unexplained proteinuria, which shows diffuse fibrillary protein deposition that shows green birefringence with polarised light. Which one of the following is the most characteristic feature of light-chain amyloidosis?

- ☑ **A** Cardiomegaly
- ☒ **B** Leukocytoclastic vasculitic rash
- ☐ **C** Nephritic syndrome
- ☐ **D** Peripheral neuropathy
- ☐ **E** Psoriatic arthropathy

7.59 A 51-year-old woman is referred to the Outpatient Department for investigation of anaemia, which was detected during a routine medical assessment. She has had no significant past illnesses, and is taking no regular medications. Investigations show Hb 87 g/l, MCV 82 fl, red cell distribution width 24%. Which one of these is the most likely explanation?

- ☐ **A** Anaemia of chronic disease
- ☐ **B** Mixed folate and vitamin B_{12} deficiency
- ☑ **C** Mixed iron and vitamin B_{12} deficiency
- ☐ **D** Myelodysplasia
- ☐ **E** Thalassaemia

7.60 A 19-year-old man is admitted via the Emergency Department in the early hours of Saturday morning with drowsiness and confusion. He appears markedly cyanosed and an arterial blood gas shows pH 7.31, PaO_2 14.5 kPa, $PaCO_2$ 4.0 kPa and lactate 3.8 mmol/l. Which of the following diagnoses should be considered most strongly?

- ☑ **A** Methaemoglobinaemia
- ☐ **B** Pulmonary embolism
- ☐ **C** Sickle cell anaemia
- ☐ **D** Tension pneumothorax
- ☐ **E** Thalassaemia

7.58 Answer: A

Cardiomegaly is present in around 50% of patients, and peripheral neuropathy is present in 10–15%. It is also associated with nephrotic syndrome and hepatosplenomegaly.

7.59 Answer: C

Normal MCV and high RDW could also suggest anaemia of chronic disease or sideroblastic anaemia; normal MCV and normal RDW found in anaemia of chronic disease or haemoglobinopathy.

7.60 Answer: A

Common causes include nitrate excess (including recreational use of amyl nitrate). Features are due to tissue hypoxia despite apparently normal PaO_2 and $PaCO_2$, and can be treated with methylene blue if methaemoglobin > 30%.

7.61 A 62-year-old woman has suffered progressively worsening angina over the past 3 days, and has been using increasingly large amounts of sublingual and buccal nitrate therapy for symptom control. On arrival in the Emergency Department she is noted to be heavily cyanosed and is found to have PaO_2 12.3 kPa, $PaCO_2$ 3.9 kPa, and methaemoglobin concentration of 45%. Which of the following is the most appropriate course of action?

- A Administer high-flow oxygen
- B Arrange for urgent exchange transfusion
- ☑ C Give intravenous methylene blue
- D Give intravenous glyceryl trinitrate to maintain systolic BP at 100 mmHg
- E Observe only and recheck arterial gases in 12 h

7.62 A 42-year-old man is admitted to the Emergency Department late on a Friday evening complaining of vague chest pain. Physical examination, resting ECG and chest X-ray are normal. Full blood count shows Hb 12.1 g/dl, MCV 103 fl and platelet count 80 × 10^9/l. What is the most likely explanation for these haematology findings?

- ☑ A Chronic alcohol excess
- B Folate deficiency
- C Hyperthyroidism
- D Iron deficiency
- E Sideroblastic anaemia

7.63 A 58-year-old woman is referred to the General Medical Outpatient Department for investigation of weight loss and abdominal bloating for the past 10 months. Investigations show Hb 10.2 g/dl, MCV 76 fl and the peripheral blood film shows hypochromic, microcytic cells and occasional Howell–Jolly bodies. What is the most likely underlying diagnosis?

- A Caecal carcinoma
- ☑ B Coeliac disease
- C Hypothyroidism
- D Ovarian carcinoma
- E Pernicious anaemia

7.61   Answer: C

Given if methaemoglobin > 30%. Exchange transfusion is used for severe, life-threatening methaemoglobinaemia (> 80%), including haemolysis, or if methylene blue is likely to be ineffective (eg G6PD deficiency).

7.62   Answer: A

The blood results suggest a simple macrocytosis, rather than a megaloblastic anaemia (in the latter Hb is usually low and MCV often > 115 fl). Typical causes also include hypothyroidism and liver disease.

7.63   Answer: B

Coeliac disease is a common cause of iron deficiency anaemia in middle-aged patients, and is often overlooked.

7.64 Which of the following factors is most useful as a prognostic indicator in patients with systemic amyloidosis?

- [ ] **A** Circulating lymphocyte count
- [ ] **B** Renal size on ultrasound scan
- [✓] **C** Serum β_2 microglobulin
- [✗] **D** Serum calcium
- [ ] **E** Weight loss

7.65 Which of the following is a recognised feature of vitamin B_{12} deficiency in elderly patients?

- [✓] **A** Can be due to inability to release cobalamin from food
- [ ] **B** Is diagnosed by Schilling's test
- [ ] **C** Is due to intrinsic factor deficiency in most cases
- [ ] **D** Present in 0.5–1.0% of patients
- [ ] **E** Rarely causes neuropsychiatric complications

7.66 Which of the following conditions most strongly indicates a need to perform thrombophilia screening?

- [✓] **A** Cerebral vein thrombosis
- [ ] **B** Family history of lower limb deep venous thrombosis
- [✗] **C** Ischaemic stroke in 47-year-old woman
- [ ] **D** Microcytic anaemia
- [ ] **E** Peripheral vascular disease in a 56-year-old man

7.67 You are asked to perform a thrombophilia screen in a 32-year-old woman who has had a number of recurrent spontaneous deep vein thromboses. Which of the following blood tests is most likely to be helpful?

- [✗] **A** Anti-protein C antibody
- [ ] **B** Anti-Scl antibody
- [ ] **C** Cysteine
- [✓] **D** Factor II Leiden
- [ ] **E** Factor IX

7.64 Answer: C

Marker of overall disease burden and linked to survival; cardiac mass is also important.

7.65 Answer: A

Probably the commonest cause, or deficiency of intestinal cobalamin transport proteins; intrinsic factor deficiency accounts for fewer than one in five cases. Neuropsychiatric and haematological complications are common, and deficiency is present in around 20% of elderly patients.

7.66 Answer: A

Venous thrombosis in unusual sites, including hepatic or portal veins, recurrent venous thrombosis, strong family history, or if there is both arterial and venous occlusion.

7.67 Answer: D

Others include antithrombin, protein C, protein S, factor V Leiden, homocysteine, lupus anticoagulant and anti-cardiolipin antibody.

Haematology and oncology answers

7.68 Which of the following features is most strongly suggestive of HELLP syndrome?

- ☑ **A** Alanine transaminase 142 IU/l
- ☐ **B** Microscopic haematuria
- ☐ **C** Platelet count 165×10^9/l
- ☐ **D** Raised serum haptoglobin concentrations
- ☐ **E** Reticulocytes 0.8%

7.69 A 56-year-old woman with chronic alcoholic liver disease is admitted with general malaise. She is deeply jaundiced, and her full blood count shows Hb 6.4 g/dl, MCV 88 fl. Which of the following findings most strongly suggests haemolysis as an explanation for her anaemia?

- ☐ **A** Dipstick urinalysis positive for bilirubin
- ☐ **B** Raised serum haptoglobin concentrations
- ☑ **C** Red cell fragments on blood film
- ☐ **D** Serum bilirubin 148 μmol/l
- ☐ **E** Serum lactate dehydrogenase 586 IU/l

7.70 A 34-year-old woman has undergone allogenic bone marrow transplantation for chronic myeloid leukaemia. Which of the following conditions is correct regarding graft-versus-host disease (GVHD)?

- ☐ **A** Acute GVHD usually appears within 6–12 hours
- ☑ **B** Can be prevented using high-dose corticosteroids
- ☐ **C** Rash is uncommon
- ☑ **D** Risks are less than autologous bone marrow transplantation
- ☐ **E** Thrombocythaemia is a common feature

7.71 A 62-year-old man is admitted to the Acute Medical Receiving Unit with progressive breathlessness. On examination, he is found to have widespread lymphadenopathy and hepatomegaly. Chest X-ray shows diffuse interstitial opacification and increased lung markings. Which of the following is the most likely diagnosis?

- ☐ **A** Acute lymphocytic leukaemia
- ☑ **B** Chronic lymphocytic leukaemia
- ☐ **C** Chronic myeloid leukaemia
- ☐ **D** Hodgkin's disease
- ☑ **E** Non-Hodgkin's lymphoma

7.68   Answer: A

Features are haemolysis, elevated liver enzymes, low platelets
(HELLP); it is seen as a subset of the antiphospholipid syndrome,
which is often characterised by recurrent spontaneous abortions.

7.69   Answer: C

Also associated with low or undetectable haptoglobin concentrations
and urinalysis positive for urobilinogen. Raised bilirubin and lactate
dehydrogenase (LDH) can be features of liver disease or haemolysis.

7.70   Answer: B

Although this can increase infection risk. Acute disease usually
presents within 2–3 weeks. Rash and thrombocytopenia are
recognised features of chronic GVHD.

7.71   Answer: B

Although difficult to distinguish from non-Hodgkin's lymphoma, the
patient's age, insidious onset and pulmonary involvement make
chronic lymphocytic leukaemia more likely.

7.72   A 21-year-old man is referred to the Haematology Clinic for investigation of night sweats and fever. He is noted to have enlarged non-tender cervical, inguinal and axillary lymph nodes, and a palpable liver edge. A lymph node biopsy is performed. Which of the following features most strongly suggests an underlying diagnosis of Hodgkin's disease?

- **A**   Howell–Jolly bodies
- **B**   Green birefringence under polarised light
- **C**   Multiple non-caseating granulomata
- ☑ **D**   Reed–Sternberg cells
- **E**   Tear-drop cells

7.73   Which of the following statements most correctly applies to non-Hodgkin's lymphoma?

- **A**   75% are derived from T lymphocytes
- **B**   Bone marrow aspiration should normally be avoided
- ☑ **C**   Prevalence is higher in patients with impaired cellular immunity
- **D**   There is less extranodal involvement than in Hodgkin's disease
- **E**   Women are more commonly affected than men

7.74   A 73-year-old woman is referred to the Medical Outpatient Department for investigation of weight loss and fatigue. She is found to have Hb 9.5 g/dl, MCV 82 fl, and ESR 98 mm/h. Which of the following would most strongly suggest an underlying diagnosis of malignant myeloma?

- ☑ **A**   High serum β_2 microglobin concentration
- **B**   Normal serum IgG concentration
- **C**   Raised serum calcium
- ☒ **D**   Serum alkaline phophatase is elevated
- **E**   Stool is negative for faecal occult blood

7.75   A 74-year-old woman is admitted for investigation of confusion associated with mild anaemia. Which of the following features most strongly suggests an underlying diagnosis of Waldenström's macroglobulinaemia?

- **A**   Cervical lymphadenopathy
- **B**   ESR of 54 mm/h
- **C**   High IgG concentration
- ☑ **D**   Impaired vision
- ☒ **E**   Leukocyte infiltration on bone marrow aspiration

7.72   Answer: D

These are large lymphoid cells, often surrounded by normal lymphocytes and plasma cells, and are pathognomonic for the disease.

7.73   Answer: C

Most are B cell in origin, and men are more often affected. Unlike Hodgkin's disease, bone marrow aspirate and trephine are often performed, and cell surface immunotyping.

7.74   Answer: A

Normally, immunoglobulin concentrations are reduced (immune paresis) in association with high paraprotein or light chain levels. Alkaline phosphatase is usually normal in the absence of fractures.

7.75   Answer: D

Due to IgM paraproteinaemia. Other features due to hyperviscosity include bruising or nosebleeds. Lymphadenopathy and splenomegaly are recognised, and bone marrow shows lymphoid cell infiltration.

8. INFECTIOUS DISEASES

8.1 A 72-year-old woman who had TB treatment 8 years ago comes to the hospital complaining of haemoptysis. She has also had night sweats over the past few months and a chronic cough. She smokes 10 cigarettes per day and has right upper lobe consolidation on examination. Her WCC is elevated at 11.5×10^9/l and *Aspergillus* precipitins are positive. The chest X-ray reveals a right upper lobe cavitating lesion. Which of the following is the most likely diagnosis?

- [ ] **A** Allergic bronchopulmonary aspergillosis
- [✓] **B** Aspergilloma
- [ ] **C** Bronchial carcinoma
- [ ] **D** Invasive aspergillosis
- [ ] **E** Reactivated tuberculosis

8.2 A 70-year-old man with a history of hypertension, diverticulosis and an inferior MI has a permanent pacemaker inserted for episodes of complete heart block. He comes back 5 days later with a fever, lower back pain and diarrhoea. Examination reveals restricted movement due to lower back pain and local tenderness over the lumbar spine. His WCC is elevated at 14.5×10^9/l and his ESR is 87 mm/h. Which of the following is the most likely diagnosis?

- [ ] **A** Ischaemic colitis
- [ ] **B** Prolapsed lumbar disc
- [ ] **C** Pyelonephritis
- [x] **D** Spinal epidural abscess
- [✓] **E** Staphlococcal discitis

8.3 You are drawing up guidelines for the use of antibiotics in your elderly care unit. When it comes to the risk of *Clostridium difficile* infection, which antibiotic is associated with the highest risk?

- [ ] **A** Amoxicillin
- [x] **B** Cefuroxime
- [✓] **C** Ciprofloxacin
- [ ] **D** Co-amoxiclav
- [ ] **E** Metronidazole

8.1 Answer: B

Aspergilloma occurs in patients who have had a previous cavitating lesion, such as tuberculosis. Management involves long-term antifungal therapy, with or without surgical excision.

8.2 Answer: E

The proximity of the infection to the pacemaker insertion suggests a link, most likely haematological spread of *Staphlococcus aureus*. Parenteral therapy for at least 6 weeks is indicated.

8.3 Answer: C

Previously, co-amoxiclav, clindamycin and cephalosporins were thought to carry the highest risk of *C. difficile* infection, but a very large Canadian cohort study found that quinolones that confer greatest risk.

8.4   A 70-year-old woman presents for a re-do of her left hip replacement 9 years after the first. Apart from a dull aching in the joint over the past year or so she has suffered no other problems. Bloods at the time of the hip replacement re-do were normal, but joint aspirate has grown a Gram-positive bacillus. Which of the following is the most likely causative organism?

- [ ] **A** *Bacillus cereus*
- [ ] **B** *Clostridium difficile*
- [ ] **C** *Clostridium perfringens*
- [x] **D** *Cornyebacterium striatum*
- [x] **E** *Propionibacterium acnes*

8.5   A 19-year-old man who is taking a short course of high-dose prednisolone therapy for exacerbation of asthma comes to the Emergency Department. He is very worried as his flatmate has just been diagnosed with chickenpox. He is absolutely certain he has never suffered from chickenpox. Which of the following is the most appropriate course of action?

- [ ] **A** Do nothing and wait to see if he becomes infected
- [ ] **B** Give the chickenpox vaccine as a matter of urgency
- [x] **C** Give VZV immunoglobulin
- [ ] **D** Start prophylactic aciclovir
- [ ] **E** Start prophylactic valciclovir

8.6   A 40-year-old man whose hobby is freshwater fishing comes to the Emergency Department. He is brought by his wife because he has become severely unwell over the past few days with a fever and is almost unable to get out of bed. On examination he is pyrexial at 38.5 °C, and looks jaundiced. He has a bandage on his leg where he cut it on some brambles at the side of the river. Bloods reveal: an elevated WCC of 15.0 × 10⁹/l and platelets of 50 × 10⁹/l; and renal failure with a creatinine of 245 µmol/l and a potassium of 6.1 mmol/l. Additional investigations reveal an ALT of 320 IU/l, bilirubin of 295 µmol/l, and a creatine kinase of 820 IU/l. Which of the following is the most appropriate treatment for him?

- [x] **A** Benzylpenicillin
- [ ] **B** Ciprofloxacin
- [x] **C** Doxycycline
- [ ] **D** Erythromycin
- [ ] **E** Fresh frozen plasma (FFP)

8.4   Answer: E

Propionibactrium acnes is a slow-growing, poorly virulent bacterium. Symptoms can occur many years after arthroplasty and the bacterium might only be found at joint revision.

8.5   Answer: C

Steroid exposure within 3 months of primary chickenpox infection puts the sufferer at greatly increased risk of severe disease. VZV immunoglobulin should be given within 3 days of exposure if possible.

8.6   Answer: A

Pyrexia, jaundice, renal failure and an elevated creatine kinase is suggestive of possible Weil's disease infection, particularly given his history of being out and about on the river. Penicillin is the treatment of choice.

8.7 A 21-year-old woman who is a rough-sleeper comes to the Emergency Department. She has been feeling very unwell over the past few days with severe fevers and rigors, and has now begun to develop a purpuric rash. On examination she is pyrexial at 38.3 °C, there are splinter haemorrhages on finger-nail examination and a generalised purpuric rash. She has injection sites and thrombosed veins on both forearms and needle marks around both femoral veins. Significant blood results include anaemia (Hb 9.8 g/dl) and a raised ESR of 72 mm/h. Her urine contains 1+ of blood and the first set of blood cultures is negative. Chest X-ray reveals cavitating lesions in both lungs. Which of the following is the next most appropriate investigation?

- ☐ **A** Autoantibody screen
- ☐ **B** CT chest
- ☐ **C** Repeat blood cultures
- ☑ **D** Transoesophageal echocardiography
- ☐ **E** Urine cultures

8.8 A 40-year-old man attends the Emergency Department with his boyfriend. He has been unwell for the past few days with a severe headache and now has right arm weakness. He is also becoming increasingly confused. He has a mild pyrexia of 37.6 °C and there is 4/5 power weakness of the right arm. He is mildly anaemic with a haemoglobin of 11.1 g/dl; his WCC is 10.0 × 10⁹/l. CSF protein is elevated and there is a mononuclear leukocytosis. Magnetic resonance imaging (MRI) of the brain reveals ventricular enlargement and a possible left-sided infarct. What is the most likely diagnosis?

- ☐ **A** Cerebral infarct
- ☑ **B** CMV encephalitis
- ☐ **C** Cryptococcal meningitis
- ☐ **D** Herpes encephalitis
- ☐ **E** Toxoplasmosis

8.7   Answer: D

The history raises the possibility of right-sided endocarditis, with seeding of multiple pulmonary abscesses. While we are not told about the presence of a murmur, an echo would be the next most logical investigation.

8.8   Answer: B

The picture seen here is typical of that seen in CMV encephalitis; intravenous ganciclovir is the treatment of choice. He should also be screened for HIV infection and started on appropriate therapy.

8.9 A 30-year-old visitor from Pakistan comes to the clinic complaining of increasing shortness of breath over the past few months. He also has a chronic cough for which a doctor has given him a salbutamol inhaler. His BMI is 20 kg/m² and he looks tired. He is hypotensive, with a BP of 105/65 mmHg, and a resting pulse of 90/min. There is bilateral ankle oedema. The WCC is slightly elevated at 11.8 × 10⁹/l, but other bloods are normal. ECG showed low-volume complexes and echo revealed a pericardial effusion which was tapped, the fluid showing a lymphocytosis. What is the most likely diagnosis?

- ☐ **A** Autoimmune pericarditis
- ☐ **B** Restrictive cardiomyopathy
- ☐ **C** Systemic amyloidosis
- ☑ **D** Tuberculous pericarditis
- ☐ **E** Viral pericarditis

8.10 A 29-year-old male sex worker presents with diarrhoea containing blood and pus. He admits to unprotected anal sex on a number of occasions over the past 2 weeks. He is slightly tender on PR; routine bloods are normal. What is the most appropriate next step?

- ☐ **A** Rectal biopsy
- ☑ **B** Stool culture on selective medium
- ☐ **C** Stool microscopy
- ☐ **D** Trial of ciprofloxacin
- ☐ **E** Trial of metronidazole

8.11 A 16-year-old boy presents to the hospital with a worsening cough productive of purulent sputum. He is known to have cystic fibrosis. He has had three previous hospital admissions over the last 5 years and is finding it increasingly difficult to maintain his weight and general health. He is pyrexial at 38.2 °C and has bilateral crackles and wheeze, particularly increased at the right base. The WCC and C-reactive protein are elevated; other bloods are unremarkable. Which of the following is the most appropriate antibiotic choice?

- ☐ **A** Benzylpenicillin
- ☐ **B** Ciprofloxacin
- ☐ **C** Erythromycin
- ☐ **D** Gentamicin
- ☑ **E** Tazocin

8.9   Answer: D

The country of origin, chronic cough, and lymphocytosis on examination of the pericardial effusion fluid all point towards tuberculous pericarditis. Aggressive management with quadruple anti-TB therapy is the treatment of choice.

8.10   Answer: B

The history is suggestive of rectal gonococcal infection. Selective culture is required to demonstrate the organism, which is normally sensitive to penicillin. He should be screened for other sexually transmitted diseases.

8.11   Answer: E

Tazocin is a combination of tazobactam and piperacillin and is specifically recommended for the treatment of cystic fibrosis exacerbations. Ciprofloxacin is no longer recommended because of resistance rates of up to 30%.

8.12 A 72-year-old man has returned from his 3-month annual winter trip to the Algarve. He has suffered from increasing cough, wheeze and shortness of breath over the past few days. By the time his son brings him to the Emergency Department he is confused and incontinent of urine, with a pyrexia of 38.8 °C, BP 105/60 mmHg and pulse 102/min. There is bilateral wheeze on auscultation of the chest. Abnormal investigations include: WCC 14.1×10^9/l, sodium 130 mmol/l, creatinine 142 µmol/l, PaO_2 7.0 kPa, $PaCO_2$ 3.9 kPa. Urine is positive for blood and protein. Which of the following is the most likely diagnosis?

- ☐ **A** Bacterial meningitis
- ☑ **B** Legionnaire's disease
- ☐ **C** *Mycoplasma* pneumonia
- ☐ **D** Pneumococcal pneumonia
- ☐ **E** Urinary sepsis

8.13 A 16-year-old girl has been doing work experience helping with the animals at a local farm. She comes to the Emergency Department with a headache, fever and diarrhoea. She is usually well, with a history only of mild asthma, and the only medication of note is the oral contraceptive pill. Her BP is elevated at 159/89 mmHg, and she is pyrexial at 37.8 °C. She has a purpuric rash and widespread petechial haemorrhages. Bloods are abnormal, with a haemoglobin of 9.2 g/dl, WCC 11.5×10^9/l, platelets 51×10^9/l, sodium 139 mmol/l, potassium 6.1 mmol/l, creatinine 209 µmol/l. Urinalysis shows: blood + +, protein + +, only 50 ml was passed. Which of the following is the most likely causative organism?

- ☐ **A** *Campylobacter*
- ☑ **B** *Escherichia coli*
- ☒ **C** *Listeria*
- ☐ **D** *Salmonella*
- ☐ **E** *Shigella*

8.12   Answer: B

The respiratory symptoms seen here, with hypoxia, haematuria and proteinuria and SIADH fit well with Legionnaire's. The infection is associated with air-conditioning systems, hence the link to the Algarve hotel.

8.13   Answer: B

The history suggests *E. coli* O157 infection, with a picture of thrombotic thrombocytopenic purpura/haemolytic uraemic syndrome. Plasmapheresis and corticosteroids are the mainstay of therapy.

8.14 A 21-year-old woman is admitted with a vesicular rash covering most of her body and a fever of 38.2 °C. She says the rash came on a few days after the symptoms of a cold. Respiratory examination is normal, the chest is clear and her oxygen saturation is 96% on air. Which of the following is the most appropriate treatment?

- ☑ **A** Aciclovir
- ☐ **B** Flucloxacillin
- ☒ **C** Ganciclovir
- ☐ **D** Paracetamol
- ☐ **E** Varicella zoster immunoglobulin

8.15 A 36-year-old gay man who is HIV-positive presents with a 10-day history of diarrhoea, originally thought to be due to *Salmonella* infection from a roast chicken, but unresponsive to ciprofloxacin. He is opening his bowels up to 10 times per day with watery diarrhoea. His WCC is raised at 10.5×10^9/l and there is renal impairment, with a creatinine of 190 µmol/l and a raised urea. Acid-fast staining of the stool reveals red oocysts against a blue–green background. What is the most likely diagnosis?

- ☑ **A** *Cryptosporidium*
- ☐ **B** Giardiasis
- ☐ **C** Isosporiasis
- ☐ **D** *Mycobacterium avium-intracellulare*
- ☐ **E** *Shigella*

8.16 A previously healthy 31-year-old aid worker has returned to the UK from Sudan in Africa. He presents with sudden onset of fever, severe myalgia and diarrhoea. On examination, there is non-suppurative pharyngitis, generalised lymphadenopathy and an erythematous rash over the trunk and limbs. Which of the following organisms is most likely to cause these features?

- ☐ **A** Adenovirus
- ☑ **B** Ebola virus
- ☐ **C** *Haemophilus influenzae*
- ☐ **D** Influenza type A virus
- ☐ **E** *Neisseria meningitides*

8.14   Answer: A

This woman has chickenpox. While the consensus in children is not to treat ordinarily, in adolescents and young adults the consensus is that treatment with aciclovir is cost-effective.

8.15   Answer: A

The patient's history and the findings on stool staining are typical of *Cryptosporidium* infection. Azithromycin partially resolves symptoms but HAART (highly active antiretroviral therapy) is equally important.

8.16   Answer: B

Recognised cause of viral haemorrhagic fever. Sporadic cases and outbreaks have been reported in Africa. There is an unknown animal reservoir, and incubation period of 5–9 days. Treatment is supportive, and mortality is high.

8.17 A 27-year-old woman has recently returned from a rural camp in West Africa, and complains of fever, nausea, backache and headache. She has facial flushing and her conjunctivae are injected. What is the most likely diagnosis?

☐ **A** Malaria

☐ **B** Meningococcal meningitis

☐ **C** Systemic lupus erythematosus

☐ **D** Trichomoniasis

☑ **E** Yellow fever

8.18 A 23-year-old man has returned to the UK from Southeast Asia, where a fever epidemic had broken out. He has suffered from malaise and headache for 3 days, and now complains of fever, arthralgia, muscle cramps and backache. Temperature is 38.1 °C, there is generalised lymphadenopathy, pulse rate 68/min and blood pressure 122/68 mmHg. What is the most likely diagnosis?

☑ **A** Dengue fever

☐ **B** Epstein–Barr viraemia

☐ **C** HIV seroconversion illness

☐ **D** Respiratory syncytial virus infection

☐ **E** Schistosomiasis

8.19 For the past 3 days, a 6-year-old boy has suffered a febrile illness with upper respiratory tract symptoms. He has now developed a maculopapular rash over the face, head and neck. Which of the following features would most strongly suggest a diagnosis of measles?

☐ **A** Consolidation on plain chest X-ray

☐ **B** Photophobia

☐ **C** Previous measles infection

☑ **D** Recent infectious measles contact

☐ **E** Recent treatment with corticosteroids

8.17 Answer: E

Later phase characterised by petechial haemorrhages and liver failure. Zoonosis caused by a flavivirus; tropical rainforests of West and Central Africa, South and Central America. Monkey pool and *Aedes* mosquito vectors.

8.18 Answer: A

Flavivirus viral haemorrhagic fever transmitted by *Aedes* mosquito vector in tropical and subtropical countries. Incubation period 2–7 days, often epidemic. May be associated with leukopenia and thrombocytopenia.

8.19 Answer: D

Highly infectious during the early catarrhal phase (day 1–2). Previous infection is associated with immunity. MMR vaccination is highly effective active immunisation. Photophobia is a non-specific feature. Pneumonia can occur due to secondary bacterial infection.

8.20 An 8-year-old girl is suspected of having measles infection. Which of the following is correct regarding the risk of this infection?

- [ ] **A** Incubation period is 12–24 h
- [ ] **B** Infection is usually via faeco–oral route
- [x] **C** Measles is caused by a paramyxovirus
- [ ] **D** MMR offers passive immunity against infection
- [ ] **E** Risk of infection greatest after morbilliform rash has developed

8.21 A 24-year-old man presents with a 2-day history of fever, malaise and painful swelling of the left parotid gland. He is suspected of having mumps. Which of the following statements is correct regarding this infection?

- [ ] **A** Encephalitis is a common complication
- [x] **B** Infection spread by droplet transmission
- [x] **C** Infectivity rate is > 90% of contacts
- [ ] **D** More than 95% of infections have clinical features
- [ ] **E** Orchitis occurs in 1–2% of post-pubescent men

8.22 You are asked to counsel a 47-year-old woman who has had HIV infection for 4 years. She is expecting her first child and is 8 months pregnant. Which of these is the most appropriate advice?

- [ ] **A** Antiretroviral treatments should be withheld in the peri-partum period
- [ ] **B** Breastfeeding does not increase transmission risk
- [x] **C** Delivery by Caesarean section reduces transmission risk
- [ ] **D** Maternal viral titres do not influence transmission likelihood
- [ ] **E** Vaginal delivery has transmission rate of 80–90%

8.23 What is the risk that a single unit of packed red blood cells available for transfusion in the UK will transmit HIV infection?

- [ ] **A** 1 in 1000
- [x] **B** 1 in 1000 if blood collected before 1992
- [x] **C** 1 in 1 000 000
- [ ] **D** None, due to heat treatment and irradiation of all donated blood
- [ ] **E** None, due to screening of all donated blood

8.20 Answer: C

Measles (rubeola) transmitted by droplets, with incubation period of 10 days. Early catarrhal stages are more infectious than when rash has developed. MMR is a highly effective live attenuated vaccine.

8.21 Answer: B

Mumps is a paramyxovirus with low infectivity, and infection is unapparent in around a third. Orchitis affects around 25% of post-pubescent men and can cause infertility if bilateral. Viral meningitis is a recognised feature.

8.22 Answer: C

There is a 15–55% risk of transmission (in utero, during parturition and breastfeeding), especially with high maternal viral load, hence prenatal screening important. Pre-partum and peri-partum anti-retrovirals reduce transmission.

8.23 Answer: C

Estimated as negligibly small but not zero. Volunteers with strong HIV risk factors are discouraged from donating, and screening involves serodiagnosis: this can be negative in early infection before seroconversion.

8.24 You are working in the Infectious Diseases Unit. One of your colleagues asks you for advice following a recent needlestick injury when drawing blood from an HIV-positive patient. Which of the following is correct regarding potential transmission of HIV infection?

☑ **A** Antiretrovirals should be taken within 1–2 h for greatest efficacy

☐ **B** Gloves do not reduce transmission after needlestick injury

☐ **C** Overall transmission risk is around 10%

☒ **D** Negative HIV antibody serology at 1 month is highly reassuring

☐ **E** Stage of HIV infection of the patient is irrelevant

8.25 A 26-year-old man presents with a 4-week history of night sweats, fever and malaise. There is generalised lymphadenopathy. Full blood count shows WCC 1.2×10^9/l and platelets 56×10^9/l, and a plain chest X-ray shows bilateral diffuse interstitial perihilar shadowing. What is the most likely diagnosis?

☑ **A** AIDS

☐ **B** Disseminated CMV infection

☒ **C** HIV seroconversion illness

☐ **D** Progressive generalised lymphadenopathy

☐ **E** Sarcoidosis

8.26 A 41-year-old woman has been diagnosed with HIV infection for 8 years. During a routine clinic appointment, she is noted to have retinitis with an appearance suggestive of CMV infection. Which of the following is true of CMV retinitis?

☐ **A** Characteristically caused by droplet transmission

☑ **B** Disseminated infection may involve the adrenal glands

☐ **C** Rarely associated with perivascular exudates

☐ **D** Typically develops despite CD4 count > 200/mm^3

☐ **E** Vision is normally preserved

8.24 Answer: A

Zidovudine reduces seroconversion rate by > 75%; current recommendation is for triple antiretroviral therapy for 1 month, started as soon as possible after exposure, eg zidovudine, lamivudine and indinavir.

8.25 Answer: A

The chest X-ray appearance strongly suggests *Pneumocystis* pneumonia, an AIDS-defining illness.

8.26 Answer: B

Uncommon unless CD4 count < 50/mm^3, can lead to rapid blindness. Perivascular exudates are typical feature, with haemorrhages in severe cases. Infection due to reactivation of latent CMV.

8.27 For the past 4 weeks, an HIV-positive man has suffered fever, weight loss and fatigue. Plain chest X-ray shows consolidation and cavitation in the right mid-zone accompanied by a small pleural effusion. Which of the following infections is most likely?

- ☐ **A** *Candida albicans*
- ☐ **B** *Mycobacterium bovis*
- ☑ **C** *Mycobacterium tuberculosis*
- ☐ **D** *Pneumocystis carinii*
- ☐ **E** *Streptococcus pneumoniae*

8.28 A 51-year-old woman has had AIDS for 18 months. She complains of fever, malaise, weight loss and breathlessness. She is found to have hepatomegaly and widespread lymphadenopathy. CD4 count is < 30/mm³, plain chest X-ray shows patchy consolidation and sputum contains numerous acid-fast bacilli. What is the most likely causative organism?

- ☐ **A** *Candida albicans*
- ☐ **B** *Chlamydia pneumoniae*
- ☐ **C** Cytomegalovirus
- ☑ **D** *Mycobacterium avium-intracellulare*
- ☐ **E** *Mycobacterium tuberculosis*

8.29 A 28-year-old man is admitted to the Emergency Department with seizures. He had been diagnosed with HIV infection 7 years earlier, and has suffered headaches, fever and malaise for the past 6 weeks. CT head scan shows a ring-enhancing mass lesion in the right cerebral hemisphere, with a rim of surrounding oedema. What is the most likely diagnosis?

- ☐ **A** Cryptococcal meningitis
- ☐ **B** Pneumococcal abscess
- ☐ **C** Staphylococcal infection
- ☑ **D** *Toxoplasma gondii* infection
- ☐ **E** Tuberculous meningitis

8.27   Answer: C

Can occur at any stage in TB, and often associated with cavitation and systemic features. *Pneumocystis carinii* pneumonia very rarely associated with effusion.

8.28   Answer: D

Usually low virulence, causes disease with very low CD4 counts. Treatment is with combinations of clarithromycin, azithromycin, rifabutin, ethambutol and amikacin.

8.29   Answer: D

Serological tests often unreliable. Diagnosis often depends on characteristic CT or MRI appearances, and brain biopsy in certain cases. Treatment is with pyrimethamine and sulfadiazine.

8.30 A 34-year-old woman has been diagnosed HIV-positive for 9 years, and recently diagnosed with Kaposi's sarcoma. Which of the following is most characteristic of this disorder?

- ☐ **A** Arises from arterial endothelium
- ☑ **B** Associated with human herpesvirus 8 (HHV-8) infection
- ☐ **C** Common feature in transfusion-acquired HIV infection
- ☐ **D** Preferentially affects the trunk and back
- ☐ **E** Skin involvement heralds poorer prognosis than lymph node infiltration

8.31 A 48-year-old man has suffered AIDS for 2 years and, over the past 4 months, has developed fever, weight loss, profuse night sweats and hepatomegaly. What is the most likely diagnosis?

- ☑ **A** B-cell lymphoma
- ☐ **B** Disseminated cytomegalovirus (CMV) infection
- ☐ **C** Kaposi's sarcoma
- ☐ **D** Systemic candidiasis
- ☐ **E** Toxoplasmosis

8.32 A 14-year-old boy presents with a pink macular rash over the head, neck and trunk. He is otherwise well, with no constitutional symptoms. A diagnosis of rubella is suspected. Which of the following is most likely to be a feature of this infection?

- ☑ **A** Diagnosis can be confirmed by serological testing
- ☒ **B** Fever and respiratory symptoms usually predominate
- ☐ **C** Incubation period is around 1–2 days
- ☐ **D** Lymphadenopathy suggests an alternative diagnosis
- ☐ **E** Recurrent rubella infection occurs in 5–10% of patients

8.33 An adult female presents with headache and fever symptoms. She is found to have a non-blanching purpuric rash overlying her trunk, neck and limbs. Which of the following infections is most likely to cause this appearance?

- ☐ **A** Enterovirus
- ☐ **B** Epstein–Barr virus
- ☐ **C** Parvovirus B19
- ☑ **D** Rubivirus
- ☐ **E** Varicella zoster virus

8.30   Answer: B

AIDS-defining. HHV-8 infection appears sexually transmitted, and Kaposi's sarcoma is uncommon in transfusion-acquired HIV infection. Arises from venules, typically involves skin on nose, penis and lower legs, mouth and hard palate.

8.31   Answer: A

Non-Hodgkin's lymphoma typically presents with 'B symptoms', and extrareticular involvement is more common than in non-HIV patients, eg gastrointestinal or bone marrow involvement. CMV less likely to cause hepatomegaly.

8.32   Answer: A

Rash most common presenting feature; children have no/mild symptoms, including suboccipital lymphadenopathy. Adults may have complications including polyarthropathy and encephalitis. Infection or MMR confer high immunity.

8.33   Answer: D

The typical rash of rubella is a pink, erythematous blanching rash. Adult infection can be complicated by thrombocytopenic purpura in some cases. The other infections listed are characteristically associated with an erythematous rash.

8.34 Which of the following statements is most accurate with regard to herpes simplex virus (HSV) infection?

- ☐ **A** Aciclovir resistance is common
- ☐ **B** Genital herpes rarely recurs
- ☑ **C** Herpes labialis may be provoked by menstruation
- ☐ **D** Prolonged aciclovir eradicates latent HSV from dorsal root ganglia
- ☐ **E** Valciclovir has direct antiviral action against HSV-1 and HSV-2

8.35 A 12-year-old boy presents with a morbilliform rash, and IgM antibody to parvovirus B19 is found to be positive. Which of the following is the most likely diagnosis?

- ☒ **A** Erysipelas
- ☑ **B** Erythema infectiosum
- ☐ **C** Erythema multiforme
- ☐ **D** Erythema nodosum
- ☐ **E** Systemic lupus erythematosus

8.36 Which of the following is most likely to be a characteristic feature of molluscum contagiosum?

- ☐ **A** Less common in immunocompromised patients
- ☐ **B** Parvovirus
- ☐ **C** Rarely resolve spontaneously
- ☐ **D** Should generally be excised to prevent malignant transformation
- ☑ **E** Transmitted via infected towelling

8.37 You review a 31-year-old visiting student in the Medical Outpatient Department. He is noted to have hyperaemia affecting the conjunctiva of his left eye, which shows numerous pale follicles. The right eye does not appear inflamed, but there is a marked entropion. Which of the following is the most likely infective organism in this condition?

- ☑ **A** *Chlamydia trachomatis*
- ☐ **B** Epstein–Barr virus
- ☐ **C** Herpes simplex virus
- ☒ **D** *Mycoplasma pneumoniae*
- ☐ **E** *Staphylococcus aureus*

8.34   Answer: C

Oral or genital infections can be caused by HSV-1 or HSV-2, and often recur. Recurrence risk is reduced by regular aciclovir administration. Valciclovir is a prodrug.

8.35   Answer: B

Also known a 'fifth disease', characterised by fever and erythematous rash ('slapped cheek'). Parvovirus B19 infection in adults often associated with arthropathy and red cell aplasia.

8.36   Answer: E

Poxvirus transmitted by direct contact or infected clothing. More common in atopic and immunocompromised individuals (incubation period 2–5 weeks). Often resolves spontaneously, but can also be treated with cryotherapy.

8.37   Answer: A

Trachoma is commonest cause of blindness. Caused by direct contact with fomites and often presents insidiously. Treated with prolonged topical or oral tetracycline. May cause scarring and entropion.

8.38 Which of the following diseases is caused by rickettsial infection in humans?

- ☐ **A** Dengue fever
- ☑ **B** Endemic typhus fever
- ☒ **C** Lassa fever
- ☐ **D** Marburg disease
- ☐ **E** Yellow fever

8.39 A 47-year-old farmer presents to the Medical Outpatient Department with flu-like symptoms, arthralgia, fever and headaches for around 4 weeks. He is found to have a soft systolic cardiac murmur. Three sets of blood cultures are negative. Which of the following organisms is the most likely to have caused his symptoms?

- ☐ **A** *Chlamydia pneumoniae*
- ☑ **B** *Coxiella burnetii*
- ☐ **C** *Haemophilus influenzae*
- ☐ **D** *Mycobacterium bovis*
- ☒ **E** *Streptococcus faecalis*

8.40 A 40-year-old woman presents to the Emergency Department with a short history of fever symptoms and a facial rash. On examination, there is well-defined, raised erythematous patch of skin overlying her left cheek, and there are a number of slightly enlarged, tender cervical lymph nodes. Which of the following is the most likely explanation?

- ☑ **A** Erythema infectiosum
- ☑ **B** Erysipelas
- ☐ **C** Kaposi's sarcoma
- ☐ **D** Staphylococcal cellulitis
- ☐ **E** Subcutaneous lymphoma

8.38   Answer: B

Caused by *Rickettsia mooseri*. Others include epidemic typhus fever (*R. prowazekii*), Rocky Mountain spotted fever (*R. rickettsii*), scrub typhus fever (*R. tsutsugamushi*), rickettsialpox and trench fever. Stems A, C, D and E are recognised causes of viral haemorrhagic fever.

8.39   Answer: B

Q-fever is a rickettsia-like organism, spread by airborne transmission from infected cattle hide, animal products or infected (unpasteurised) milk. Diagnosed by rising antibody titres, and treated with tetracycline.

8.40   Answer: B

Streptococcal in majority of cases. Often spread from the nose and therefore involves the face. Raised, oedematous lesions and well-defined margin distinguishes it from common bacterial cellulitis. Responds well to penicillin.

8.41 A 54-year-old patient with diabetes mellitus is admitted for treatment of an infected skin ulcer. Culture of wound swab demonstrates multiple colony-forming units of *Staphylococcus aureus*. Which of the following would be the most appropriate treatment?

- [ ] A Benzylpenicillin
- [ ] B Ciprofloxacin
- [ ] C Erythromycin
- [x] D Flucloxacillin
- [ ] E Vancomycin

8.42 A 32-year-old woman is admitted for investigation of chronic fever symptoms, recent weight loss and a murmur that fluctuates in its site and intensity. *Staphylococcus epidermidis* is grown from blood culture bottles taken on two separate occasions. Which of the following statements is most likely to be true?

- [ ] A Culture findings are likely to be due to skin contamination
- [ ] B Endocarditis may be eradicated with short courses of antibiotics
- [ ] C Skin colonisation requires antibiotic treatment for eradication
- [x] D *S. epidermidis* may be resistant to flucloxacillin
- [ ] E This bacterium characteristically causes acne

8.43 A 13-year-old boy attends the Infectious Diseases Unit for assessment of laryngitis, mild fever and nasal discharge. On examination, he is found to have diffuse neck swelling, an injected throat and tonsils, with an overlying grey membrane. Which of the following diagnoses requires most urgent consideration?

- [ ] A Acute Epstein–Barr virus infection
- [x] B Diphtheria
- [ ] C Epiglottitis
- [ ] D Peritonsillar abscess
- [ ] E Primary herpes simplex infection

8.44 Which of the following statements is correct in relation to infection with *Corynebacterium diphtheriae*?

- [ ] A Erythromycin is ineffective treatment
- [ ] B Is becoming less prevalent due to passive immunity
- [ ] C Nasal infection does not require treatment
- [ ] D Only exotoxin-positive cases require public health notification
- [x] E Serum sickness is a recognised complication of antiserum treatment

8.41   Answer: D

More than 90% of *S. aureus* are resistant to penicillin (eg amoxicillin). Most are sensitive to flucloxacillin, but an increasing proportion are resistant to this and other antimicrobials (methicillin-resistant *S. aureus*, MRSA) and may necessitate vancomycin treatment.

8.42   Answer: D

Methicillin-resistant strains are now recognised. Common skin commensal that can cause endocarditis in patients with valvular lesions or immunocompromise. Notoriously difficult to eradicate.

8.43   Answer: B

Incubation period 2–4 days. Early symptoms may be mild. May be followed by exotoxin-mediated neuropathy, laryngeal paralysis and myocarditis. Requires urgent antitoxin administration and intravenous benzylpenicillin while confirmation is awaited.

8.44   Answer: E

Erythromycin eradicates organisms in carriers. Intravenous benzylpenicillin is given in acute infection; antiserum is used to prevent life-threatening exotoxin-mediated complications (myocarditis and neuropathy). All cases should be reported to the Public Health Department.

8.45 Which of the following clinical features is most likely to be a feature of infection by *Bordetella pertussis*?

- ☑ **A** Bouts of coughing followed by vomiting
- ☐ **B** Commonly associated with neurological complications
- ☐ **C** Diagnosis is by electron microscopy of nasopharyngeal secretions
- ☐ **D** Lymphopenia on full blood count
- ☐ **E** Onset between 10 and 20 years of age

8.46 Which of the following organisms characteristically causes food poisoning mediated by toxin production?

- ☐ **A** *Bacillus cereus*
- ☐ **B** *Campylobacter jejuni*
- ☐ **C** Norwalk virus
- ☑ **D** *Staphylococcus aureus*
- ☐ **E** Wootbot virus

8.47 Which one of the following organisms is believed to cause gastroenteritis due to local infection, ie non-toxin-mediated infection?

- ☑ **A** *Campylobacter jejuni*
- ☐ **B** Ciguatoxin
- ☐ **C** *Clostridium botulinum*
- ☐ **D** *Clostridium perfringens*
- ☐ **E** *E. coli* O157

8.48 A 26-year-old woman is admitted with a 48-h history of severe vomiting and profuse watery diarrhoea. She is dehydrated, tachycardic and her temperature is 38.6 °C. Which one of the following steps is most appropriate in her initial management?

- ☐ **A** High-dose corticosteroids intravenously for at least 48 h
- ☐ **B** Intravenous ciprofloxacin is indicated
- ☐ **C** Paracetamol should be given to reduce pyrexia
- ☑ **D** Rapid intravenous hydration with 0.9% saline
- ☐ **E** Restrict fluid intake until diarrhoea settling

8.45   Answer: A

Pathognomonic of the paroxysmal stage. Most infectious during the earlier catarrhal stage. Typically occurs in young children. Diagnosis is established by demonstration culture of nasopharyngeal swabs, and treatment is with erythromycin.

8.46   Answer: D

Wootbot does not cause human disease. The others are recognised causes of non-toxin-mediated gastroenteritis. Other toxin-mediated food poisoning causes are *E. coli* O157, *Clostridium botulinum* and *Clostridium perfringens*.

8.47   Answer: A

Ciguatoxin is a recognised cause of non-infective gastroenteritis, sourced from tropical fish. The others listed in stems C, D and E are recognised causes of toxin-mediated food poisoning.

8.48   Answer: D

In the absence of heart failure, very rapid hydration can be tolerated. This should aim to quickly restore normal hydration status, and meet the requirements of ongoing fluid loss. In hydration, saline interferes less with potassium homeostasis than, for example, 5% dextrose administration.

8.49 A 28-year-old traveller presents to the Emergency Department with persistent fever, sweating, headache and muscle cramps for 2 weeks. On examination, he is found to have a palpable spleen and his temperature is 38.1 °C. Which of the following is most likely to account for his symptoms?

- A Bacterial meningitis
- ☑ B Brucellosis
- C Leptospirosis
- ☒ D Scurvy
- E Tuberculosis

8.50 A 28-year-old nurse has returned from a 3-week trip to Asia. She has suffered 3 days of fever, profuse watery diarrhoea and colicky abdominal pain. Over the past 24 h she has started vomiting, and is becoming increasingly dehydrated. Which of the following infections is most likely to account for these symptoms?

- A Brucellosis
- ☑ B Cholera
- C HIV seroconversion illness
- D Malaria
- E Primary tuberculosis

8.51 Which of the following measures is most likely to be effective in limiting the spread of a cholera epidemic?

- A Antiserum administration
- B Bedrest and avoidance of swimming pools
- ☑ C Ensuring good sanitation and hygiene
- D Oral co-trimoxazole administration
- E Oral tetracycline administration

8.52 Which of the following clinical features is most strongly indicative of lepromatous leprosy?

- A Absence of *Mycobacterium leprae* on tissue biopsy
- ☑ B Involvement of nasopharyngeal mucosa
- C Loss of sensation overlying skin lesions
- D Marked skin hypopigmentation
- ☒ E Prominent involvement of peripheral nerves

8.49   Answer: B

Now uncommon in UK, and can be spread via unpasteurised milk. More common in farmers and animal workers. In Mediterranean and Far East is transmitted from infected goats and sheep. Treated with tetracycline plus rifampicin, or tetracycline plus streptomycin.

8.50   Answer: B

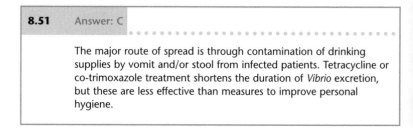

Vibrio cholerae causes severe acute gastrointestinal infection. Faeco–oral transmission is through contaminated water, unwashed hands or infection of food via flies.

8.51   Answer: C

The major route of spread is through contamination of drinking supplies by vomit and/or stool from infected patients. Tetracycline or co-trimoxazole treatment shortens the duration of *Vibrio* excretion, but these are less effective than measures to improve personal hygiene.

8.52   Answer: B

In lepromatous leprosy, there is widely disseminated skin and nerve involvement, with poorly demarcated skin lesions; nerve enlargement is a late feature. The natural outcome is progression, and other tissues and organs may be involved. Immune-complex-mediated reactions are a recognised feature.

8.53 Which of the following treatments is most likely to be useful in the treatment of leprosy?

- ☐ **A** Amoxicillin
- ☐ **B** Clarithromycin and amoxicillin
- ☐ **C** Dapsone
- ☐ **D** Rifampicin
- ☑ **E** Rifampicin, clofazimine and dapsone

8.54 A 43-year-old veterinary surgeon is admitted with sudden onset of fever, jaundice and hepatitis. A diagnosis of Weil's disease is suspected. Which of the following is the most useful diagnostic test in this condition?

- ☒ **A** Blood cultures
- ☐ **B** CSF microscopy and culture
- ☐ **C** Liver biopsy
- ☑ **D** Rising specific leptospiral antibody titres
- ☐ **E** Urine microscopy

8.55 A 56-year-old forestry worker presents with a 4-week history of fever, erythematous rash overlying trunk and limbs, neck stiffness and photophobia. There is tenderness and mild swelling affecting the small joints of both ankles, wrists and hands. Which of the following is the most likely diagnosis?

- ☐ **A** Brucellosis
- ☐ **B** Echovirus infection
- ☐ **C** Leptospirosis
- ☑ **D** Lyme disease
- ☐ **E** Primary tuberculosis

8.56 A 23-year-old student is referred by her GP with a scaly erythematous rash over her left forearm. The appearance is strongly suggestive of ringworm. Which of these factors is most likely to have predisposed to ringworm infection in this patient?

- ☑ **A** Eczema
- ☐ **B** History of hay fever
- ☑ **C** Inhaled corticosteroids
- ☐ **D** Menstruation
- ☐ **E** Recent course of amoxicillin

8.53   Answer: E

Rifampicin is the most effective, and need be given only 1 day per month because of the slow *Mycobacterium leprae* turnover. Clofazimine and dapsone are given daily in combination to reduce resistance, and treatment is usually for 2 years.

8.54   Answer: D

Liver function tests often indicate a hepatitis (high AST and ALT), often with some degree of biliary obstruction (high GGT and ALP). Renal involvement is signified by raised serum creatinine and red cells and granular casts on urine microscopy. Treatment is with high-dose intravenous penicillin or macrolide antibiotics.

8.55   Answer: D

Around one in four forestry workers are seropositive. Caused by *Borrelia burgdorferi*, a spirochaete transmitted by the *Ixodes ricinus* tick from infested sheep and deer. Erythema chronicum migrans is an early feature, followed by neurological and cardiac involvement. Late features are arthropathy and neuropathy.

8.56   Answer: A

Due to loss of skin integrity. Other factors include diabetes, pregnancy, malignancy, topical or systemic corticosteroids and HIV infection.

8.57 A 24-year-old woman with a history of asthma presents to the Emergency Department with fever and breathlessness. A plain chest X-ray shows diffuse interstitial opacification in both lung fields. Which of the following is the most probable diagnosis?

- [ ] **A** Acute exacerbation of asthma
- [ ] **B** Acute pulmonary oedema
- [✓] **C** Allergic bronchopulmonary aspergillosis
- [ ] **D** Corticosteroid-induced cardiomyopathy
- [ ] **E** Fibrosing alveolitis

8.58 A 34-year-old man with long-standing asthma suffers an exacerbation of his respiratory symptoms. A chest X-ray shows diffuse pulmonary infiltration, and a diagnosis of allergic bronchopulmonary aspergillosis is suspected. Which of these findings would be most helpful in establishing the diagnosis?

- [ ] **A** Allergic response to amoxicillin administration
- [✓] **B** Demonstration of *Aspergillus fumigatus* on sputum microscopy
- [✗] **C** Elevated serum IgE concentrations
- [ ] **D** High peripheral blood eosinophil count
- [ ] **E** Skin hypersensitivity to *A. fumigatus* extract

8.59 A 32-year-old man with HIV infection presents with a short history of fever, photophobia and neck stiffness. Meningitis is suspected, and a lumbar puncture shows mildly turbid CSF with spores seen on microscopy. What is the most likely infective organism?

- [ ] **A** *Candida albicans*
- [ ] **B** *Chlamydia trachomatis*
- [✓] **C** *Cryptococcus neoformans*
- [ ] **D** *Cryptosporidium parvum*
- [ ] **E** Cytomegalovirus

8.57 Answer: C

Commonest systemic fungal infection in UK, more common in patients with asthma. Treatment includes antifungal therapy (eg amphotericin) but often this cannot be given long-term. Corticosteroids are used to suppress local inflammation, and physiotherapy aids expectoration and prevents collapse.

8.58 Answer: B

C, D and E are associated features, but less specific. Additionally, the presence of serum precipitating antibodies to *A. fumigatus* helps confirm the diagnosis.

8.59 Answer: C

Cryptococcal meningitis is much more common in immunocompromised patients. Diagnosis is made by demonstration of spores in CSF, or demonstration of serum cryptococcal antigen.

8.60 A 31-year-old man has recently returned to the UK from a 4-week holiday in Kenya. He is complaining of headache, nausea and fever. Investigations show haemoglobin 8.9 g/dl. Examination shows icteric sclera and temperature 38.3 °C. A diagnosis of malaria is suspected. What is the most likely explanation for anaemia in this patient?

- ☑ **A** Acute haemolysis of infected red blood cells
- ☐ **B** Autoimmune anaemia
- ☐ **C** Bone marrow suppression
- ☐ **D** Hepatomegaly and red cell sequestration
- ☐ **E** Vitamin B_{12} depletion

8.61 A 36-year-old woman has recently been in Tanzania and is complaining of headache, fever and rigors. On examination, she is mildly jaundiced, and temperature is 38.6 °C. Which of these most strongly suggests a diagnosis of malaria?

- ☐ **A** Anaemia
- ☐ **B** Haemoglobinuria
- ☐ **C** Raised serum alanine transaminase
- ☑ **D** Ring forms seen on peripheral blood film
- ☐ **E** Splenomegaly

8.62 A 48-year-old previously healthy businessman has returned from a 4-week trip to Indonesia. He is admitted via the Emergency Department after a witnessed generalised seizure. He is mildly jaundiced, there is palpable splenomegaly, and his temperature is 39.2 °C. What organism is most likely to be responsible?

- ☐ **A** *Entamoeba histolytica*
- ☐ **B** *Mycobacterium tuberculosis*
- ☑ **C** *Plasmodium falciparum*
- ☐ **D** *Plasmodium malariae*
- ☐ **E** *Treponema pallidum*

8.60   Answer: A

Haemolysis of infected red cells and, to a lesser extent, non-infected red cells is the major cause. Other contributing factors include impaired erythropoiesis, splenic sequestration and folate depletion. Jaundice is a common feature due to haemolysis and hepatic involvement.

8.61   Answer: D

Feature of early *Plasmodium falciparum* infection; direct visualisation of parasites is pathognomonic. A, B, C and E are characteristic findings in malaria, but less specific.

8.62   Answer: C

The features are consistent with malaria infection; the *falciparum* strain is more likely to be associated with severe anaemia, intravascular haemolysis, shock and organ damage than others. *P. malariae* is usually associated with mild fever every 3rd day, and fewer systemic complications.

8.63 A 34-year-old woman has recently returned to the UK after a vacation in Egypt. She is complaining of abdominal cramps and fever, associated with intermittent constipation and diarrhoea with offensive-smelling stool. What is the most likely diagnosis?

- ✓ ☒ **A** Amoebic dysentery
- ☒ **B** *Campylobacter* infection
- ☐ **C** *Clostridium difficile* gastroenteritis
- ☐ **D** Malaria
- ☐ **E** Schistosomiasis

8.64 A 41-year-old man presents to the Emergency Department with a history of intermittent fever, malaise and right upper quadrant pain for 6 weeks after returning to the UK from India. On examination, his temperature is 37.7 °C and a tender, enlarged liver is palpable. Which of the following is the most likely explanation for these findings?

- ☐ **A** Bacterial overgrowth syndrome
- ☐ **B** Chronic cholecystitis
- ☐ **C** Crohn's disease with secondary abscess
- ☑ **D** Hepatic amoebiasis
- ☐ **E** Tropical sprue

8.65 A 24-year-old medical student has recently returned from a medical elective in India. He is complaining of persistent diarrhoea, vomiting and abdominal pain, and 8 kg weight loss over the past 4 weeks. Which of the following diagnoses is most likely?

- ☐ **A** Amoebic dysentery
- ☒ **B** *Campylobacter* gastroenteritis
- ☑ **C** Giardiasis
- ☐ **D** Schistosomiasis
- ☐ **E** Typhoid

8.63   Answer: A

Caused by ingestion of *Entamoeba histolytica* cysts in contaminated water, or food contamination by infected faeces. Often runs a chronic course, responds quickly to oral metronidazole or tinidazole. Diloxanide furoate eliminates intestinal cysts.

8.64   Answer: D

Symptoms are often vague. Large abscesses can rupture and cause secondary complications in the pleural or abdominal cavities. Treatment is with metronidazole or tinidazole.

8.65   Answer: C

Caused by the parasite *Giardia lamblia*, common in the tropics, spread by contaminated water supplies. Cysts remain viable in water for several months. Symptoms last between several days and months, and can be associated with malabsorption and steatorrhoea. Treated with metronidazole or tinidazole.

8.66 Which of the following features is most closely associated with schistosomiasis?

- ☐ **A** Cercariae are unable to penetrate skin or mucous membranes
- ☑ **B** Larval migration can cause myositis and hepatitis
- ☐ **C** Peripheral blood neutrophil count is usually raised
- ☐ **D** Sheep and goats are the natural host for this infection
- ☐ **E** Typically spread by ixodes mosquito vector

8.67 A 58-year-old Asian farmworker is visiting his daughter in the UK. He attends the Emergency Department after sustaining a fall when climbing a set of stairs. Pelvic X-rays show two discrete calcified cystic lesions of the left quadriceps muscle. Which of the following is most likely to account for these?

- ☐ **A** Amyloidosis
- ☑ **B** Cysticercosis
- ☐ **C** Haemarthrosis
- ☐ **D** Tuberculosis
- ☐ **E** Weil's disease

8.68 A 43-year-old man complains of abdominal pain and intermittent diarrhoea. He is found to have a raised peripheral blood eosinophil count. Which of the following is the most likely explanation?

- ☐ **A** Cysticercosis
- ☒ **B** Cryptosporidiosis
- ☐ **C** Giardiasis
- ☐ **D** Oropharyngeal candidiasis
- ☑ **E** Strongyloidiasis

8.66   Answer: B

The helminiths *Schistosoma mansoni, S. japonicum* and
S. haematobium can also cause pneumonitis, serum sickness and
eosinophilia. Egg deposition in the bladder causes cystitis and
haematuria; cysts passed into water by urine or faeces multiply in
freshwater snails that release cercariae into water; these cause
infection after penetrating skin. Praziquantel is effective treatment.

8.67   Answer: B

Taenia solium (pork tapeworm) is common in Central Europe, Asia
and South America, often acquired by ingesting undercooked pork.
Cysts can eventually die and become calcified. Neurological
involvement can cause seizures, abnormal gait and raised intracranial
pressure.

8.68   Answer: E

Other conditions associated with eosinophilia are trichinosis
(myositis), onchocerciasis (skin involvement) and cysticercosis
(muscle and CNS involvement).

8.69 A 16-year-old boy had unsuccessfully attempted to pierce his own ear using a long pin. Twelve hours later he is admitted to hospital with fever, reduced conscious level and rash. Temperature is 39.9 °C, BP 88/60 mmHg and heart rate 146/min in sinus rhythm. Several sets of blood cultures are negative. What is the most likely diagnosis?

- [ ] **A** Anaphylaxis
- [ ] **B** MRSA infection
- [ ] **C** Staphylococcal septicaemia
- [ ] **D** Streptococcal sepsis
- [x] **E** Toxic shock syndrome

8.70 Which of the following is most commonly recognised as a feature of gonorrhoea infection?

- [ ] **A** > 98% of organisms are sensitive to penicillin
- [x] **B** Bacteraemia is a more common complication in men
- [x] **C** Ceftriaxone is a recognised effective treatment
- [ ] **D** Pharyngeal or rectal infection is rarely asymptomatic
- [ ] **E** Organism responsible is a spirochaete

8.71 Which of the following statements is most correct with respect to syphilis?

- [ ] **A** Blood transfusion is not recognised as a mode of transmission
- [x] **B** Diagnosis can be made by serology
- [ ] **C** HIV-positive patients are less likely to develop CNS complications
- [ ] **D** Penicillin treatment is curative for tertiary complications
- [ ] **E** Urine microscopy is a highly sensitive diagnostic technique

8.72 A 34-year-old woman is undergoing investigation because she and her husband have been unsuccessful in their attempts to conceive over the past 2 years. Which of the following organisms is most likely to be responsible for infertility?

- [ ] **A** Adenovirus
- [x] **B** *Chlamydia trachomatis*
- [ ] **C** Herpes simplex
- [ ] **D** Recurrent *E. coli* urinary tract infections
- [ ] **E** *Treponema pallidum*

8.69 Answer: E

Diagnosis can be confirmed by demonstration of TSS-1 toxin in serum. *Staphylococcus aureus* is the most likely causal organism, which can be a localised rather than systemic infection. More commonly associated with staphylococcal infection introduced via tampons in young females.

8.70 Answer: C

Caused by *Neisseria gonorrhoeae*, most strains (90%) sensitive to penicillin; third-generation cephalosporins and ciprofloxacin are alternative agents. Bacteraemia is more common in women, and the disease is often asymptomatic.

8.71 Answer: B

Either ELISA or EIA tests can be confirmatory. Dark-ground microscopy can allow direct demonstration of spirochaetes in chancre or rash biopsy specimens. HIV patients have a higher risk of neurosyphilis as a complication.

8.72 Answer: B

This is the commonest cause of pelvic inflammatory disease in the UK, and is often asymptomatic in women. It is often asymptomatic in men but is a recognised cause of prostatitis and epididymitis. Treatment is with a macrolide or tetracycline.

8.73 Which of the following statements is most correct with respect to current methods of HIV testing employed in the UK?

- [ ] **A** Antibody tests can now detect infection within 2 weeks of inoculation
- [ ] **B** Antibody titre is a good indicator of overall viral load
- [✓] **C** Detection of p24 antigen can allow an earlier diagnosis
- [ ] **D** HIV-1 but not HIV-2 can be detected
- [ ] **E** Seroconversion illness makes the test redundant

8.74 Which of the following features most strongly supports a clinical diagnosis of *Pneumocystis carinii* pneumonia?

- [ ] **A** Bilateral lower zone shadows on plain chest X-ray
- [ ] **B** Clinical response to co-trimoxazole treatment
- [ ] **C** Hypoxia at rest
- [✓] **D** Identification of sputum cysts that are positive after silver staining
- [ ] **E** Positive HIV antibody test

8.75 A 16-year-old girl who has been helping at a local farm is admitted with a diarrhoeal illness. She is vomiting increasingly and passing smaller and smaller amounts of urine. Blood testing reveals: Hb 10.1 g/dl, WCC 12.2 × 10⁹/l, platelets 562 × 10⁹/l, potassium 5.9 mmol/l and creatinine is 650 μmol/l. Which of the following is most likely to be responsible?

- [ ] **A** *Salmonella typhi*
- [ ] **B** *Salmonella paratyphi*
- [✓] **C** *E. coli* O157
- [ ] **D** *Shigella*
- [ ] **E** *Campylobacter*

8.73 Answer: C

Seroconversion can take several months after infection, and antibody tests are unreliable before then. Seroconversion illness consists of non-specific features (fever, diarrhoea, sore throat, lymphadenitis, sore throat) and affects around two-thirds of patients. HIV polymerase chain reaction (PCR) can also be positive before seroconversion takes place.

8.74 Answer: D

Usually requires specimen to be obtained by broncho-alveolar lavage for positive confirmation. Treatment is with high-dose oral co-trimoxazole, or intravenous pentamidine (alternatively: clindamycin and primaquine, dapsone and trimethoprim). Prophylactic treatment may be needed if CD4 count < 200/mm^3.

8.75 Answer: C

This patient has a blood picture consistent with haemolysis and renal failure, which would fit with a haemolytic uraemic syndrome/TTP picture. Unfortunately the incidence of permanent renal impairment is high in this population.

9. NEPHROLOGY

9.1 A 55-year-old man was admitted with an acute MI. His past history includes hypertension controlled with three agents. He was taken straight to the Catheter Lab where a left main-stem stenosis was diagnosed and stented. He appeared to make a good recovery, but you are asked to review him about 30 h later. His legs look dusky in colour and his toes are turning blue, he has splinter haemorrhages on both feet and a loud right femoral bruit. Blood testing reveals a potassium of 6.0 mmol/l and a creatinine of 645 µmol/l. He has blood and protein in his urine. What is the most likely diagnosis?

- ☑ **A** Cholesterol embolism
- ☐ **B** Fat embolism
- ☐ **C** Femoral artery embolism
- ☐ **D** Renal artery stenosis
- ☒ **E** Renal vein thrombosis

9.2 A 60-year-old woman presents to the Emergency Department with new-onset atrial fibrillation. She has known ischaemic cardiomyopathy and a dilated left atrium. Her creatinine is elevated at 199 µmol/l. Which of the following determines the loading dose of digoxin required in this patient?

- ☐ **A** Bioavailability
- ☐ **B** First-pass metabolism
- ☐ **C** Plasma-binding proteins
- ☑ **D** Renal clearance
- ☐ **E** Volume of distribution

9.3 A 78-year-old man was found lying on the floor unconscious, with an empty bottle of temazepam tablets lying next to him. There is a history of hypertension for which he has recently been started on an angiotensin-converting enzyme (ACE) inhibitor. It appeared to his home help that he was there for most of the night. On examination his temperature is 34 °C, his BP is 100/60 mmHg, and his pulse is 51/min. His WCC is elevated at 12.1 × 10⁹/l, his potassium is 6.1 mmol/l and his creatinine is 290 µmol/l. He is catheterised, the urine showing blood ++. What is the most likely diagnosis?

- ☐ **A** ACE inhibitor-related renal failure
- ☐ **B** Occult transitional cell carcinoma
- ☐ **C** Renal carcinoma
- ☑ **D** Rhabdomyolysis
- ☐ **E** Urinary sepsis

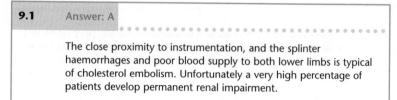

9.1   Answer: A

The close proximity to instrumentation, and the splinter haemorrhages and poor blood supply to both lower limbs is typical of cholesterol embolism. Unfortunately a very high percentage of patients develop permanent renal impairment.

9.2   Answer: D

Digoxin is highly water-soluble, so in a low renal clearance patient the half-life is considerably prolonged.

9.3   Answer: D

This patient has been unconscious on the floor for some hours. With significant myonecrosis, his urine is positive for blood on dipstick, but microscopy will be negative as it is myoglobin which is present.

9.4 A 42-year-old man who has bilateral renal artery stenosis diagnosed on renal angiography is medicated with 20 mg of lisinopril and 5 mg of amlodipine that he has been taking for the past 7 months. His most recent creatinine level is 120 µmol/l and his BP is 159/101 mmHg. An echo prior to discharge showed a normal ejection fraction. What is the next appropriate treatment?

- ☒ **A** Add atenolol to the regime
- ☐ **B** Add doxazosin to the regime
- ☐ **C** Add indapamide to the regime
- ☑ **D** Bilateral renal artery stenting
- ☐ **E** Stop the lisinopril

9.5 A 40-year-old man with hepatitis B is referred to the Renal Outpatient Department with worsening peripheral oedema. His transaminases are only just above the normal range, but he can't maintain his serum albumin – most recently it had fallen to 25 g/l. On examination his BP is 125/72 mmHg, his pulse is 70/min, and he has marked peripheral oedema but no signs of left ventricular failure. His creatinine is 110 µmol/l, but the 24-h urinary protein is 4.2 g and his urine contains hyaline casts. What is the next most appropriate treatment?

- ☐ **A** ACE inhibition
- ☐ **B** Calcium antagonist therapy
- ☐ **C** Corticosteroids
- ☒ **D** Cyclophosphamide
- ☑ **E** Hepatitis B antiviral therapy

9.6 A 56-year-old man with type 2 diabetes managed with a bd mixed insulin regime has significant proteinuria. He failed to tolerate ACE inhibition due to hyperkalaemia. Which one of the following additional medications has been shown to reduce proteinuria in diabetes?

- ☐ **A** Amlodipine
- ☐ **B** Atenolol
- ☑ **C** Diltiazem
- ☐ **D** Doxazosin
- ☒ **E** Indapamide

9.4   Answer: D

This is a young patient with still uncontrolled hypertension. Given his age, his prognosis over the longer term would be poor with medical treatment alone, and so bilateral stenting is the best option.

9.5   Answer: E

He is most likely to have focal segmental glomerulosclerosis and subsequent nephrotic syndrome. It is related to hepatitis B infection, and could partially resolve after antiviral therapy.

9.6   Answer: C

Evidence from one randomised controlled trial (RCT) suggests an effect of diltiazem on proteinuria over and above that expected by its blood pressure-lowering effect.

9.7 A 60-year-old man who has had type 1 diabetes for 50 years comes to the Renal Outpatient Department. He has mild chronic renal impairment and he takes a basal-bolus insulin regime. He takes ramipril, indapamide and amlodipine but recently had to reduce his ramipril because of hyperkalaemia. His BMI is 22 kg/m² and his BP is 155/92 mmHg. His potassium is 6.0 mmol/l, his creatinine 182 µmol/l and his bicarbonate is 22 mmol/l. What is the most likely diagnosis?

- [ ] **A** Addison's disease
- [ ] **B** Hyporeninaemic hypoaldosteronism
- [ ] **C** Renal tubular acidosis type 1
- [X] **D** Renal tubular acidosis type 2
- [✓] **E** Renal tubular acidosis type 4

9.8 A 60-year-old woman with end-stage renal failure and type 2 diabetes comes to the Renal Outpatient Department. She has a number of bony aches and pains. Medication includes three antihypertensives, atorvastatin and aspirin. Her BP is 150/90 mmHg and her creatinine is 215 µmol/l. Her calcium is low at 2.05 mmol/l and her PTH is 2.5 times the upper limit of normal. What is the most appropriate management?

- [ ] **A** Calcium supplementation
- [ ] **B** Cinacalcet
- [X] **C** Etidronate
- [ ] **D** Lanthanum carbonate
- [✓] **E** Vitamin D supplementation

9.9 A 45-year-old woman presents with lethargy, nausea and, most recently, haemoptysis, which is causing her great concern. She is awaiting plastic surgery for collapse of her nasal bridge. Her BP is elevated at 167/92 mmHg, she has bilateral inspiratory crackles and decreased breath sounds. She has a raised WCC of 12.5 × 10⁹/l, a creatinine of 230 µmol/l, and blood and protein in her urine. Which of the following is the most appropriate therapy?

- [ ] **A** Azathioprine
- [ ] **B** Corticosteroids
- [ ] **C** Cyclophosphamide
- [✓] **D** Cyclophosphamide and corticosteroids
- [ ] **E** Methotrexate

9.7 Answer: E

Type 4 renal tubular acidosis (RTA) can occur in response to a number of chronic diseases, including diabetes, HIV and SLE. Renal tubular responsiveness to aldosterone is diminished.

9.8 Answer: E

This patient will have low levels of 25-hydroxy-vitamin D, leading to the development of secondary hyperparathyroidism. Guidelines for intervention are that it is appropriate when the PTH is more than twice the upper limit of normal.

9.9 Answer: D

This woman has Wegener's granulomatosis and this must be managed aggressively with dual immunosuppressive therapy.

9.10 A 78-year-old man is referred by his GP for management of hyperkalaemia. He has a history of severe headaches, and ischaemic pain in his fingers and toes which seems to get better if he keeps them cold or if he takes an aspirin tablet. Abnormal bloods include platelets of 825 × 10⁹/l and a potassium of 6.2 mmol/l. Which of the following is the best way to deal with his hyperkalaemia?

- A   Reassure the patient it is a spurious result
- ☑ B   Re-check at the hospital
- C   Start a small dose of furosemide
- D   Start him on calcium resonium
- ☑ E   Stop his ACE inhibitor

9.11 A 60-year-old man with chronic renal failure and a creatinine of 220 µmol/l comes to the Renal Outpatient Department complaining of tiredness. His Hb is 9.2 g/dl and his ferritin is 210 µg/l. Which of the following is the most appropriate treatment?

- A   Arrange an intravenous iron transfusion
- B   No intervention and review in 3 months
- ☑ C   Start EPO and target an Hb of 10.5–12.5 g/dl
- D   Start erythropoietin (EPO) and target an Hb of ≥ 13.5 g/dl
- E   Start oral ferrous sulphate

9.12 A 19-year-old student presents to the Renal Outpatient Department very concerned because he is has frank haematuria after a recent upper respiratory tract infection. He says that he has had this once before after a sore throat. His BP is 142/82 mmHg; examination is otherwise normal. His creatinine is elevated at 132 µmol/l and there is blood and protein in his urine. Which one of the following investigations is most likely to confirm the diagnosis?

- A   Anti-streptolysin-O titre (ASOT)
- B   Cystoscopy
- ☑ C   Renal biopsy
- ☒ D   Serum IgA levels
- E   Urine culture

9.10 Answer: B

While pseudohyperkalaemia related to essential thrombocytosis is the most likely diagnosis, it still needs to be confirmed. The best way to do this is to take a sample at the hospital and process it straightaway.

9.11 Answer: C

A Cochrane review on EPO in chronic renal failure suggests that targeting a range of 10.5–12.5 g/dl for haemoglobin is more appropriate than the higher target, which can be associated with seizures.

9.12 Answer: C

This history and clinical picture is very typical of IgA nephropathy. Renal biopsy would be expected to show diffuse mesangial proliferation and extracellular matrix expansion.

9.13 A 40-year-old man is reviewed 2 weeks after receiving a live kidney transplant from his brother. The transplant appeared to go well, his notes show a flick-up in temperature to 37.5 °C the day after surgery, but nil else of note. His creatinine is 160 μmol/l (it was 145 μmol/l just after the transplant) and his ciclosporin level is 310 ng/ml (normally this should be less than 300 ng/ml). Renal ultrasound and angiography are within acceptable limits. Which of the following is the most likely cause of the deterioration in his creatinine?

- ☐ **A** Acute rejection
- ☐ **B** Anastomotic stenosis
- ☑ **C** Ciclosporin toxicity
- ☐ **D** CMV infection
- ☐ **E** Delayed graft rejection

9.14 An 18-year-old man goes out for his birthday and drinks 10 pints of beer. He suffers from polyuria and comes to the Emergency Department after passing huge volumes of urine. His bloods reveal: sodium 145 mmol/l, potassium 4.5 mmol/l, urea 14.9 mmol/l, creatinine 198 μmol/l. Which of the following is the most likely underlying process?

- ☐ **A** Increased GFR
- ☐ **B** Increased vasopressin levels
- ☐ **C** Reduced angiotensin levels
- ☑ **D** Reduced expression of renal aquaporin channels
- ☐ **E** Reduced glomerular filtration rate (GFR)

9.15 A 73-year-old man with a history of hypertension presents to the Emergency Department with an episode of paroxysmal nocturnal dyspnoea. He was commenced on ramipril 5 mg daily by his GP a short time ago. On examination his BP is 182/105 mmHg and he is in left ventricular failure. His creatinine is 210 μmol/l (it was 135 μmol/l a month earlier). Echocardiography reveals mild left ventricular hypertropy. What is the most likely cause of his presentation with pulmonary oedema?

- ☐ **A** Aortic stenosis
- ☐ **B** Coronary artery disease
- ☐ **C** Hypertensive heart disease
- ☐ **D** Hypertrophic obstructive cardiomyopathy
- ☑ **E** Renal artery stenosis

9.13 Answer: C

A transient rise in temperature is to be expected after the transplant and the normal blood flow, coupled with a ciclosporin level above the normal range, makes ciclosporin toxicity the most likely diagnosis.

9.14 Answer: D

Reduced expression of renal aquaporin channels leads to increased water excretion and reduces the response of the kidney to vasopressin.

9.15 Answer: E

The episode of flash pulmonary oedema and the rapidly worsening creatinine in response to ACE inhibition is typical of renal artery stenosis.

9.16 A 41-year-old woman is referred to the Renal Outpatient Department for investigation of polyuria. She reports passing large volumes of dilute urine, and drinks around 3 l per day to avoid thirst. Which of the following conditions might account for her symptoms?

- [ ] **A** Addison's disease
- [ ] **B** Adverse effect of sertraline
- [x] **C** Cranial diabetes insipidus
- [ ] **D** Hypocalcaemia
- [ ] **E** SIADH

9.17 In which one of the following situations would renal biopsy be most helpful in establishing the underlying cause of presumed kidney disease?

- [ ] **A** c-ANCA positive
- [x] **B** Chronic renal failure with normal-sized kidneys
- [ ] **C** Recurrent proteinuria on dipstick urinalysis
- [ ] **D** Severe hypertension and renal impairment
- [ ] **E** Strong family history of nephrotic syndrome

9.18 A 45-year-old man undergoes renal biopsy during investigation of unexplained chronic renal failure. Which of the following is *not* a typical early complication of the procedure and would most strongly suggest an alternative diagnosis?

- [ ] **A** Bladder tenderness
- [ ] **B** Colicky back pain
- [x] **C** Epigastric pain and vomiting
- [ ] **D** Haematuria with clots
- [x] **E** Hypotension

9.19 You are asked to 'check over' a 36-year-old man who has been admitted for renal biopsy later in the day. Which of the following would be most strongly associated with an increased risk of complications?

- [ ] **A** Creatinine > 300 µmol/l
- [x] **B** INR 2.5
- [ ] **C** Persistent haematuria
- [ ] **D** Proteinuria +++ on dipstick urinalysis
- [ ] **E** Systolic BP 146 mmHg

9.16   Answer: C

Diabetes insipidus is associated with polyuria and polydipsia. Other causes include nephrogenic diabetes insipidus, psychogenic polydipsia and drugs (eg lithium).

9.17   Answer: B

Note that severe hypertension is a contraindication to renal biopsy.

9.18   Answer: C

Recognised complications include local pain, external bleeding, haematuria and clots, which can lead to ureteric colic and bladder outflow obstruction.

9.19   Answer: B

Due to increased bleeding risk. Normally deferred until INR ≤ 1.5 in most cases.

9.20 A 19-year-old man has noticed occasional dark urine, and is concerned that he may be suffering from haematuria. Dipstick urinalysis is negative. Which of the following statements is correct?

- ☐ **A** A renal ultrasound should be considered
- ☐ **B** Cystoscopy should be performed irrespective of urinalysis result
- ☐ **C** Dipstick urinalysis has a high false-negative rate
- ☑ **D** Test should be repeated
- ☑ **E** The patient should be reassured

9.21 A 24-year-old woman is found to have blood +++ and protein + on dipstick urinalysis. Urine microscopy shows 14 000 neutrophils/mm³, but no organisms are seen. Blood pressure is 118/62 mmHg, and serum urea, creatinine and electrolytes are normal. Which of the following offers the most likely explanation for these findings?

- ☐ **A** Acute tubular necrosis
- ☑ **B** Cystitis
- ☐ **C** Early glomerulonephritis
- ☐ **D** Renal carcinoma
- ☐ **E** Systemic lupus erythematosus

9.22 A 23-year-old man is found to have microscopic haematuria during a routine medical screen. There is no proteinuria, and blood pressure and renal function are normal. Which of the following underlying disorders should be considered?

- ☐ **A** Acute nephritis
- ☑ **B** IgA nephropathy
- ☐ **C** Mesangioproliferative glomerulonephritis
- ☐ **D** Renal cell carcinoma
- ☐ **E** Renal tubular acidosis

9.23 A 22-year-old woman is found to have proteinuria ++ during a routine medical screening. Subsequent 24-h urine collection showed total protein amount of 2.6 g. Which of these is the most likely site of the renal abnormality to account for these findings?

- ☐ **A** Bladder mucosa
- ☐ **B** Distal convoluted tubule
- ☑ **C** Glomerulus
- ☐ **D** Loop of Henle
- ☐ **E** Proximal convoluted tubule

9.20   Answer: E

There are a number of innocent causes of dark urine. Dipstick urinalysis is highly sensitive, and a negative result is very reassuring. Occasional haematuria does not mandate investigation, whereas persistent haematuria may do.

9.21   Answer: B

Despite lack of demonstrable organisms, recent or current infection is the most likely explanation. Culture may identify organisms.

9.22   Answer: B

In the vast majority of cases, there will be no underlying significant pathology and observation is sufficient. Haematuria may be an early marker of IgA nephropathy, which is also associated with recurrent respiratory infections.

9.23   Answer: C

Heavy proteinuria is pathognomonic of glomerular dysfunction, particularly if albumin content is high.

9.24 A 56-year-old patient is found to have dipstick urinalysis protein + and haemoglobin negative. Which one of the following conditions is *least* likely to cause proteinuria, and therefore most suggestive of the need for further investigation?

- [ ] **A** Chronic heart failure
- [ ] **B** Diabetes mellitus
- [x] **C** Febrile illness
- [x] **D** Severe asthma
- [ ] **E** Vigorous exercise

9.25 A 56-year-old woman is undergoing assessment for unexplained weight loss and fever symptoms. Investigations show the presence of Bence Jones protein in the urine. Which of the following is most likely to account for this?

- [x] **A** Amyloidosis
- [ ] **B** Chronic bronchitis
- [ ] **C** Chronic lymphocytic leukaemia
- [ ] **D** Nephrotic syndrome
- [ ] **E** Sarcoidosis

9.26 A 61-year-old woman complains of weight loss, fever and generalised malaise for around 3 months. Clinical examination is normal. Haemoglobin is 9.5 g/dl, MCV 84 fl and ESR 88 mm/h, and you suspect a diagnosis of multiple myeloma. Which of the following findings on urinalysis would most strongly support this diagnosis?

- [ ] **A** Albuminuria > 1.5 g/24 h
- [x] **B** Bence Jones protein
- [ ] **C** Dipstick urinalysis protein +++ and haemoglobin –
- [ ] **D** Red cell casts on microscopy
- [ ] **E** Tamm–Horsfall protein

9.27 Which of the following provides the most sensitive means of assessing renal protein loss?

- [ ] **A** 24-h urinary albumin measurement
- [x] **B** 24-h urinary protein:creatinine ratio
- [x] **C** 24-h urinary protein measurement
- [ ] **D** Dipstick urinalysis
- [ ] **E** Serum albumin:protein ratio

9.24 Answer: D

The other conditions can be associated with mild, transient proteinuria, which disappears on resolution of the provoking condition.

9.25 Answer: A

Other causes include plasma cell dyscrasias and, most importantly, myeloma.

9.26 Answer: B

Found in plasma cell dyscrasia and systemic amyloidosis. Urinalysis dipstick tests are characteristically insensitive to Bence Jones proteins and laboratory quantification is required.

9.27 Answer: B

This allows variation in dilution to be taken into account, although will be subject to variability in creatinine generation (eg muscle bulk, diet and exercise).

9.28 A 38-year-old man is found to have hypoalbuminaemia, fluid retention and peripheral oedema, and a diagnosis of nephrotic syndrome is suspected. Which of the following would most strongly support this diagnosis?

- ☐ **A** Dipstick urinalysis shows protein +++
- ☐ **B** Urinary 24-h protein:creatinine ratio 3 mg/mmol
- ☐ **C** Urinary albumin excretion 500 mg/24 h
- ☐ **D** Urine osmolality 282 mOsm/l
- ☑ **E** Urinary protein excretion 4 g/24 h

9.29 A 29-year-old man is found to have serum albumin 27 g/l, urinary protein excretion of 3.8 g/24 h. Which of the following is most likely to explain these abnormalities?

- ☐ **A** Acute tubular necrosis
- ☐ **B** Diabetic nephropathy
- ☑ **C** Focal segmental glomerulosclerosis
- ☐ **D** Renal cell carcinoma
- ☐ **E** Type 2 renal tubular acidosis

9.30 A 31-year-old woman has proteinuria and hypoalbuminaemia, and a diagnosis of nephrotic syndrome is suspected. Which of the following features would strongly suggest an alternative diagnosis?

- ☐ **A** Hypercholesterolaemia
- ☐ **B** Hypogammaglobulinaemia
- ☐ **C** Pneumococcal infection
- ☑ **D** Urinary protein excretion 1.2 g/24 h
- ☐ **E** Venous thromboembolism

9.31 A 27-year-old woman attending the Renal Outpatient Department for investigation of proteinuria and oedema is diagnosed with nephrotic syndrome. Which of the following is *least* likely to be useful in her subsequent management?

- ☐ **A** Amiloride
- ☑ **B** Atenolol
- ☐ **C** Furosemide
- ☐ **D** Simvastatin
- ☐ **E** Warfarin

9.28 Answer: E

Typically, nephrotic syndrome is associated with protein excretion of > 3.5 g/24 h, and serum albumin < 30 g/l.

9.29 Answer: C

Other causes of nephrotic syndrome are minimal-change nephropathy, membranous nephropathy, mesangiocapillary glomerulonephritis, SLE, diabetic nephropathy (less common) and amyloidosis.

9.30 Answer: D

Nephrotic syndrome is characteristically associated with urinary protein excretion of > 3.5 g/24 h.

9.31 Answer: B

Nephrotic syndrome is less likely to cause hypertension than most other chronic renal disease. Hypercholesterolaemia and increased risk of venous thromboembolism are recognised features. The mainstay of treatment is diuretics and salt restriction; hypotension is often a complication.

9.32 Which of the following mechanisms is most likely to influence glomerular filtration pressure in an elderly patient?

- ☐ **A** Afferent arteriolar constriction by prostaglandin E_2
- ☑ **B** Angiotensin II-mediated vasoconstriction of the efferent arteriole
- ☐ **C** Baroreceptor reflex insensitivity
- ☐ **D** Increased permeability of the loop of Henle
- ☐ **E** Relaxation of bladder tone

9.33 A 49-year-old woman is complaining of general malaise and lethargy. She is found to have serum urea 28.5 mmol/l and creatinine 348 μmol/l. Which of the following would most strongly indicate 'pre-renal' acute renal impairment?

- ☐ **A** Blood pressure 107/65 mmHg
- ☐ **B** Dipstick urinalysis shows blood +++
- ☒ **C** Urine osmolality < 280 mOsm/kg
- ☑ **D** Urinary sodium < 20 mmol/l
- ☐ **E** Urine:plasma urea ratio < 5:1

9.34 Which of the following treatments is most appropriate for preventing osteodystrophy in patients with chronic renal failure?

- ☑ **A** 1-α-hydroxycholecalciferol
- ☒ **B** 25-α-hydroxycholecalciferol
- ☒ **C** Calcium carbonate
- ☐ **D** Cholecalciferol
- ☐ **E** Magnesium silicate

9.35 Which of the following strategies is most likely to prevent or delay the progression of renal osteodystrophy?

- ☑ **A** Aluminium hydroxide
- ☐ **B** Aluminium silicate
- ☒ **C** Calcium chloride
- ☐ **D** High-phosphate diet
- ☐ **E** Thyroid replacement therapy

9.32 Answer: B

This is an important mechanism for maintaining glomerular filtration rate (GFR) in the setting of reduced afferent arteriolar pressure; hence, blockade by ACE inhibitors or angiotensin II-receptor blockers can precipitate acute renal failure.

9.33 Answer: D

Hypotension is suggestive but not specific. Typically, concentrated urine is produced in small quantities. Osmolality is > 600 mOsm/kg and urine:plasma urea ratio > 10:1.

9.34 Answer: A

Vitamin D normally undergoes 1-α-hydroxylation by the kidney and 25-α-hydroxylation by the liver to its biologically active form 1,25-dihydroxycholecalciferol.

9.35 Answer: A

Calcium carbonate and aluminium hydroxide have phosphate-binding properties, so reduce gut absorption, coupled with a low-phosphate diet.

9.36 Which of the following statements is correct regarding renal replacement therapy in chronic renal failure?

☐ A Continuous ambulatory peritoneal dialysis (CAPD) is used in fewer than 5% of patients with end-stage renal failure

☐ B Haemodialysis has been available to NHS patients for 15 years

☒ C Home dialysis has increased in prevalence in the past 10 years

☐ D Number of haemodialysis patients has fallen over the past 5 years

☑ E Renal transplantation rates are progressively increasing

9.37 A 52-year-old woman is transferred to the Renal Unit for haemodialysis for acute renal failure. Which of the following is most accurate in relation to haemodialysis?

☐ A Can be performed using single-lumen femoral catheter

☐ B Causes less cardiovascular instability than continuous haemofiltration

☑ C Effectiveness may be assessed by the urea reduction ratio

☐ D Heparin must be infused to reduce thrombosis risk

☐ E Treatment should be administered for 3–4 h every day

9.38 Which of the following statements is correct regarding the use of peritoneal dialysis in end-stage renal failure?

☑ A Causes less haemodynamic disturbance than haemodialysis

☐ B Dialysis fluid is normally instilled and drained 1–2 times per day

☐ C Fluid exchange must be performed manually

☐ D Patients should switch to haemodialysis if peritonitis occurs

☐ E Sterile dialysis fluid is normally hypertonic

9.39 A 56-year-old man has developed acute renal failure 3 days after initiation of enalapril treatment for hypertension. Which underlying condition is most likely to have caused acute renal failure?

☐ A Bladder outflow obstruction

☑ B Extensive renal artery atherosclerosis

☐ C Previous nephrectomy

☐ D Renal sarcoidosis

☐ E Retroperitoneal fibrosis

9.36 Answer: E

CAPD is used in around 20% of patients with end-stage renal failure (ESRF). Haemodialysis has been available for more than 40 years, and the number of patients receiving regular treatment is progressively increasing.

9.37 Answer: C

A double-lumen catheter is used. Daily treatment is reserved for catabolic patients; otherwise, treatment on alternate days is normally adequate. Prostacyclin is an alternative to heparin and may be associated with lower bleeding risk.

9.38 Answer: A

Isotonic dialysate is instilled for around 6 h then drained, 3–4 times per day. Automated peritoneal devices allow dialysis exchange to take place overnight.

9.39 Answer: B

ACE inhibitors and angiotensin-receptor antagonists can precipitate acute renal failure where there is reduced renal blood flow because angiotensin II constricts the efferent arteriole to maintain GFR. They should be used only with great caution in patients who have undergone previous nephrectomy.

9.40 You are considering introducing an ACE inhibitor for blood pressure control in a patient with uncontrolled hypertension and mild renal impairment. In which of the following situations is treatment most likely to be associated with worsening of renal function?

- ☐ **A** Already receiving nifedipine
- ☐ **B** Anaphylactic reaction to contrast media in the past
- ☐ **C** Associated haematuria ++ on urinalysis
- ☑ **D** Asymmetric kidneys on ultrasound examination
- ☐ **E** Atrial fibrillation

9.41 A 51-year-old woman is found to have serum urea 18 mmol/l and creatinine 344 μmol/l. Full blood count shows Hb 9.8 g/dl, MCV 82 fl and red cell fragments are seen on the peripheral blood film. Which of these is the most likely cause of her renal impairment?

- ☐ **A** Acute pyelonephritis
- ☐ **B** Acute tubular necrosis
- ☑ **C** Microscopic polyangiitis
- ☐ **D** Scleroderma
- ☐ **E** Tuberculosis

9.42 Which of the following statements is correct in relation to Alport syndrome?

- ☐ **A** Associated with conductive hearing loss
- ☐ **B** Autosomal dominant inheritance
- ☐ **C** Contraindication to renal transplantation
- ☑ **D** End-stage renal failure usually develops in late teens or twenties
- ☐ **E** Renal impairment due to anti-GBM antibodies

9.43 A 24-year-old patient with Alport syndrome has been receiving haemodialysis treatment for 3 years. He is being considered for renal transplantation. Which complication of transplantation occurs more commonly in Alport syndrome than in other types of end-stage renal failure?

- ☐ **A** Acute graft artery occlusion
- ☑ **B** Anti-GBM disease
- ☐ **C** Ciclosporin toxicity
- ☒ **D** Graft ureteric occlusion
- ☐ **E** Pyelonephritis

9.40 Answer: D

This is strongly suggestive of renovascular disease, which is often asymmetrical.

9.41 Answer: C

The features suggest small-vessel disease, which can be caused by DIC, systemic sclerosis, accelerated hypertension, cholesterol embolism, thrombotic microangiopathy and small-vessel vasculitis (eg microscopic polyangiitis).

9.42 Answer: D

X-linked and autosomal recessive patterns. Abnormalities of basement membrane collagen (type IV), hence renal GBM abnormalities, sensorineuronal deafness and ocular defects.

9.43 Answer: B

Some patients develop antibodies to normal type IV collagen in the donor kidney, which can cause anti-GBM disease in a small number.

9.44 A 38-year-old woman has had fever symptoms and malaise for 6 weeks. She is found to have impaired renal function, low C3 complement, and red cell casts on urine microscopy. Which is the most likely cause of these findings?

- ☐ **A** Acute tubular necrosis
- ☐ **B** Drug-induced nephritis
- ☑ **C** Mesangiocapillary glomerulonephritis
- ☐ **D** Systemic sclerosis
- ☐ **E** Tuberculosis

9.45 A 28-year-old man has suffered intermittent haematuria over the past 18 months. He has recently been treated with amoxicillin for a suspected chest infection, and found to have urea 19 mmol/l and creatinine 288 μmol/l, and dipstick urinalysis shows blood +++. Which is the most likely cause of his renal impairment?

- ☐ **A** Acute pyelonephritis
- ☐ **B** Alport syndrome
- ☐ **C** Disseminated intravascular coagulation
- ☐ **D** Drug-induced SLE
- ☑ **E** IgA nephropathy

9.46 A renal biopsy is undertaken in a 37-year-old woman with unexplained chronic renal failure. Which appearance would most strongly suggest a diagnosis of membranous glomerulonephritis?

- ☐ **A** Deposition of amorphous fibrillary material in glomeruli
- ☐ **B** Disruption of epithelial cell architecture
- ☐ **C** Focal glomerulosclerosis
- ☒ **D** Immunoglobulin light chains deposited in the glomerular basement membrane
- ☑ **E** Thickened glomerular basement membrane

9.44 Answer: C

Features suggest glomerular disease associated with low serum complement. Other causes are SLE, post-infective glomerulonephritis, subacute bacterial endocarditis (SBE) and cryoglobulinaemia.

9.45 Answer: E

History also suggestive of acute post-infectious glomerulonephritis and Goodpasture syndrome.

9.46 Answer: E

Focal glomerulosclerosis is a feature of diabetic nephropathy, Ig deposition in light-chain disease and amorphous fibrillary deposition suggests amyloidosis.

9.47 A 34-year-old man with cystic fibrosis is found to have heavy proteinuria and hypoalbuminaemia associated with mild chronic renal impairment. Renal biopsy shows deposition of fibrillary material throughout the glomeruli which takes up Congo red stain. Which is the most likely cause of these findings?

- [ ] **A** Acute interstitial nephritis
- [ ] **B** Primary amyloidosis
- [x] **C** Reactive amyloidosis
- [ ] **D** Retroperitoneal fibrosis
- [ ] **E** Tuberculosis

9.48 A 56-year-old woman has recently commenced a new anti-hypertensive drug. She develops impaired renal function, which is thought due to acute interstitial nephritis. Which of the following would most strongly suggest an alternative diagnosis?

- [x] **A** Anuria
- [ ] **B** Eosinophilia
- [x] **C** Fever
- [ ] **D** Generalised erythematous rash
- [ ] **E** Urine microscopy shows eosinophils

9.49 A 46-year-old man has developed acute renal failure shortly after initiation of lansoprazole therapy. There is associated fever and an erythematous rash over his trunk and arms, and peripheral blood shows an eosinophilia. What is the most likely explanation for these findings?

- [x] **A** Acute interstitial nephritis
- [ ] **B** Acute pancreatitis
- [ ] **C** Acute pyelonephritis
- [ ] **D** Acute tubular necrosis
- [ ] **E** Drug-induced urinary calculus formation

9.50 Which of the following statements is correct regarding adult polycystic kidney disease?

- [ ] **A** Inherited in autosomal recessive manner
- [ ] **B** Male:female prevalence is around 10:1
- [ ] **C** *PKD-1* gene is encoded on chromosome 1
- [x] **D** *PKD-2* gene is associated with more aggressive form of the disease
- [x] **E** Polycystin appears to mediate pathological features

9.47   Answer: C

Primary amyloidosis involves deposition of immunoglobulin light chains. In reactive amyloidosis there is deposition of amyloid A component (AA), which is an acute-phase protein, and occurs in chronic infectious or inflammatory disorders.

9.48   Answer: A

Acute interstitial nephritis may be associated with moderate to severe renal impairment, but oliguria is not a prominent feature. The other features listed are characteristic of drug-induced nephritis.

9.49   Answer: A

Other features include eosinophils in urine. Other causes include allopurinol, ciprofloxacin, penicillin, NSAIDs, diuretics, aciclovir, H_2-receptor blockers.

9.50   Answer: E

Autosomal dominant inheritance, so men and women are equally affected. The *PKD-1* gene on chromosome 16 encodes polycystin. The *PKD-2* gene on chromosome 4 is associated with a milder disease form.

9.51 A 34-year-old man presents with vague loin pain and haematuria. He is found to have: blood pressure 168/94 mmHg, a ballotable right kidney and serum creatinine 424 μmol/l. Which is the most likely diagnosis?

- [ ] **A** Acute interstitial nephritis
- [x] **B** Adult polycystic kidney disease
- [ ] **C** Hypertensive encephalopathy
- [ ] **D** NSAID-induced nephropathy
- [ ] **E** Renal cell carcinoma

9.52 A 24-year-old woman is found to have glucose ++ on dipstick urinalysis during a routine health check. What is the most likely cause?

- [ ] **A** Factitious glycosuria
- [ ] **B** False positive
- [x] **C** Renal glycosuria
- [ ] **D** Type 1 diabetes
- [ ] **E** Type 2 diabetes

9.53 Which of the following is most likely to cause renal failure as a consequence of underlying malignancy?

- [ ] **A** Hypercalcaemia due to lung carcinoma
- [x] **B** Hyperviscosity associated with myeloma
- [ ] **C** Interstitial nephritis due to methotrexate
- [ ] **D** Light-chain deposition in patients with colonic carcinoma
- [x] **E** Obstructive uropathy immediately after chemotherapy

9.54 A 33-year-old woman has suffered recurrent lower urinary tract infections. Which of the following steps would most effectively lower the risk of future infection?

- [ ] **A** Avoid excess fluid intake
- [ ] **B** Avoid passing small urine volumes
- [x] **C** Emptying bladder before and after intercourse
- [ ] **D** Partial bladder voiding
- [ ] **E** Regular sodium bicarbonate intake

9.51   Answer: B

Renal cell carcinoma should also be considered, and IgA nephropathy. The diagnosis can be confirmed by demonstration of multiple bilateral renal cysts.

9.52   Answer: C

This is the commonest cause of glycosuria detected by dipstick urinalysis in otherwise healthy individuals, accompanied by normal plasma glucose. Due to reduced renal threshold, which is subject to high inter-individual variablity.

9.53   Answer: E

Due to urate crystal deposition in tumour lysis syndrome. Methotrexate may cause interstitial and retroperitoneal fibrosis (obstructive nephropathy). Myeloma is associated with light-chain deposition.

9.54   Answer: C

Other steps include oral fluid intake > 2.5 l/day, regular and complete bladder voiding and prophylactic oral antibiotics in some cases.

9.55 A 27-year-old woman has symptoms suggestive of urethritis, but mid-stream urine culture is negative. What is the most likely explanation of her symptoms?

- [ ] **A** Bladder carcinoma
- [✓] **B** *Chlamydia* urethritis
- [✗] **C** *Klebsiella* cystitis
- [ ] **D** Pregnancy
- [ ] **E** Trauma secondary to regular vigorous jogging

9.56 Culture of a mid-stream urine specimen from an apparently well 65-year-old woman shows growth of > 10^6 organisms/ml. Which is the correct statement?

- [ ] **A** Antibiotic treatment is indicated
- [✓] **B** Asymptomatic bacteriuria occurs in 2–5% of adult women
- [ ] **C** Is associated with acute pyelonephritis in 30% of cases
- [ ] **D** Renal ultrasound is indicated
- [ ] **E** This is diagnostic of bacterial cystourethritis

9.57 A 22-year-old man is admitted with fever, rigors and right flank pain. On examination, there is tenderness overlying the right lumbar region and suprapubic area. Urinalysis reveals blood ++ and protein +. What is the most probable cause of his fever?

- [✗] **A** Acute appendicitis
- [ ] **B** Aortic dissection
- [ ] **C** Cystitis
- [✓] **D** Pyelonephritis
- [ ] **E** Ureteric colic

9.58 A 57-year-old man complains of loin pain, malaise and fever. An ultrasound scan shows left-sided hydronephrosis with dilatation of the left ureter, and normal bladder appearance. Which is the most likely diagnosis?

- [ ] **A** Bladder outflow obstruction
- [ ] **B** Pelvi-ureteric obstruction
- [ ] **C** Prostatic encroachment on the urethral lumen
- [ ] **D** Retroperitoneal fibrosis
- [✓] **E** Vesico-ureteric junction (VUJ) obstruction

9.55   Answer: B

Infection due to organisms not easily grown by routine culture methods; *Klebsiella* could usually be detected. Other causes include trauma associated with intercourse and chemical irritation.

9.56   Answer: B

Asymptomatic bacteriuria requires no further investigation or treatment unless found in infants or pregnant women (risk of scarring).

9.57   Answer: D

Suprapubic pain suggests additional cystitis (30% of cases), but this alone would be less likely to cause systemic features.

9.58   Answer: E

Lack of dilatation of the right collecting system suggests the obstruction is proximal to the bladder. VUJ blockage will cause dilatation along the whole length of the ureter. Retroperitoneal fibrosis can cause stricturing of the ureter and obstruction at any level.

9.59 Ultrasonography of the renal tract indicates dilatation of both ureters and renal pelvises. Which statement regarding subsequent investigations is correct?

- [ ] **A** Antegrade pyelography should be avoided
- [ ] **B** Intravenous urography can distinguish the cause of the obstruction
- [x] **C** Nephrostomy should be performed in acute renal failure
- [ ] **D** Retrograde pyelography can identify the cause of the obstruction
- [ ] **E** Transurethral cystoscopy should be performed

9.60 A 65-year-old man is admitted with back pain and acute renal failure. What is the correct initial treatment for this condition?

- [ ] **A** Finasteride if prostatic hypertrophy suspected
- [ ] **B** High-dose furosemide
- [ ] **C** Intravenous hydrocortisone
- [x] **D** Percutaneous nephrostomy if hydronephrosis present
- [ ] **E** Suprapubic catheter insertion if urethral blockage suspected

9.61 What is the commonest component of urinary calculi occurring in patients in the UK?

- [ ] **A** Calcium chloride
- [x] **B** Calcium oxalate
- [ ] **C** Calcium pyruvate
- [ ] **D** Glycosaminoglycan
- [ ] **E** Urate

9.62 Which one of the following disorders is most strongly associated with an increased risk of ureteric calculus formation?

- [ ] **A** Alport syndrome
- [x] **B** Amiloride treatment
- [x] **C** Chronic lymphocytic leukaemia
- [ ] **D** Hypoparathyroidism
- [ ] **E** Wegener's granulomatosis

9.59 Answer: C

Obstructive uropathy may be the cause of acute renal failure; nephrostomy insertion can restore renal function, and allow antegrade pyelography. The listed investigations identify the site, but not the cause of obstruction in most cases.

9.60 Answer: D

Treatment of suspected urethral blockage (eg prostatism) should be with transurethral catheter insertion in the first instance. Finasteride has no role in acute treatment.

9.61 Answer: B

Around a third are predominantly calcium oxalate, and a further third involve predominantly calcium or magnesium salts (but not calcium pyruvate!).

9.62 Answer: C

Myeloproliferative disorders increase the risk of urate nephropathy and ureteric calculi due to tumour lysis syndrome. Hyperparathyroidism is associated with increased risk of calcium-based calculus formation.

9.63 A 61-year-old man presents with haematuria and loin pain, and is found to have a palpable mass in his left flank, and renal cell carcinoma is suspected. Which of these would most strongly suggest an alternative cause?

- A Anaemia
- B Hypertension
- C Raised ESR
- ☑ D Strong family history of dialysis-dependent renal failure
- E Weight loss

9.64 Which of the following disorders is most likely to be associated with hypercalcaemia and hypercalciuria?

- A Cushing syndrome
- B Familial hypercalciuria
- C High dietary calcium intake
- D Renal tubular acidosis
- ☑ E Sarcoidosis

9.65 Which statement is correct in relation to renal stone formation?

- ☒ A Bile salt malabsorption is associated with urate stone formation
- ☑ B Dehydration predisposes to all types of ureteric calculi
- C Hypocalciuria predisposes to calcium oxalate stones
- D Urinary tract infection is associated with calcium oxalate stones
- E Xanthinuria is associated with urate stone formation

9.66 A 38-year-old male smoker presents with recurrent haemoptysis and progressive renal impairment. Anti-GBM antibody is detected. What is the most likely diagnosis?

- A Alport syndrome
- ☑ B Goodpasture syndrome
- C IgA nephropathy
- D SLE
- E Wegener's granulomatosis

9.63   Answer: D

This might suggest adult polycystic kidney disease (APKD) instead. Other features of renal cell carcinoma include pyrexia, raised alkaline phosphatase, hypercalcaemia, polycythaemia and neuropathy.

9.64   Answer: E

Other causes include hyperparathyroidism, myeloma and vitamin D intoxication. The other listed stems are associated with hypercalciuria and normal serum calcium concentrations.

9.65   Answer: B

Bile salt malabsorption is associated with increased colonic oxalate absorption and calcium oxalate calculi formation; hypocitraturia and hypercalciuria also predispose to these. Xanthinuria and cystinuria are associated with xanthine and cystine stones respectively.

9.66   Answer: B

Alport syndrome is associated with defective type IV collagen. Renal transplantation can give rise to anti-GBM antibodies and, in some patients, features similar to Goodpasture syndrome.

9.67 A 34-year-old man presents with recurrent haemoptysis and progressive renal failure. A diagnosis of Goodpasture syndrome is suspected. Which treatment is the most likely to be effective?

- ☐ **A** Azathioprine
- ☐ **B** Ceftriaxone
- ☑ **C** Plasma exchange
- ☒ **D** Prednisolone
- ☐ **E** Smoking cessation

9.68 A 14-year-old boy presents with colicky abdominal pain and a purpuric rash overlying the anterior aspect of both lower limbs. Investigations show serum urea 19 mmol/l and creatinine 236 µmol/l. What is the most likely diagnosis?

- ☐ **A** Acute appendicitis
- ☐ **B** Bacterial peritonitis
- ☑ **C** Henoch–Schönlein purpura
- ☐ **D** Renal tuberculosis
- ☐ **E** Sarcoidosis

9.69 A 42-year-old woman presents with arthralgia, nail-fold infarcts and is found to have significantly impaired renal function; p-ANCA is positive. What is the most likely cause of renal impairment?

- ☐ **A** Cryoglobulinaemia
- ☑ **B** Microscopic polyangiitis
- ☐ **C** Polyarteritis nodosa
- ☐ **D** Sarcoidosis
- ☐ **E** Wegener's granulomatosis

9.70 A 67-year-old woman is recovering from a viral gastroenteritis, but is found to have rapidly declining renal function. Investigations show Hb 9.7 g/dl and multiple red cell fragments on microscopy. What is the most likely cause of her renal impairment?

- ☐ **A** Ciprofloxacin-induced acute interstitial nephritis
- ☑ **B** Haemolytic uraemic syndrome
- ☐ **C** Pseudomembranous colitis
- ☐ **D** Ulcerative colitis
- ☐ **E** Vancomycin-induced nephrotoxicity

9.67   Answer: C

Removes the anti-GBM antibody, often used in combination with
immunosuppressive cytotoxics and high-dose corticosteroids.
Haemoptysis is more common in smokers and cessation advice seems
sensible.

9.68   Answer: C

Characteristic features also include raised serum IgA concentrations in
some patients and focal segmental glomerulosclerosis.

9.69   Answer: B

ANCA is characteristically negative in polyarteritis nodosa; c-ANCA is
positive in Wegener's granulomatosis.

9.70   Answer: B

Characterised by intravascular haemolysis, red cell fragmentation,
thrombocytopenia and renal impairment. TTP has similar features,
with more prominent neurological involvement.

9.71 A patient with loin pain and suspected ureteric colic is referred for intravenous urography. Which factor will most increase the likelihood of contrast-mediated nephropathy?

- ☐ **A** Asthma
- ☐ **B** Diabetes mellitus
- ☐ **C** Hypercholesterolaemia
- ☑ **D** Hypovolaemia
- ☐ **E** Male gender

9.72 Which of the following factors is most likely to cause chronic tubulo-interstitial nephritis?

- ☒ **A** Amyloidosis
- ☑ **B** Diabetes
- ☐ **C** Heart failure
- ☐ **D** Hypertension
- ☐ **E** Tuberculosis

9.73 A 56-year-old woman undergoes abdominal X-ray for investigation of constipation, which shows diffuse calcification of both renal parenchyma. Which disorder is most likely to account for this appearance?

- ☒ **A** Chronic glomerulonephritis
- ☐ **B** Nephrotic syndrome
- ☐ **C** Osteomalacia
- ☐ **D** Osteoporosis
- ☑ **E** Renal tubular acidosis

9.71   Answer: D

Risk also enhanced by renal impairment, especially diabetic nephropathy (not diabetes alone). Risk reduced by intravenous hydration.

9.72   Answer: B

Others include NSAID use, sickle cell disease, reflux nephropathy and hyperuricaemic nephropathy.

9.73   Answer: E

This appearance is consistent with nephrocalcinosis, which can also be caused by hypercalcaemia, medullary sponge kidney and tuberculosis.

10. NEUROLOGY

10.1   A 40-year-old man comes to the Neurology Outpatient Department complaining because he has been banging into door frames and most recently crashed his car into a parked vehicle. He has been increasingly tired over the past few weeks and has found it difficult to cope with work. On examination he has a bitemporal hemianopia. Routine bloods are unremarkable. Which of the following is the most likely site of the lesion leading to his visual disturbance?

☐   **A**   Frontal lobe

☑   **B**   Optic chiasm

☐   **C**   Occipital lobe

☐   **D**   Optic nerve

☐   **E**   Temporal lobe

10.2   A 30-year-old woman collapses at work. When she reaches the Emergency Department she is drowsy and complaining of a severe headache. The only medication of note is the oral contraceptive pill. She is hypotensive at 90/60 mmHg, there is no visual response in her left eye, her right eye shows a peripheral temporal field loss and and a third nerve palsy. Her sodium is 134 mmol/l and her potassium is 5.3 mmol/l; otherwise her bloods are unremarkable. Which of the following is the most likely diagnosis?

☑   **A**   Basilar artery thrombosis

☐   **B**   Extradural haemorrhage

☑   **C**   Pituitary apoplexy

☐   **D**   Posterior communicating artery aneurysm

☐   **E**   Subarachnoid haemorrhage

10.1 Answer: B

The visual field defect and symptoms of tiredness raise the possibility of a pituitary tumour, with compression at the optic chiasm. MRI of the pituitary is the investigation of choice.

10.2 Answer: C

Collapse with headache and hypotension is very typical of pituitary apoplexy. Her hyponatraemia and relatively high potassium raises the possibility of adrenocorticotropic hormone (ACTH) deficiency, again supporting the diagnosis.

10.3 A 69-year-old man is admitted by ambulance, having collapsed in front of his wife after complaining of a severe occipital headache. He has a history of hypertension, for which he takes ramipril and amlodipine. His BP on admission is 190/105 mmHg, his pupils are pinpoint but are reactive to light. He is comatose, with his eyes in mid-position, and there is no movement on head turning. Bilateral tone is increased; plantars are upgoing. Bloods are unremarkable. Which of the following is the most likely diagnosis?

- ☒ **A** Lacunar haemorrhage
- ☐ **B** Lateral medullary syndrome
- ☐ **C** Left middle cerebral artery infarct
- ☑ **D** Pontine haemorrhage
- ☐ **E** Thalamic haemorrhage

10.4 A 54-year-old man with a history of type 2 diabetes who has been playing badminton in a bid to lose weight presents with sudden loss of the upper field of vision of his left eye part-way through a game. The right eye shows evidence of moderate hypertensive retinopathy; the left reveals a swollen optic disc and retinal haemorrhages in all four quadrants, and there is an afferent pupillary defect. His BP is 159/91 mmHg. Bloods are normal apart from the cholesterol, which is 6.3 mmol/l; his HbA1c is 7.8%. Which of the following is the most likely diagnosis?

- ☒ **A** Anterior ischaemic optic neuropathy
- ☐ **B** Branch retinal vein occlusion
- ☐ **C** Central retinal artery occlusion
- ☑ **D** Central retinal vein occlusion
- ☐ **E** Optic neuritis

10.5 A 40-year-old man comes to the Neurology Outpatient Department with his 70-year-old father, who is treated with a dopamine agonist for Parkinson's disease. His aunt also has Parkinson's and he is very worried about developing the disease himself. Which one of the following signs is an important early pointer to the development of Parkinson's disease?

- ☐ **A** Excessive daytime sleepiness
- ☐ **B** Hypnagogic hallucinations
- ☐ **C** Insomnia
- ☑ **D** REM sleep behaviour disorder
- ☐ **E** Sleep walking

| 10.3 | Answer: D |

The prognosis is appalling – massive pontine haemorrhage is almost invariably fatal, with a mortality of 80% at the 48-h stage.

| 10.4 | Answer: D |

The history and clinical appearance are typical of central retinal vein occlusion. The area of visual field loss is variable in the early stages; blood flow can be assessed with retrobulbar colour flow Doppler.

| 10.5 | Answer: D |

This occurs when muscle tone is incompletely abolished, when patients can be seen to act out their dreams – kicking, screaming, moving, even laughing while asleep.

10.6   A 56-year-old man with bronchial carcinoma and one brain
metastasis presents 12 days after cranial radiotherapy. His wife
comes with him and says he is sleeping all day, is clumsy, and has
significant mental slowing. His BP is normal, there is no
papilloedema and no focal neurological signs. Which of the
following is the most likely diagnosis?

- [ ] **A**   Cerebral oedema around the existing metastasis
- [ ] **B**   Further cerebral metastasis
- [ ] **C**   Lethargy due to anaemia and poor nutrition
- [x] **D**   Post-cranial irradiation somnolence syndrome
- [ ] **E**   Post-irradiation hypercalcaemia

10.7   A 21-year-old medical student is falling behind in his studies because
he keeps on falling asleep in the daytime. His nights are disturbed
and he feels constantly restless. He falls asleep suddenly during a
class, when he is stressed, debating, or even when he is with his
girlfriend. He is using larger and larger amounts of alcohol to try
and sleep at night and a friend has suggested he use amphetamines
to stay awake in the day. Bloods are normal apart from a urinary
tox. screen which is positive for amphetamines. Which of the
following is the most likely diagnosis?

- [ ] **A**   Alcohol abuse
- [ ] **B**   Amphetamine addiction
- [x] **C**   Narcolepsy
- [ ] **D**   REM sleep disorder
- [ ] **E**   Restless legs syndrome

10.8   A 72-year-old man comes to the ENT clinic for hearing assessment.
He complains that he is significantly more deaf after a recent illness.
Recent medication history includes furosemide, aciclovir, amoxicillin,
co-amoxiclav and intravenous erythromycin. Which of these agents
is the most likely cause of hearing loss?

- [ ] **A**   Aciclovir
- [ ] **B**   Amoxicillin
- [ ] **C**   Co-amoxiclav
- [x] **D**   Intravenous erythromycin
- [ ] **E**   Oral furosemide

10.6 Answer: D

Post-cranial irradiation somnolence syndrome tends to occur 11–21 days after radiotherapy. No mechanism has been postulated but it might be due to post-irradiation demyelination.

10.7 Answer: C

Daytime sleepiness, hypnagogic hallucinations, cataplexy and sleep paralysis are the symptoms and signs of narcolepsy. Amphetamine-related agents and modafinil are the treatments of choice.

10.8 Answer: D

Although intravenous furosemide has been identified as a cause of sensorineural deafness, particularly in special care baby units, intravenous erythromycin is the more likely cause here.

10.9 A 19-year-old woman from the British triathlon team comes to the Neurology Outpatient Department. She is very worried as over the past few months she has noticed involuntary fasciculations, particularly in her forearms and thighs after a particularly strenuous period of training. She looks fit, has very well-demarcated limb muscles, and a normal neurological examination. Which of the following is the most likely diagnosis?

- ☑ **A** Benign fasciculations
- ☐ **B** Dermatomyositis
- ☐ **C** McArdle's disease
- ☐ **D** Motor neurone disease
- ☐ **E** Polymyositis

10.10 A 78-year-old woman has severe temporal headaches and jaw ache towards the end of her main meal. She presents to the Emergency Department with sudden loss of vision in her right eye. There is a past history of hypertension. On examination there is bilateral temporal tenderness, no vision detected in the right eye, and 6/12 vision in the left eye. Which of the following is the most likely diagnosis?

- ☐ **A** Mastoiditis
- ☐ **B** Right carotid stenosis
- ☒ **C** Right optic neuritis
- ☐ **D** Thromboembolic disease
- ☑ **E** Vasculitis

10.11 A 39-year-old Indian woman comes to the Emergency Department with a 6-month history of low-grade fever, tiredness and intermittent confusion. She has a past history of asthma and has suffered a number of grand mal seizures which have been increasing in frequency over the past few months. She has an eosinophila on blood testing and wavy linear lesions seen bilaterally on her CT head scan. Which of the following is the most likely diagnosis?

- ☑ **A** Churg–Strauss syndrome
- ☒ **B** Cysticercosis
- ☐ **C** Hydatid disease
- ☐ **D** SLE
- ☐ **E** Tuberculous meningitis

10.9   Answer: A

Benign fasciculations are relatively common in people who undergo strenuous training, or after excessive alcohol binging. Carbamazepine and phenytoin can reduce the fasciculations, but most patients elect to receive no treatment.

10.10   Answer: E

This woman has a history which is typical of temporal arteritis. Temporal artery biopsy confirms the diagnosis, but the response to high-dose corticosteroids is often diagnostic in itself.

10.11   Answer: A

Asthma and peripheral blood eosinophilia are typical features of Churg–Strauss syndrome, with neurological symptoms occurring in some patients. Corticosteroids are the mainstay of therapy.

10.12 A 59-year-old woman is seen in the Pain Clinic for chronic back pain. She also has bipolar disorder and a chronic skin condition. Her home help has realised that she is becoming increasingly confused. Physical examination is unremarkable, but her sodium is reduced at 116 mmol/l. Which one of the following medications should she discontinue?

- ☑ **A** Citalopram
- ☐ **B** Codeine phosphate
- ☐ **C** Diazepam
- ☐ **D** Lisinopril
- ☐ **E** Oxytetracycline

10.13 A 29-year-old farmer was admitted with a severe post-influenza pneumonia, characterised by multiple associated cutaneous abscesses and possible cavitating lung lesions. He was neurologically normal on admission but deteriorated 48 h after commencing gentamicin and flucloxacillin, complaining of limb weakness. The nurses notice that he has a bilateral ptosis and lack of facial expression. Which of the following is the most likely diagnosis?

- ☒ **A** *Clostridium botulinum*
- ☐ **B** *Clostridium difficile*
- ☑ **C** Gentamicin-related neuromuscular blockade
- ☐ **D** Guillain–Barré syndrome
- ☐ **E** Organophosphate poisoning

10.14 A 45-year-old man presents with increasing tiredness. By the end of the day he even finds it difficult to eat his dinner and he can hardly keep his eyes open. On examination he has bilateral ptosis, which is worse when you ask him to look up, he has weakness in his upper arms when you ask him to hold them outstretched, and he is short of breath when he lies down. Clinical examination is otherwise normal and there is no muscle tenderness. Bloods, including creatine kinase, are normal. What is the most likely diagnosis?

- ☐ **A** Congenital myotonic dystrophy
- ☐ **B** Dermatomyositis
- ☐ **C** Guillain–Barré syndrome
- ☑ **D** Myaesthenia gravis
- ☐ **E** Polymyositis

10.12 Answer: A

Citalopram is associated with syndrome of inappropriate ADH secretion (SIADH) in some patients. Oxytetracycline is associated with renal diabetes insipidus and is actually used as a treatment for SIADH resistant to fluid restriction.

10.13 Answer: C

Gentamicin-related neuromuscular blockade is rare, but the timing of the onset of neurological symptoms does point towards this diagnosis in this case. Confusion, drowsiness and hallucinations can also occur.

10.14 Answer: D

The slow onset of weakness, with increasing fatiguability during the day, is typical of myasthenia gravis. Recovery of motor activity and reduction in fatiguability can be tested with the edrophonium test.

10.15 A 31-year-old woman with increasing migraines comes to the Neurology Outpatient Department. She also has a history of asthma, for which she takes a Seretide inhaler. Which of the following agents is most likely to be effective for migraine prophylaxis in this patient?

- ☑ **A** Amitryptiline
- ☐ **B** Ibuprofen
- ☐ **C** Paracetamol
- ☐ **D** Propanolol
- ☐ **E** Sumatriptan

10.16 A 48-year-old man is referred to the Neurology Clinic with a history of four blackout episodes in the past year. These start with a feeling that he is going to pass out, and he does so within a few seconds. The attacks are unrelated to postural change, and he is not aware of any change in his heart rate or breathing, or tongue biting or loss of continence. After the attacks, he usually sleeps for around 2 h, then feels completely well. Which of the following is the most likely diagnosis?

- ☒ **A** Absence attacks
- ☐ **B** Autonomic neuropathy
- ☐ **C** Cardiac arrhythmia
- ☑ **D** Generalised seizures
- ☐ **E** Recurrent hypoglycaemia

10.17 A 68-year-old man attends the Emergency Department complaining of sudden onset of profound weakness affecting his right upper limb. On examination, there is a flaccid paresis and impaired sensation affecting his right upper limb. Physical examination is otherwise normal. Which of the following is the most likely diagnosis?

- ☑ **A** Partial anterior circulation stroke
- ☒ **B** Partial focal seizure
- ☐ **C** Posterior circulation stroke
- ☐ **D** Subacute combined degeneration of the cord
- ☐ **E** Total anterior circulation stroke

10.15   Answer: A

Tricyclic antidepressants and β-blockers are the drugs of choice for migraine prophylaxis; the asthma history here means propanolol should be avoided.

10.16   Answer: D

Lack of cardiorespiratory symptoms and absence of any postural trigger make a cardiac cause of blackout less likely. Somnolence is consistent with a post-ictal state.

10.17   Answer: A

Depending on timing, the diagnosis might be stroke or transient ischaemic attack (TIA), but the clinical features suggest a left cerebral anterior circulation distribution. Total anterior circulation stroke would additionally involve dysphasia, visual field loss, cranial nerve and/or lower limb involvement.

10.18 A 72-year-old woman attends the Emergency Department after a fall in the street. She remembers feeling faint and dizzy, then losing consciousness for an uncertain duration. She now feels completely well. There is a laceration over the left side of her forehead, and examination is otherwise normal. Which of the following is the most likely explanation for her collapse?

- ☑ **A** Episode of complete heart block
- ☐ **B** Subarachnoid haemorrhage
- ☐ **C** Subdural haematoma
- ☐ **D** Total anterior circulation stroke
- ☐ **E** Transient ischaemic attack

10.19 A 58-year-old man presents to the Emergency Department 4 h after sudden onset of severe dizziness, vomiting and occipital headache. He is found to have coarse nystagmus on left lateral gaze, and marked incoordination of all four limbs. Which of the following is the best explanation for his symptoms and signs?

- ☐ **A** Bacterial meningitis
- ☐ **B** Partial complex seizures
- ☑ **C** Posterior circulation stroke
- ☐ **D** Total anterior circulation stroke
- ☐ **E** Viral encephalitis

10.20 A 72-year-old woman is admitted as an acute medical emergency after a sudden collapse and weakness affecting her left arm and leg. She does not report loss of consciousness, and her weakness is already beginning to improve 12 h after her collapse. Which of these is the best explanation for her limb weakness?

- ☐ **A** Compression of the cervical spine
- ☒ **B** Partial anterior circulation stroke (PACS)
- ☐ **C** Post-ictal phenomenon
- ☑ **D** Total anterior circulation stroke (TACS)
- ☐ **E** Vertebrobasilar ischaemia

10.18 Answer: A

Loss of consciousness is *not* a typical feature of TIA or stroke. Subdural haematoma does not cause collapse, but can complicate a head injury. Loss of consciousness and rapid recovery after syncope are characteristic of an underlying cardiac cause.

10.19 Answer: C

The symptom and sign clusters indicate a peripheral cerebellar lesion. The sudden onset suggests posterior circulation TIA or stroke; prominent headache suggests vertebrobasilar dissection.

10.20 Answer: D

Involvement of upper and lower limbs makes TACS more likely than PACS. It is unlikely that spine compression would manifest so suddenly, and resolve spontaneously. Seizure is unlikely, given no loss of consciousness.

10.21 A 65-year-old man is referred to the Medical Admissions Unit after a sudden collapse and right arm and leg weakness which has now resolved 8 h later. He has previously had a TIA and has been taking aspirin 75 mg and simvastatin 40 mg daily. Which of the following treatment options would be most appropriate?

- [ ] **A** Add clopidogrel 75 mg daily
- [✓] **B** Add dipyridamole MR 200 mg twice daily
- [ ] **C** Stop aspirin and introduce clopidogrel 75 mg daily
- [ ] **D** Stop aspirin and introduce dipyridamole MR 200 mg twice daily
- [ ] **E** Stop aspirin and introduce warfarin

10.22 A 52-year-old woman presents to the Emergency Department with sudden onset of severe occipital headache. There is marked dysarthria and incoordination of her upper and lower limbs. Blood pressure is 168/102 mmHg, and examination is otherwise normal. Which of the following diagnoses would be most important to consider?

- [ ] **A** Anterior circulation infarction
- [ ] **B** Central pontine haemorrhage
- [ ] **C** Parietal lobe haemorrhage
- [ ] **D** Undisclosed phenytoin overdose
- [✓] **E** Vertebral artery dissection

10.23 A 69-year-old man attends the Neurovascular Outpatient Clinic for assessment. He has experienced two short-lived episodes of right arm weakness and dysarthria, and his GP has commenced aspirin 75 mg daily and simvastatin 20 mg nocte. On examination, heart rate is regular and 82/min, and BP is 172/86 mmHg. Which of the following statements is most accurate regarding cardiovascular risk reduction?

- [ ] **A** Atenolol is the first-line antihypertensive of choice
- [ ] **B** Calcium-channel blockers reduce risk stroke in elderly patients
- [ ] **C** Diastolic BP is a more important treatment target
- [✓] **D** Dipyridamole should be added to aspirin in all patients
- [ ] **E** Target systolic BP is 160 mmHg

10.21 Answer: B

There is good evidence that long-term aspirin reduces stroke incidence in high-risk patients, and clopidogrel appears at least as effective. Addition of dipyridamole to aspirin appears to be effective in recurrent stroke; substitution of clopidogrel might be effective in some patients, but evidence of this is less convincing.

10.22 Answer: E

Typically causes severe occipital headache, complicated by cerebellar ischaemia/infarction. Can be precipitated by cervical spine hyperextension, eg leaning head backwards into hair washbowl. Can be diagnosed by four-vessel neck Doppler scans, and CT or MR angiography.

10.23 Answer: B

Dihydropyridine calcium-channel blockers (eg nifedipine) or a thiazide diuretic should be first-line treatment in patients > 60 years. Target systolic BP should be ≤130 mmHg in patients with established cerebrovascular disease.

10.24 A 58-year-old woman presents to the Emergency Department with sudden onset of right-sided facial numbness and weakness affecting her left arm and leg. She is found to have nystagmus and ataxia affecting her right upper limb. Which of the following is the most likely diagnosis?

☐ **A** Acute infarction of the left cerebellar lobe

☐ **B** Acute infarction of the right cerebellar lobe

☐ **C** Acute infarction of the cerebellar vermis

☒ **D** Internal capsule infarction

☑ **E** Lateral medullary syndrome

10.25 A 71-year-old man attends the Emergency Department with sudden onset of visual impairment. On examination, there is a right homonymous hemianopia. Physical examination appears otherwise normal. Which of the following is the most likely explanation?

☐ **A** Lacunar infarction

☐ **B** Middle cerebral artery occlusion

☑ **C** Partial anterior circulation stroke

☐ **D** Posterior cerebral artery occlusion

☐ **E** Total anterior circulation infarction

10.26 A 27-year-old woman is admitted to the Emergency Department with a short history of fever, headache and photophobia. A lumbar puncture (LP) is performed, and CSF shows 80 lymphocytes/mm³, protein 0.5 g/l and glucose 3.2 mmol/l (plasma glucose 5.1 mmol/l). Which of the following is the most likely diagnosis?

☐ **A** Cryptococcal meningitis

☐ **B** Herpes simplex virus (HSV) encephalitis

☑ **C** Enterovirus meningitis

☐ **D** Pneumococcal meningitis

☐ **E** Tuberculous meningitis

10.24 Answer: E

Also called Wallenberg syndrome; caused by thrombosis of the posterior inferior cerebellar artery or vertebral artery.

10.25 Answer: C

Other features of anterior circulation stroke are hemiparesis, hemisensory loss and aphasia (dominant hemisphere). Posterior circulation strokes can cause hemianopia, but are typically associated with other features, eg diplopia, vertigo, ataxia and nystagmus.

10.26 Answer: C

History indicates meningism, and modestly raised or normal protein, and glucose > 50% of plasma concentrations and lymphocytosis suggest a viral cause. Commonest causes are enteroviruses (eg echovirus and coxsackievirus), or mumps, HSV, HIV or Epstein–Barr virus.

10.27 You are telephoned by the ward staff to tell you the results of CSF analyses of a patient admitted earlier in the day with headache. These show 168 neutrophils/mm³, protein 0.7 g/l and glucose 2.3 mmol/l (plasma glucose 4.9 mmol/l). Which one of the following is the most likely diagnosis?

- ☐ **A** *Cryptococcus neoformans* meningitis
- ☐ **B** Herpes simplex meningitis
- ☐ **C** *Mycobacterium tuberculosis* cerebral abscess
- ☐ **D** Sarcoidosis with neurological involvement
- ☑ **E** *Staphylococcus aureus* meningitis

10.28 You are looking after a 23-year-old woman who presented 3 days earlier with meningococcal meningitis. Which of the following prophylactic measures is most appropriate?

- ☐ **A** Amoxicillin should be offered to suspected contacts
- ☐ **B** Contacts with headache should undergo lumbar puncture
- ☑ **C** Public Health Department must be notified
- ☐ **D** Rifampicin treatment should be offered to all next of kin
- ☐ **E** Steps should be taken to prevent faeco-oral transmission

10.29 Which of the following meningitis infections can most effectively be prevented by the use of vaccines?

- ☐ **A** Epstein–Barr virus
- ☐ **B** *Listeria monocytogenes*
- ☐ **C** *Staphylococcus aureus*
- ☑ **D** *Streptococcus pneumoniae*
- ☐ **E** *Treponema pallidum*

10.27   Answer: E

Polymorph leukocytosis, raised protein concentration and CSF glucose < 50% plasma concentration strongly suggest bacterial infection. TB is typically associated with a higher protein concentration and lymphocytosis.

10.28   Answer: C

Potential contacts should be offered rifampicin, and vaccination with a meningococcal C conjugate should be considered.

10.29   Answer: D

Particularly in patients with recurrent pneumococcal meningitis, eg after a skull fracture and CSF leak. Other vaccines used to prevent meningitis include Hib (*Haemophilus influenzae*) and MenC (*Neisseria meningitidis*).

10.30 A 39-year-old woman has recently returned to the UK from a holiday in the tropics. She presents with a short history of headache, neck stiffness and photophobia, and a diagnostic lumbar puncture is performed. Which of the following is most accurate regarding the differential diagnosis in this patient?

A Cryptococcal meningitis is diagnosed by direct microscopy

B Normal microscopy excludes bacterial meningitis

C Polymerase chain reaction (PCR) techniques are ineffective in detecting *Neisseria meningitidis*

D Relief of headache after LP is characteristic of viral meningitis ✓

E Ziehl–Neelsen staining is highly sensitive for tuberculous meningitis ✗

10.31 A 52-year-old woman presents with a rapidly progressive history of lower limb weakness and urinary retention. MRI scan of the spine shows some white matter changes and diffuse swelling at the T12 level. Which of the following diagnoses offers the best explanation for these findings?

A HSV encephalitis

B Meningioma

C Neuroma with spinal cord compression

D Spinal abscess with cord infiltration ✗

E Transverse myelitis due to varicella ✓

10.32 A 69-year-old man is found to have a rash overlying the left side of his chest with early vesicle formation. Which of the following features is most strongly suggestive of shingles?

A Erythema surrounding the vesicles

B History of chickenpox earlier in life

C Recent contact with patient with chickenpox infection

D Recent treatment with oral prednisolone ✓

E Tenderness overlying the rash ✗

10.30   Answer: D

PCR is highly sensitive for detecting meningococcal and other bacterial infections; microscopy alone can be insensitive. Cryptococcal and other fungal infections can be detected using India ink.

10.31   Answer: E

Transverse myelitis involves inflammation of the spinal cord, causing paraparesis or tetraparesis depending on the level of involvement. This occurs due to varicella zoster virus (VZV) or post-infective encephalomyelitis (eg after measles, VZV, mumps or rubella).

10.32   Answer: D

Dorsal root ganglion VZV re-activation, often many years after primary infection. Patients can acquire chickenpox from people with shingles, but not the other way around.

10.33 Which of the following neurotransmitters is most likely to raise the seizure threshold in adults?

- [ ] **A** Acetylcholine
- [ ] **B** Dopamine
- [✓] **C** Gamma-aminobutyric acid (GABA)
- [✗] **D** Glutamate
- [ ] **E** Noradrenaline

10.34 A 24-year-old man is referred for electroencephalography (EEG) for suspected generalised epilepsy. Which of these statements is correct in relation to the EEG?

- [ ] **A** Alpha rhythm is provoked by visual stimulation
- [✓] **B** Benzodiazepines increase β-waveform activity
- [ ] **C** It is effective as a means of diagnosing epilepsy
- [ ] **D** It is less good than CT for identifying an electrical focus in epilepsy
- [✓] **E** Scalp electrodes detect more than 90% of brain electrical activity

10.35 A 32-year-old woman has complained of transient visual loss affecting the right eye, and is suspected of having suffered retrobulbar neuritis. Which of the following tests would most strongly confirm this diagnosis?

- [ ] **A** CT scan through the orbits
- [✓] **B** Delayed visual-evoked responses
- [ ] **C** Diffuse cerebral white matter changes noted on MRI scan
- [ ] **D** Temporal lobe atrophy on CT scanning
- [ ] **E** Widened cerebral sulci

10.36 A 21-year-old man attends the Neurology Outpatient Clinic for investigation of chronic headache. Which of the following is correct regarding lumbar puncture investigation?

- [ ] **A** A standard 20-gauge needle should routinely be used
- [ ] **B** Bedrest is important to prevent headache
- [ ] **C** Fluid restriction is important in the first 24 h after the procedure
- [✓] **D** May relieve headache in benign intracranial hypertension
- [ ] **E** No more than 10 ml CSF should be withdrawn

10.33   Answer: C

GABA is an inhibitory neurotransmitter whose effects are enhanced by a number of anti-epileptic drugs (eg vigabatrin and gabapentin). The others are stimulatory neurotransmitters.

10.34   Answer: B

As with other sedative drugs. Resting β rhythms are abolished by eye opening. EEG can be useful in distinguishing the type of epilepsy and source of abnormal electrical activity. Scalp electrodes detect < 1% of all brain electrical activity.

10.35   Answer: B

Delayed visual-evoked responses can detect involvement of any part of the visual pathway from eye to occipital cortex. Often, the structural appearance on CT or even MRI scanning can be normal.

10.36   Answer: D

Also a characteristic feature in viral meningitis. Up to 100 ml CSF can leak over 24 h after lumbar puncture, and maintaining hydration can prevent post-lumbar puncture headache. Bedrest can exacerbate headache on mobilising, and is not necessary.

10.37 A 32-year-old woman is admitted via the Emergency Department with sudden onset of headache. A lumbar puncture is performed, and CSF is clear and microscopy shows 1500/mm³ lymphocytes and glucose 4.1 mmol/l. Plasma glucose is 5.3 mmol/l. What is the most likely diagnosis?

- A   Bacterial meningitis
- B   Multiple sclerosis
- C   Sarcoidosis
- D   Tuberculous meningitis
- ☑ E   Viral meningitis

10.38 A 29-year-old woman has suffered from headaches for the past 9 weeks, thought to be simple tension headaches. Which of the following would most strongly suggest an alternative underlying diagnosis?

- ☒ A   Brisk plantar reflex responses
- B   Local scalp tenderness
- ☑ C   Photophobia
- D   Poor response to analgesia
- E   Urinary frequency

10.39 For the past 9 months, a 27-year-old woman has suffered from intermittent episodes of severe headache associated with vomiting and transient visual disturbance. Which of the following is the most likely diagnosis?

- A   Benign intracranial hypertension
- B   Glioblastoma multiforme
- ☑ C   Migraine
- D   Retinal detachment
- E   Temporal arteritis

10.40 Which of the following is correct with regard to migraine?

- A   Attacks typically occur at times of intense emotional stress
- B   Female:male prevalence is around 1.5:1
- C   Headache phase is associated with extracranial vasoconstriction
- ☑ D   May be provoked by dietary chocolate in some patients
- E   Vomiting suggests an alternative diagnosis

10.37 Answer: E

Lymphocytosis, normal glucose (> 60% plasma glucose) and normal or slightly high protein (< 0.5 g/l).

10.38 Answer: C

Brisk, symmetrical reflexes are a common finding in healthy young women. Local scalp tenderness is a common feature of tension headache, and can also be found in trigeminal neuralgia and temporal arteritis.

10.39 Answer: C

Lifetime prevalence is 20% in women, 5% in men; presents before age 40 years in > 90%.

10.40 Answer: D

Migraine may occur *after* periods of stress. Female:male prevalence is around 4:1, and the headache phase is associated with vasodilatation of extracranial vessels.

10.41 Over the past 10 days, a 22-year-old man has suffered severe intermittent left-sided frontal headache associated with lacrimation of his left eye. He reports similar headaches occurring 1 year before. Which is the most likely diagnosis?

- [ ] **A** Allergic conjunctivitis
- [✓] **B** Cluster headache
- [ ] **C** Temporal lobe epilepsy
- [ ] **D** Tension headache
- [ ] **E** Viral meningitis

10.42 A previously well 45-year-old man presents to the Emergency Department with sudden onset of severe headache during sexual intercourse. The pain intensity gradually diminished over 45 min, and there are no residual neurological symptoms or signs. What is the most likely explanation?

- [✓] **A** Coital cephalgia
- [ ] **B** Subarachnoid haemorrhage
- [ ] **C** Subdural haematoma
- [ ] **D** Temporal arteritis
- [ ] **E** Transient ischaemic attack

10.43 A 61-year-old man complains of severe, sharp, right-sided facial pain associated with facial twitching. The pain is exacerbated by chewing food. Which is the most likely diagnosis?

- [ ] **A** Cluster headache
- [ ] **B** Migraine
- [ ] **C** Tension headache
- [ ] **D** Toothache
- [✓] **E** Trigeminal neuralgia

10.41 Answer: B

Also known as migrainous neuralgia, this is uncommon and occurs mostly in men. Characteristically, pain is peri-orbital and can be associated with an ipsilateral Horner syndrome and nasal congestion.

10.42 Answer: A

No vomiting, neck stiffness or photophobia. Unlikely to recur, but can be prevented with simple analgesia or treatments for migraine prophylaxis. Needs CT and lumbar puncture to distinguish it from subarachnoid haemorrhage.

10.43 Answer: E

Can also be precipitated by touching facial trigger zones.

10.44 A 38-year-old woman presents to the Emergency Department with an 18-h history of severe vertigo, ataxia and vomiting. Vertigo is exacerbated by sudden head movements. Tone, power and reflexes appear normal in upper and lower limbs. What is the most likely diagnosis?

- ☐ **A** Acute gastritis
- ☑ **B** Labyrinthitis
- ☐ **C** Meningioma
- ☐ **D** Otitis media
- ☐ **E** Transient ischaemic attack

10.45 A 42-year-old heavy goods vehicle driver is admitted via the Emergency Department following a generalised seizure lasting < 2 min, terminated with rectal diazepam administered by paramedics. There is no past history of seizures. Clinical examination and CT head scan are normal. What advice should he be given regarding driving?

- ☐ **A** Advise to inform DVLA and avoid all driving for 6 weeks
- ☐ **B** Advise to inform DVLA and avoid vocational driving for 1 year
- ☑ **C** Advise to inform DVLA and avoid vocational driving lifelong
- ☐ **D** Advise to inform DVLA and continue driving until further notice
- ☒ **E** No specific precautions after an isolated seizure

10.46 A 28-year-old man is admitted to the Acute Medical Admissions Unit after a short-lived generalised seizure that terminated spontaneously on arrival at hospital. There are no signs of neurological deficit, and an outpatient CT head scan has been arranged. What advice is it most important to give before discharge from hospital?

- ☐ **A** Advise to avoid swimming or boating for 1 week
- ☑ **B** Avoid cycling for 6 months
- ☐ **C** Avoid taking a bath for 1 year
- ☐ **D** Inform DVLA and continue driving until further notice
- ☒ **E** No specific precautions after an isolated seizure

10.44 Answer: B

Also known as vestibular neuronitis; assumed to be viral in origin, usually self-limiting. Can also be associated with nystagmus.

10.45 Answer: C

No PSV or HGV licence permitted if any seizure has occurred after 5 years of age, unless seizure-free for 10 years off anti-epileptic medications and there is no structural epileptogenic focus.

10.46 Answer: B

Advise to inform DVLA and avoid driving for 1 year; licence can be restored if seizure-free. Should be advised to take only shallow baths, and to be accompanied if undertaking swimming or boating activities. If the patient insists on cycling, then they should be accompanied if possible, heavy traffic avoided and a helmet must be worn.

10.47 A 33-year-old woman has had recurrent generalised seizures and has been diagnosed with epilepsy. What treatment would be most appropriate?

- ☑ **A** Carbamazepine
- ☐ **B** Clonazepam
- ☐ **C** Ethosuximide
- ☐ **D** Gabapentin
- ☒ **E** Phenytoin

10.48 A 32-year-old man has suffered from three separate generalised seizures over the past 4 months, and is commenced on sodium valproate. Which of the following is the most likely clinical course?

- ☐ **A** 50% mortality at 20 years after diagnosis
- ☑ **B** 50% seizure-free off medications at 20 years after diagnosis
- ☐ **C** 80% prevalence of alcoholism at 20 years after diagnosis
- ☒ **D** 90% seizure-free on medications at 20 years after diagnosis
- ☐ **E** 95% seizure-free off medications at 20 years after diagnosis

10.49 A 55-year-old man complains of weakness affecting his right arm. On examination, there is marked weakness of elbow and wrist extension and brisk biceps and triceps reflexes on the right side. Which of the following is the most likely cause?

- ☑ **A** Cerebral metastases
- ☐ **B** Guillain–Barré syndrome
- ☐ **C** Myasthenia gravis
- ☐ **D** Parkinson's disease
- ☒ **E** Thoracic spine compression

10.50 For 6 weeks, a 57-year-old woman has noticed progressive weakness of her arms, particularly affecting elbow, wrist and finger extension. On examination, there is marked muscle wasting and fasciculation in the upper limbs, associated with diminished reflexes. Which of the following is the most likely cause?

- ☐ **A** Cerebral metastases
- ☑ **B** Myasthenia gravis
- ☐ **C** Parkinson's disease
- ☐ **D** Recent stroke
- ☐ **E** Thoracic spine compression

10.47 Answer: A

Or sodium valproate. Phenytoin also effective, but more adverse effects (acne, facial coarseness, osteomalacia and gingival hyperplasia). Ethosuximide used for absence seizures, gabapentin for partial seizures and clonazepam is an adjunctive treatment.

10.48 Answer: B

At 20 years after diagnosis, around a third will have persisting seizures despite ongoing anti-epileptic treatment.

10.49 Answer: A

Signs indicate weakness in a pyramidal distribution; hyperreflexia suggests an upper motor neurone lesion. Thoracic spine compression may cause upper motor neurone signs in the lower limbs.

10.50 Answer: B

Signs indicate weakness in a pyramidal distribution; hyporeflexia and muscle wasting and fasciculation suggest a lower motor neurone or neuromuscular junction lesion.

10.51 A 65-year-old man complains of weakness and incoordination affecting his left arm. On examination, there is minimal muscle wasting in both upper limbs, coarse resting tremor affecting his left hand and increased tone in his upper limbs, particularly noticeable on the left side. What is the most likely cause?

- [ ] **A** Cerebral metastases
- [ ] **B** Guillain–Barré syndrome
- [ ] **C** Myasthenia gravis
- [x] **D** Parkinson's disease
- [ ] **E** Thoracic spine compression

10.52 A 64-year-old woman presents with increasing gait instability. When walking on flat surfaces, her legs are noted to be hyperextended, her toes scuff along the ground and there is circumduction at the hips. What is the most likely underlying diagnosis?

- [ ] **A** Cerebral metastases
- [ ] **B** Guillain–Barré syndrome
- [ ] **C** Myasthenia gravis
- [x] **D** Parkinson's disease
- [x] **E** Thoracic spine compression

10.53 A 57-year-old man is noted to have a tremor at rest, affecting only his right forearm and hand. It diminishes with focused movements of the right arm, such as picking up a cup. What is the most likely cause?

- [ ] **A** Alcoholic myopathy
- [ ] **B** Cerebellar ataxia
- [ ] **C** Motor neurone disease
- [x] **D** Parkinsonism
- [ ] **E** Wernicke's encephalopathy

10.51 Answer: D

Increased tone and tremor (combined, give cog-wheel rigidity), typically affecting upper more than lower limbs, are characteristic of parkinsonism. Muscle wasting is usually mild, reflexes may be slightly increased or decreased and there is bradykinesia.

10.52 Answer: E

These features are strongly suggestive of upper motor neurone lesions affecting both lower limbs ('pyramidal' gait), ie spastic paraparesis. Cerebral metastases may be accompanied by upper motor neurone lesions affecting the upper and lower limbs (often asymmetric), seizures and features of raised intracranial pressure (ICP).

10.53 Answer: D

Rest tremor is pathognomonic of parkinsonism, lessened by concentration, and worsened by augmentation/distraction techniques.

10.54 A 48-year-old woman is noted to have a fine, rapid tremor affecting both upper limbs that is most pronounced when the fingers and arms are outstretched. Which of the following is the most likely explanation?

- [ ] **A** Alcohol toxicity
- [ ] **B** Atenolol therapy
- [x] **C** Cerebellar ataxia
- [✓] **E** Theophylline treatment
- **D** Parkinsonism

10.55 A 59-year-old man complains of sudden onset of sensory loss affecting his right arm and leg, and the left side of his face. Involvement of which anatomical site is most likely to cause these findings?

- [x] **A** Left side of the medulla
- [✓] **B** Left side of the midbrain
- [ ] **C** Left side of the thoracic spine
- [ ] **D** Right side of the midbrain
- [ ] **E** Right side of the medulla

10.56 A 41-year-old man is rushed to the Emergency Department after a motor vehicle accident. His conscious level is reduced. On examination, he opens his eyes in response to pain, demonstrates abnormal flexor responses to pain, and is making incomprehensible sounds. What is his Glasgow Coma Scale (GCS) score?

- [ ] **A** 2
- [ ] **B** 4
- [✓] **C** 6
- [ ] **D** 8
- [ ] **E** 10

10.54 Answer: E

Action tremor can be physiological, and exaggerated by anxiety, thyrotoxicosis, drugs (eg salbutamol, theophylline, caffeine), fatigue and alcohol withdrawal.

10.55 Answer: B

Spinothalamic and dorsal column fibres have crossed the midline at this site, so there is hemisensory loss of all modalities in the arm and leg.

10.56 Answer: C

GCS allows serial comparison of consciousness, and is a useful prognostic indicator in trauma patients. Other scoring systems might be more appropriate in different patient groups, eg poisoning severity score (PSS) after drug overdose.

10.57 A 66-year-old left-handed man is admitted with sudden onset of expressive dysphasia and mild right arm weakness. What is the most likely anatomical site giving rise to these findings?

- [ ] **A** Left side of the midbrain
- [✓] **B** Left temporoparietal lobe
- [ ] **C** Right medullary
- [ ] **D** Right temporal lobe
- [ ] **E** Right-sided midbrain

10.58 A 63-year-old man has had progressively worsening memory problems over the past 8 months. A diagnosis of Alzheimer's disease is suspected. Which of the following would most strongly suggest an alternative explanation for his symptoms?

- [ ] **A** Apathy and poor food intake
- [✓] **B** Ataxia and urinary incontinence
- [ ] **C** Inability to recall home address
- [ ] **D** Preservation of long-term memory
- [ ] **E** Social isolation

10.59 A 51-year-old man is admitted with sudden onset of dysarthria associated with head tremor and truncal ataxia. What is the most likely cause of his speech defect?

- [✗] **A** Basal ganglia infarction
- [ ] **B** Bulbar palsy
- [✓] **C** Cerebellar infarct
- [ ] **D** Pseudobulbar palsy
- [ ] **E** Pyramidal tract lesion at midbrain level

10.60 A 57-year-old woman is admitted for investigation of progressive dysphagia and dysarthria. On examination, the tongue appears wasted and there is fasciculation. What is the most likely diagnosis?

- [ ] **A** Basal ganglia infarction
- [✓] **B** Bulbar palsy
- [ ] **C** Cerebellar infarct
- [ ] **D** Pseudobulbar palsy
- [ ] **E** Pyramidal tract lesion at midbrain level

10.57   Answer: B

Dysphasia indicates a dominant temporal (receptive) or parietal (expressive) lobe lesion. This is the left cerebral cortex in virtually all right-handed people and in around two-thirds of left-handed people. Simultaneous right arm weakness confirms involvement of the left anterior circulation.

10.58   Answer: B

Suggest the possibility of normal-pressure hydrocephalus. Apathy, poor self-caring and social isolation are common features, but may also suggest the possibility of depression.

10.59   Answer: C

Also associated with limb ataxia, nystagmus and incoordination.

10.60   Answer: B

Bilateral involvement of cranial nerves IX–XII can cause dysphagia and dysarthria. Bulbar palsy arises from a lower motor neurone lesion. Pseudobulbar palsy (upper motor neurone lesion) causes brisk jaw jerk and a small, contracted tongue.

10.61 A 56-year-old woman complains of impairment of her vision. Confrontational visual field assessment shows that there is a bitemporal hemianopia. What is the most likely cause for this disturbance?

- ☐ **A** Bilateral optic neuritis
- ☐ **B** Dominant occipital lobe tumour
- ☑ **C** External compression of the optic chiasm
- ☐ **D** Parietal lobe infarction
- ☐ **E** Wernicke's encephalopathy

10.62 A 46-year-old man complains of visual disturbance. He is found to have a partial ptosis of his left eye, with lateral and inferior deviation of left eye gaze. Pupil sizes and reactions appear normal. What is the most likely diagnosis?

- ☒ **A** Complete left IIIrd nerve palsy
- ☐ **B** Complete right IIIrd nerve palsy
- ☐ **C** Graves' ophthalmopathy
- ☑ **D** Partial left IIIrd nerve palsy
- ☐ **E** Retro-orbital tumour

10.63 A 63-year-old woman is admitted in an acute confusional state. She is noted to have a small, irregular pupil on the left, which accommodates normally but fails to constrict on direct illumination. What is the most likely diagnosis?

- ☑ **A** Argyll Robertson pupil
- ☐ **B** Glaucoma
- ☐ **C** Holmes–Adie syndrome
- ☐ **D** Partial left IIIrd nerve palsy
- ☐ **E** Previous trauma to the left eye

10.64 A 48-year-old man is complaining of excess sweating and occasional palpitations. On examination, he is found to have swelling of the optic disc. Which of the following is the most likely explanation for this sign?

- ☐ **A** Amyloidosis
- ☐ **B** Cerebral abscess
- ☐ **C** Non-Hodgkin's lymphoma
- ☐ **D** Sarcoidosis
- ☑ **E** Severe hypertension

10.61   Answer: C

Often caused by pituitary lobe tumours.

10.62   Answer: D

Sparing of pupil responses indicates partial, rather than complete ipsilateral IIIrd nerve palsy (autonomic pupillary innervation remains intact).

10.63   Answer: A

Lesion is at the dorsal midbrain region, and usually due to tertiary syphilis. Holmes–Adie syndrome gives a dilated pupil that fails to accommodate but usually reacts to light.

10.64   Answer: E

The others are recognised causes, albeit uncommon. Optic disc swelling is often a sign of raised intracranial pressure. Alcohol excess is a very common cause of unexplained sweating, and often contributes to hypertension.

10.65 A 41-year-old woman with established multiple sclerosis is complaining of a burning pain sensation across both legs and lower back. On examination, light touch is exquisitely tender. Which of the following is most likely to be effective in controlling her symptoms?

- ☒ **A** Baclofen
- ☑ **B** Carbamazepine
- ☒ **C** Clonazepam
- ☐ **D** Methylprednisolone
- ☐ **E** Physiotherapy

10.66 A 45-year-old woman with established multiple sclerosis has been suffering from progressively declining mobility over the past 6 weeks due to increasing lower limb spasticity. Which of the following is most likely to be effective in reducing her spasticity?

- ☐ **A** Amitriptyline
- ☐ **B** Carbamazepine
- ☑ **C** Intrathecal baclofen
- ☐ **D** Methylprednisolone
- ☐ **E** Phenytoin

10.67 A 46-year-old woman has been diagnosed with multiple sclerosis for 8 years. Over the past 2 days, she has had rapidly progressive leg weakness that is affecting her ability to live independently. Which one of the following statements is correct in relation to the use of corticosteroid treatment?

- ☑ **A** Acute dysphoria is a recognised adverse effect
- ☐ **B** Chronic administration reduces relapse rate
- ☐ **C** High-dose treatment reduces relapse severity but not duration
- ☐ **D** Short-term treatment reduces long-term morbidity
- ☐ **E** Treatment should normally be given for 1–2 weeks

10.65   Answer: B

Dysaesthesia may also respond to phenytoin, amitriptyline or gabapentin.

10.66   Answer: C

Although oral treatment is almost as effective, with fewer complications; physiotherapy, benzodiazepine and dantrolene may also be effective.

10.67   Answer: A

A short course of high-dose corticosteroids (eg methylprednisolone 1 g daily for 3 days) can lessen the duration of relapses, thereby minimising functional impairment. Multiple courses should be avoided due to the long-term adverse effects, eg osteoporosis, obesity, type 2 diabetes and increased susceptibility to infection.

10.68 A 45-year-old man has been diagnosed with multiple sclerosis, with a relapsing–remitting pattern over the past 6 years. Which one of the following statements is true regarding long-term treatment of this condition?

- [ ] **A** Azathioprine increases 5-year survival by around 30%
- [ ] **B** Beta-interferon substantially reduces long-term disability
- [ ] **C** Ciclosporin reduces relapse rate by around 50%
- [x] **D** Hyperbaric oxygen reduces relapse rate by around 25%
- [x] **E** Linoleic acid diet supplements have no effect on relapse rate

10.69 A 47-year-old man presents with rigidity of his upper limbs, associated with bradykinesia and a coarse resting tremor. Which of the following is the most important investigation for a possible underlying cause?

- [x] **A** 24-h urinary copper estimation
- [ ] **B** CT head scan
- [ ] **C** Early morning urinary lead concentration
- [x] **D** MRI head scan
- [ ] **E** Serum iron concentration

10.70 A 68-year-old man complains of progressive limb weakness and difficulty swallowing. He has been treated for pneumonia on two recent occasions. On examination, he has increased muscle tone and brisk reflexes in all four limbs, and both plantar responses are extensor. Which of the following is the most likely diagnosis?

- [x] **A** Amyotrophic lateral sclerosis
- [ ] **B** Multiple sclerosis
- [ ] **C** Polymyositis
- [ ] **D** Progressive bulbar palsy
- [ ] **E** Progressive muscular atrophy

10.68 Answer: E

Immune modulation can reduce relapse rate, eg up to 30% reduction with β-interferon, but has a minimal effect on long-term outcome/disability. A number of other treatments and special diets offer no proven benefits.

10.69 Answer: A

In a young patient (< 50 years), differential diagnoses of Parkinson's disease should be investigated, including Wilson's disease (high serum caeruloplasmin and 24-h urinary copper excretion).

10.70 Answer: A

Form of motor neurone disease in which upper motor neurone pyramidal tract signs predominate. In progressive bulbar palsy, dysarthria and dysphagia are early features, while in progressive muscular atrophy there is predominant spinal neurone involvement with prominent wasting and fasciculation.

10.71 Over the past 6 months, a 35-year-old woman has noticed intermittent drooping of both eyelids, and progressive facial weakness on speaking and upper limb weakness while typing. A diagnosis of myasthenia gravis is suspected. Which of these investigations would most strongly establish the diagnosis?

- **A** Abnormal spike activity on resting electromyography (EMG)
- ☒ **B** Anti-acetylcholine receptor antibodies
- **C** Anti-skeletal muscle antibodies
- **D** Inducible fatigue on repetitive upper limb exercise
- ☑ **E** Rapid improvement in muscle power after edrophonium chloride

10.72 A 45-year-old man has been treated for HIV infection for 8 years, and was treated for *Pneumocystis carinii* infection 8 months ago. He now presents with progressive memory impairment, weakness of his right arm and leg and marked dysphasia. MRI head scan shows diffuse white matter abnormalities. What is the most likely diagnosis?

- **A** Cryptococcal meningitis
- **B** Herpes simplex encephalitis
- **C** HIV encephalitis
- **D** *Pneumocystis carinii* cerebral abscess
- ☑ **E** Progressive multifocal leukoencephalopathy

10.73 For the past 6 weeks, a 54-year-old woman has received co-amoxiclav treatment for chronic sinusitis. She is admitted via the Emergency Department complaining of severe pain over the right maxilla, and is observed to have a short-lived, self-limiting generalised seizure shortly after arrival. What is the most likely explanation for the seizure?

- **A** Adverse drug reaction
- **B** Febrile convulsion
- **C** Herpes simplex encephalitis
- ☑ **D** Subdural empyema
- **E** Tricyclic antidepressant overdose

10.71   Answer: E

Anti-ACh antibodies present in 85% of cases; anti-skeletal muscle antibodies often positive, especially if thymoma present. Resting EMG typically normal, but characteristic decremental response with repetitive stimulation. Edrophonium is a short-acting cholinesterase inhibitor that potentiates neuromuscular ACh concentrations.

10.72   Answer: E

Due to oligodendrocyte infection by JC human polyomavirus, a complication of AIDS, carcinomatosis, leukaemia and lymphoma. Often rapidly progressive with high mortality.

10.73   Answer: D

Often arises as a complication of chronic sinusitis, osteomyelitis, middle ear disease or trauma. Focal signs suggest abscess formation; requires contrast CT head for detection.

10.74 A 41-year-old man with established AIDS presents with progressive headache, drowsiness, nausea and vomiting. On examination, his temperature is 37.8 °C, pulse rate 48/min and BP 188/90 mmHg. Which of the following is most likely to account for his symptoms?

- ☐ **A** Acute pancreatitis
- ☐ **B** Bacterial meningitis
- ☐ **C** Fungal meningitis
- ☐ **D** Migraine
- ☑ **E** Raised intracranial pressure

10.75 Which of the following is the most characteristic feature of type 2 neurofibromatosis?

- ☐ **A** Axillary freckling
- ☑ **B** Bilateral acoustic neuromas
- ☐ **C** Multiple cutaneous café au lait spots
- ☒ **D** Prominent cutaneous neurofibromas
- ☐ **E** Scoliosis

10.76 A 59-year-old woman has previously received treatment for small-cell lung carcinoma. Over the past 6 weeks she has developed progressive ataxia and vertigo, and is found to have vertical nystagmus. Which antibody test most strongly suggests paraneoplastic cerebellar degeneration?

- ☐ **A** Anti-double-stranded DNA antibody
- ☐ **B** Anti-Jo 1 antibody
- ☐ **C** Anti-nuclear antibody
- ☐ **D** Anti-Ro antibody
- ☑ **E** Anti-Yo antibody

10.74 Answer: E

Characteristic features include headache, impaired consciousness, papilloedema, vomiting, bradycardia and hypertension. This could be due to obstruction of CSF flow by fungal meningitis, or a mass lesion, eg lymphoma or cerebral abscess.

10.75 Answer: B

Type 1 accounts for around 75% of cases, and involves predominantly peripheral features, whereas type 2 is characterised by acoustic neuroma, optic nerve glioma, meningioma and spinal neuromas, with few or no cutaneous features.

10.76 Answer: E

Anti-Yo and anti-Hu antibodies are strongly suggestive; anti-Hu antibody is also detectable in a number of other paraneoplastic syndromes, eg subacute motor neuropathy, myelitis and sensory neuropathy. Anti-Jo 1 is associated with dermatomyositis and polymyositis, which may be associated with underlying lung, breast or ovarian cancer.

11. OPHTHALMOLOGY

11.1 A 55-year-old man with a history of type 2 diabetes comes to the Ophthalmology Outpatient Department complaining of blue vision. He has a number of other health problems, including hypertension, chronic atrial fibrillation and erectile dysfunction. Which of the following agents is most likely to be responsible?

- [ ] **A** Atorvastatin
- [ ] **B** Bendroflumethiazide
- [ ] **C** Digoxin
- [ ] **D** Ramipril
- [x] **E** Sildenafil

11.2 A 29-year-old woman was noted to have unequal pupils. The left one is more dilated than the right, with no constriction to light. Dark adaptation didn't improve the reaction to light, but the pupil did constrict to accommodation. What is the most likely diagnosis?

- [x] **A** Adie's pupil
- [x] **B** Argyll Robertson pupil
- [ ] **C** Fourth cranial nerve palsy
- [ ] **D** Horner syndrome
- [ ] **E** Sixth cranial nerve palsy

11.3 A 50-year-old man with a history of SLE presents with sudden loss of vision in his right eye. His BP is 160/95 mmHg and fundoscopy reveals flame-shaped retinal haemorrhages and retinal oedema on the temporal side. What is the most likely cause of his symptoms?

- [ ] **A** Branch retinal artery occlusion
- [x] **B** Branch retinal vein occlusion
- [ ] **C** Central retinal artery occlusion
- [x] **D** Central retinal vein thrombosis
- [ ] **E** Vitreous haemorrhage

11.1 Answer: E

Sildenafil is a PDE-5 inhibitor, but at high doses there is some crossover with PDE-6 inhibition. PDE-6 is involved in the functioning of the retina, and inhibition leads to blue vision. Digoxin toxicity may be associated with yellow vision due to CNS effects.

11.2 Answer: A

Adie's pupil does not react to light but does to accommodation. Argyll Robertson pupil is usually bilateral. The Adie pupil is caused by damage to the ciliary ganglion.

11.3 Answer: B

Inflammatory conditions such as SLE increase the risk of retinal vein occlusion, as do pro-thrombotic conditions such as protein C deficiency or protein S deficiency. Anticoagulants and antithrombotics have no effect on prognosis.

11.4 A 41-year-old gay man presents with rapid deterioration of vision in his left eye. He has been feeling unwell for some months and has lost a considerable amount of weight and suffered from a chronic cough. On examination his left eye has a 'cheese pizza' appearance, with evidence of haemorrhage and formation of considerable amounts of white material. His BP is elevated at 155/98 mmHg. Which of the following is the most likely diagnosis?

- [ ] **A** Branch retinal artery occlusion
- [ ] **B** Central retinal artery occlusion
- [ ] **C** Central retinal vein occlusion
- [✓] **D** CMV retinitis
- [ ] **E** Hypertensive retinopathy

11.5 Which of the following extraocular muscles is most likely to be affected by a lesion involving the fourth cranial nerve?

- [ ] **A** Inferior oblique
- [ ] **B** Lateral rectus
- [ ] **C** Medial rectus
- [✓] **D** Superior oblique
- [ ] **E** Superior rectus

11.6 A 49-year-old woman presents to the Emergency Department with sudden deterioration of the vision in her right eye. Fundoscopy shows changes characteristic of retinal vein occlusion. Which of the following is most likely to predispose to this condition?

- [ ] **A** Asthma
- [ ] **B** Breast cancer
- [✗] **C** Diabetes
- [✓] **D** Hypertension
- [ ] **E** Varicose veins

11.7 A 63-year-old man attends the Emergency Department with a history of dizziness, headache and blurred vision. On examination, he is found to have loss of his superior temporal visual field in his right eye. What is the most likely cause?

- [ ] **A** Acute conjunctivitis
- [ ] **B** Acute stroke
- [✓] **C** Branch retinal artery occlusion
- [ ] **D** Episcleritis
- [ ] **E** Glaucoma

11.4 Answer: D

This man has a number of clinical pointers towards end-stage HIV infection, of which CMV retinitis is a feature. Management involves the use of intravenous ganciclovir.

11.5 Answer: D

The others listed are supplied by the third cranial nerve (IO, IR, MR, SR) and sixth cranial nerve (LR).

11.6 Answer: D

Diabetes is also recognised, albeit less commonly. Other causes are hyperviscosity states (myeloma, Waldenström's macroglobulinaemia) and vasculitides.

11.7 Answer: C

Often painless, this can cause variable visual field defects depending on the extent of retinal involvement. Unlike stroke, the visual field loss is uniocular, rather than bitemporal.

11.8 A 54-year-old woman is referred to the Hypertension Clinic, having been found by her employer to have BP readings of 182/86 mmHg and 184/82 mmHg. On examination, dipstick urinalysis is positive for glucose and protein, and fundoscopy shows multiple tiny haemorrhages and a small number of cotton-wool spots. What is the most likely diagnosis?

- **A** Accelerated hypertension
- **B** Aortic valve incompetence
- **C** Diabetic retinopathy
- ☒ **D** Grade II hypertensive retinopathy
- ☑ **E** Grade III hypertensive retinopathy

11.9 A 56-year-old man attends an annual follow-up appointment in the Diabetes Outpatient Clinic. On fundoscopy, you find haemorrhages and exudates in a pattern suggestive of diabetic retinopathy. Which of the following statements is correct regarding this condition?

- **A** It is a macrovascular complication of poorly controlled diabetes
- **B** Platelet adhesiveness is generally diminished
- **C** Rare cause of blindness in adults
- ☑ **D** Risk of retinopathy is related to the duration of diabetes
- **E** Smoking cessation does not delay progression

11.10 A 57-year-old woman attends the Medical Outpatient Department for follow-up assessment of her diabetes. The presence of which feature is most strongly indicative of background retinopathy?

- **A** Absence of exudates
- **B** Impaired central visual acuity
- ☒ **C** Multiple exudates involving and around the macula
- **D** Neovascularisation around the optic disc
- ☑ **E** Only microaneurysms present

11.8   Answer: E

Grade I is characterised by arteriolar narrowing, grade II is associated with AV nipping, whereas grade IV (accelerated hypertension) is associated with papilloedema.

11.9   Answer: D

Commonest cause of blindness in young adults. Present in 80% of patients who have had type 2 diabetes for 20 years. Treatment involves good control of blood pressure and diabetes and smoking cessation advice.

11.10   Answer: E

Non-proliferative (background) retinopathy is usually associated with normal vision and is therefore only detected by fundoscopy screening. Characteristic features include microaneurysms and exudates. Diabetic maculopathy involves extensive exudates around the macula.

11.11 A 62-year-old diabetic man is referred to the Ophthalmology Outpatient Department for assessment of cataracts, which have caused impaired vision over the past year. Which one of the following would most strongly indicate the need for corrective surgery?

- [ ] **A** Bilateral cataracts
- [ ] **B** Family history of cataract disease
- [x] **C** Fundus cannot be seen to assess progression of diabetic retinopathy
- [ ] **D** History of corticosteroid treatment
- [ ] **E** White reflex

11.12 A 21-year-old man is referred to the Ophthalmology Clinic because his GP thought he had 'unusual looking eyes' during a routine check-up for asthma. Slit-lamp examination shows downward dislocation of both lenses. What is the most likely diagnosis?

- [ ] **A** Corticosteroid treatment
- [ ] **B** Diabetes mellitus
- [x] **C** Homocystinuria
- [x] **D** Marfan syndrome
- [ ] **E** Trauma

11.13 A 37-year-old woman is referred to the General Medical Outpatient Department for assessment of blurred vision and generalised weakness. The GP did not find any physical abnormality, and has requested a second opinion. On examination, there is reduced visual acuity affecting the left eye associated with a central field defect. Pupil sizes are equal, but there is a relative afferent pupillary defect on the left. What is the most likely diagnosis?

- [ ] **A** Acute glaucoma
- [ ] **B** Acute stroke
- [ ] **C** Graves' ophthalmopathy
- [x] **D** Optic neuritis
- [ ] **E** Retinal artery occlusion

11.11 Answer: C

An additional indication is severe functional impairment, eg recurrent falls.

11.12 Answer: C

Also seen in Ehlers–Danlos syndrome, with uveal tumours and after trauma (less likely cause in absence of history). Marfan syndrome is typically associated with upward, outward dislocation of the lens.

11.13 Answer: D

The other possible causes listed are retinal artery occlusion (less likely in young adult with no predisposing factors) or acute glaucoma (less likely in absence of other signs.

11.14 A 24-year-old woman is referred for investigation of long-standing headaches. Seated BP is 128/72 mmHg and pulse 74/min. Fundoscopy shows bilateral papilloedema. What is the most likely cause of this appearance?

- ☑ **A** Benign intracranial hypertension
- ☐ **B** Carbon dioxide retention
- ☐ **C** Diabetes mellitus
- ☐ **D** Multiple sclerosis
- ☐ **E** Posterior fossa tumour

11.15 A 47-year-old man self-presents to the Ophthalmology Emergency Department with an acutely painful left eye. On examination, the left eye looks red and inflamed with excess lacrimation. What is the most likely diagnosis?

- ☐ **A** Acute bacterial conjunctivitis
- ☐ **B** Acute viral conjunctivitis
- ☑ **C** Anterior uveitis
- ☐ **D** Graves' ophthalmopathy
- ☐ **E** Optic neuritis

11.16 A 56-year-old man is referred as an urgent case to the Ophthalmology Clinic by his GP because of reduced vision in his left eye. He is otherwise asymptomatic. He has a history of hypertension and smoking. On examination, pupils appear normal-sized but there is a relative afferent pupillary defect affecting the left eye. What is the most likely underlying diagnosis?

- ☐ **A** Acute glaucoma
- ☐ **B** Acute scleritis
- ☑ **C** Branch retinal artery occlusion
- ☐ **D** Keratoconjunctivitis
- ☐ **E** Posterior uveitis

11.14 Answer: A

Most commonly found in young females, especially if co-existent obesity. Carbon dioxide retention can cause papilloedema in severe cases, eg sleep apnoea, but conscious level would be expected to be reduced. Posterior fossa tumour can increase ICP, but less likely in the absence of other clinical features.

11.15 Answer: C

Conjunctivitis is rarely uniocular, even if asymmetric, and such a diagnosis should raise suspicion. Anterior uveitis can be a feature of ankylosing spondylitis, sarcoidosis, inflammatory bowel disease and Reiter's disease.

11.16 Answer: C

All of the above conditions can cause acute deterioration in visual acuity, but A, B and D are generally painful, and his vascular risk factors point to C as the most likely event.

11.17 A 46-year-old woman with long-standing Graves' disease is referred to the Ophthalmology Outpatient Department because of deterioration in vision affecting her left eye. Examination findings include a relative afferent pupillary defect affecting the left eye, and pallor of the left optic disc. What is the cause of these findings?

- ☒ **A** Branch retinal artery occlusion
- ☐ **B** Keratoconjunctivitis
- ☑ **C** Optic nerve compression
- ☐ **D** Proptosis
- ☐ **E** Superior sagittal sinus thrombosis

11.18 A 27-year-old man with long-standing respiratory symptoms has recently been diagnosed with sarcoidosis. He is referred to the Ophthalmology Department for review. What is the most likely ocular manifestation in this disease?

- ☐ **A** Cataract formation
- ☑ **B** Granulomatous infiltration of the lacrimal glands
- ☐ **C** Mononeuritis multiplex causing palsy of cranial nerves III, IV or VI
- ☐ **D** Optic nerve atrophy
- ☐ **E** Retinal artery branch occlusion

11.19 A 52-year-old woman self-presents to the Emergency Department with an acutely painful and inflamed right eye. The Emergency Department doctor considers a diagnosis of acute glaucoma, and contacts the Ophthalmology Department for advice. What feature most strongly supports the diagnosis of glaucoma?

- ☐ **A** Established bilateral cataracts
- ☐ **B** History of short-sightedness
- ☐ **C** Homonymous visual field defect
- ☐ **D** Intraocular pressure of 18 mmHg
- ☑ **E** Severe eye pain and vomiting

11.20 Which one of the following medications is most likely to increase the risk of developing cataracts in later life?

- ☑ **A** Chlorpromazine
- ☐ **B** Ethambutol
- ☐ **C** Isoniazid
- ☐ **D** Quinine
- ☐ **E** Thyroxine

11.17   Answer: C

This can be a complication of Graves' ophthalmopathy due to retrobulbar soft tissue inflammation and swelling, or may be due to lymphoma (increased incidence in Graves' disease).

11.18   Answer: B

Therefore associated with sicca syndrome, and patients should be treated with 'artificial tears' lubrication to preserve corneal integrity. Cataract is more prevalent, and may be a late complication of sarcoidosis.

11.19   Answer: E

This is more often encountered in acute glaucoma than other causes of a painful red eye. Patients with long-sightedness are at greater risk, and intraocular pressure is usually significantly higher than normal (> 22 mmHg).

11.20   Answer: A

Also corticosteroid treatment, particularly if prolonged courses at high dose. Quinine is a recognised cause of retinal toxicity, isoniazid can cause optic neuritis, and ethambutol can cause retrobulbar neuritis.

12. PSYCHIATRY

12.1 A 17-year-old girl is taken to the Emergency Department after slashing at her arms with a kitchen knife. She has previously taken paracetamol overdoses in response to rows with her boyfriend and has been arrested by the police on two occasions for being drunk and disorderly. She moved out of the original family home due to increasing domestic violence. On examination there are multiple fresh and healed forearm scars, she is abusive and tearful, but otherwise seems fine. Which of the following is the most likely diagnosis?

- A   Bipolar disorder
- ☑ B   Borderline personality disorder
- C   Depression
- D   Post-traumatic stress disorder
- E   Schizophrenia

12.2 A 71-year-old woman presents with worsening dementia. She has a history of hypertension and type 2 diabetes and had an MI 8 years ago. A psychiatrist diagnoses her with Lewy body dementia. Which of the following is the strongest pointer to this type of dementia?

- A   Auditory hallucinations
- B   Characteristic appearance on EEG
- ☑ C   Fluctuating mental state
- D   Poor concentration
- E   Rapid deterioration

12.3 A 40-year-old woman comes to the Psychiatric Outpatient Department complaining that her ears are too large for her head. She has visited 12 doctors over the past year and they have all told her she is normal. On examination her ears are clearly completely normal. She has no other medical history of note and holds down a job as an office administrator. Which of the following is the most likely diagnosis?

- ☑ A   Body dysmorphia
- B   Depression
- C   Munchausen syndrome
- D   Obsessive-compulsive disorder
- E   Somatisation disorder

12.1   Answer: B

She should be offered behavioural interventions to prevent self-harm episodes. Increased community support and planning should reduce the frequency of presentation to acute services.

12.2   Answer: C

Fluctuating mental state, with varying levels of alertness and significant daytime somnolence are typical of Lewy body dementia. There is also a strong association with visual hallucinations and parkinsonian features.

12.3   Answer: A

Psychotherapy is the mainstay of therapy for body dysmorphia, although selective serotonin reuptake inhibitors (SSRIs) can be of value in some patients. Patients with body dysmorphia have an increased incidence of obsessive-compulsive disorder.

12.4 A 29-year-old woman attends the Psychiatric Outpatients Department with chronic diarrhoea and a low BMI. She is unable to complete a day's work at the pharmacy and is now on long-term sick pay. On examination her BMI is 17 kg/m². Her potassium is low at 2.6 mmol/l on routine blood testing. Stool volumes are normal during an inpatient stay, and melanosis coli is seen on colonoscopy. Which of the following is the most likely diagnosis?

- ☐ **A** Coeliac disease
- ☐ **B** Diuretic abuse
- ☐ **C** Irritable bowel syndrome
- ☑ **D** Laxative abuse
- ☐ **E** Lymphocytic colitis

12.5 A 29-year-old man presents with depression, weight loss and chorea. He informs you that both his father (at age 50) and his grandfather (at age 70), died of a similar neurological disease. Which of the following is the most likely diagnosis?

- ☐ **A** Creutzfeld–Jakob disease (CJD)
- ☐ **B** Friedreich's ataxia
- ☑ **C** Huntingdon's disease
- ☐ **D** Lewy body dementia
- ☐ **E** Pick's disease

12.6 A 40-year-old man with advanced HIV presents with difficulties with short-term memory, generalised weakness and gait disturbance. He has weakness of the left arm and the right leg. His CD4 count is 71/mm³, he has a raised CSF protein, and his MRI shows hyperintense white-matter lesions, mostly in the frontal and parietal regions. Which of the following is the most likely diagnosis?

- ☐ **A** CJD
- ☐ **B** Focal cerebritis
- ☐ **C** Herpes simplex encephalitis
- ☐ **D** HIV encephalopathy
- ☑ **E** Progressive multifocal leukoencephalopathy (PML)

12.4   Answer: D

This patient has access to the pharmacy, a history of diarrhoea that is not reflected in monitoring during her hospital stay, hypokalaemia and low body weight. The most likely diagnosis is therefore laxative abuse.

12.5   Answer: C

Huntingdon's disease shows this type of picture with genetic anticipation, as evidenced by the fact that successive generations suffer from the disease at younger and younger ages.

12.6   Answer: E

PML is thought to be caused by the JC virus, which infects oligodendrocytes, the cells which maintain the myelin sheath. Ultimately the condition is fatal, but progression can be slowed by HAART.

12.7 A 60-year-old man who was recently made redundant from his job at a bank presents to the Psychiatry Outpatient Department accompanied by his wife. He has low mood, early-morning wakening and poor short-term memory. He is constantly worried about money but his wife assures you they have no financial problems. Clinical examination is normal and his mini-mental state examination (MMSE) score is 26/30. Which of the following is the most likely diagnosis?

- [ ] **A** Alzheimer's disease
- [ ] **B** CJD
- [x] **C** Depression
- [ ] **D** Multi-infarct dementia
- [ ] **E** Pick's disease

12.8 A 23-year-old who has been intermittently out of work since leaving university is picked up by the police trying to kick in the window of a television shop. He says that two voices are talking about him in a negative way, and that they are being transmitted through the TVs in the shop. He was admitted 2 weeks ago with an overdose and has had a history of Emergency Department attendances for heroin, cannabis and alcohol abuse. On examination he is unkempt and dirty, and he constantly mumbles to himself, looking very agitated. What is the most likely diagnosis?

- [ ] **A** Cannabis-related delusions
- [ ] **B** Depression
- [ ] **C** Hypomanic episode
- [ ] **D** Personality disorder
- [x] **E** Schizophrenia

12.9 A 48-year-old woman with a past history of mania attends the Outpatient Department for review. Which of the following statements is most accurate with regard to this condition?

- [x] **A** Delusions and hallucinations are recognised features
- [ ] **B** Increased somnolescence is a characteristic feature
- [ ] **C** It is the commonest mood disorder in Western societies
- [ ] **D** Mood is typically low during acute episodes
- [x] **E** Patients often experience only a single episode

12.7   Answer: C

The proximity of this episode to his recent job loss makes depression the most likely diagnosis here. Patients with depression can have a decreased mental state score, mimicking dementia.

12.8   Answer: E

This presentation is typical of schizophrenia, with auditory hallucinations in the third person, delusions and loss of insight. As initial therapy, anti-psychotics are usually combined with anxiolytics.

12.9   Answer: A

Mania and hypomania (milder variant) are characterised by abnormally elevated mood, overactivity and reduced need for sleep. Most patients have recurrent episodes, and often develop depressive episodes. Unipolar depression is the commonest mood disorder.

12.10 One of the patients attending your Diabetic Outpatient Department has symptoms suggestive of unipolar depression. You are contemplating initiation of antidepressant treatment. Which of the following would most strongly indicate that referral to a specialist psychiatric service is indicated?

- ☑ **A** Auditory hallucinations
- ☐ **B** Depressive symptoms have persisted more than 9 months
- ☐ **C** Family history of suicide
- ☐ **D** Sleep disturbance
- ☐ **E** Symptoms and signs suggestive of co-existent anxiety

12.11 You are asked to review a 24-year-old man in the Emergency Department, who presented with evidence of deliberate self-harm. On examination, he is found to have superficial cuts across both wrists. In determining his suicide risk, which of the following factors is *least* likely to be of importance?

- ☐ **A** History of alcohol abuse
- ☐ **B** History of personality disorder
- ☑ **C** Low socio-economic class
- ☐ **D** Recent loss of a job
- ☐ **E** Recent split from his girlfriend

12.12 You are asked by one of your psychiatry colleagues to medically assess a 46-year-old man with a major depressive disorder before he undergoes electroconvulsive therapy (ECT). Which of the following statements is correct regarding ECT?

- ☐ **A** Administrations of ECT should separated by at least 1 week
- ☐ **B** Antidepressant medications should be stopped for 1 week before ECT
- ☐ **C** It is an alternative to antidepressant medication in elderly patients
- ☑ **D** It is associated with early remission in around 70–75% of patients
- ☐ **E** Psychotic symptoms are a contraindication

12.10 Answer: A

Referral to a psychiatrist is recommended when the patient is at risk of suicide, psychotic symptoms are present or if they have bipolar depression.

12.11 Answer: C

This is less important than a recent fall in socio-economic class or employment status. Established psychiatric illness, family history of suicide, previous suicide attempts, and drug abuse are other important factors.

12.12 Answer: D

ECT is generally reserved for severe depression, not responsive to medication, and usually repeated administration is required (eg bicranial three times in 1 week). Heart failure, raised ICP, severe COPD, recent stroke and severe ischaemic heart disease are associated with greater adverse effects of ECT.

12.13 You are asked to review a 46-year-old man by the Emergency Department doctor, who thought that the patient's long-standing symptoms and signs suggested a diagnosis of schizophrenia. Which one of the following symptoms is most *unlikely* to be a feature of schizophrenia, and might suggest an alternative diagnosis?

☒ A Delusions of grandeur

☐ B Disorganised thinking

☐ C Impairment of attention

☐ D Social withdrawal

☑ E Visual hallucinations

12.14 Which of the following features is a 'negative' symptom characteristic of schizophrenia?

☐ A Auditory hallucinations

☐ B Disordered speech

☐ C Inability to focus on tasks

☑ D Loss of interest in academic pursuits

☐ E Persecutory delusions

12.15 A 32-year-old man has suffered from periodic auditory hallucinations and depressive episodes over the past 9 months, and has become increasingly socially isolated. He is diagnosed with schizophrenia, and commenced on treatment. Which of the following statements is correct regarding this condition?

☐ A A combination of typical and atypical antipsychotics is the optimal initial treatment

☑ B Around 10% of patients commit suicide

☐ C Clinical course is typically one of progressive deterioration

☐ D Substance misuse is present in around 5% of patients

☐ E There is no need for the patient to inform the DVLA

12.16 You review a 39-year-old woman with suspected anxiety disorder. Which of the following features would most strongly suggest an alternative underlying physical diagnosis?

☐ A Breathlessness

☐ B Chest pain

☑ C Heat intolerance

☐ D Insomnia

☐ E Palpitations

12.13 Answer: E

Delusions and auditory hallucinations are characteristic features ('positive' symptoms). Visual hallucinations can occur in organic brain disease, eg alcohol withdrawal, encephalopathy. Other features include cognitive and affective symptoms. Grandiose delusions might also suggest mania.

12.14 Answer: D

'Positive' (type 1) symptoms are abnormal by their presence (eg delusions, hallucinations), 'negative' (type 2) symptoms are the *absence* of normal behaviours (eg social withdrawal, flat affect). Impaired attention is a recognised sign of cognitive impairment.

12.15 Answer: B

Suicide is common, particularly during the active phase of the illness. Cardiovascular and accidental deaths are also more common. Substance misuse is present in around 30%, and most patients have a relapsing–remitting course. The DVLA must be informed in all cases.

12.16 Answer: C

Heat intolerance suggests hyperthyroidism. Other symptoms of anxiety disorder include tremor, sweating, headache, dizziness, diarrhoea and poor concentration.

12.17 You are asked to review a 43-year-old woman in the Emergency Department who is complaining that she is unable to move her left arm. Reflexes are normal and symmetrical in her upper limbs, and other examination findings are entirely normal. Her behaviour seems somewhat odd, and she is comparatively unconcerned about this disability. Which one of the following diagnoses might most fully account for her symptoms?

- A Brachial plexus compression
- ☑ B Dissociative disorder
- C Partial anterior circulation stroke
- D Phobic anxiety disorder
- E Somatisation disorder

12.18 A 19-year-old man is admitted for assessment after taking a deliberate drug overdose. Which of the following factors most strongly indicates risk of future suicide?

- ☒ A Alcohol ingestion at the time of overdose
- B Antisocial personality disorder
- ☑ C Background depressive illness
- D Family history of drug dependence
- E Recent bereavement

12.19 A 68-year-old man is brought to the Emergency Department by the police, having been found confused and disorientated in the street late at night. Which of the following features would most strongly suggest underlying dementia, rather than an acute confusional state?

- A Decreased attention span
- B Delusional thoughts
- ☑ C Flat affect
- D Fluctuating conscious level
- E Visual hallucinations

12.17 Answer: B

Dissociative (conversion) disorder commonly presents with gait disturbance, loss of limb function, aphonia, pseudoseizures or blindness. Characteristically there is apparent unconcern, despite significant physical disability.

12.18 Answer: C

Background psychiatric illness is a major risk factor. Other risk factors include recent unemployment, bereavement, social withdrawal, previous self-harm, drug or alcohol dependence, chronic physical illness, age > 45 years and violent means.

12.19 Answer: C

Dementia is often associated with blunted affect and depressive features. Fluctuating conscious level strongly suggests an acute confusional state.

12.20 A 42-year-old woman presents to her GP with a history suggestive of generalised anxiety disorder. Which one of the following features would be most strongly supportive of this diagnosis?

- ☑ **A** Breathlessness and palpitations
- ☐ **B** Early morning wakening
- ☐ **C** Fatigue and lack of interest
- ☐ **D** Loss of libido
- ☐ **E** Excessive sweating

12.21 A 52-year-old woman regularly drinks 8–12 units of alcohol daily. She is admitted to hospital for an elective laparoscopic sterilisation procedure, and you consider the possibility of alcohol withdrawal. Which one of the following is most accurate with regard to alcohol withdrawal-related seizures?

- ☐ **A** Epilepsy does not confer increased risk
- ☐ **B** Risk is greater in females than males
- ☐ **C** Risk is greatest at 12–24 h after withdrawal
- ☐ **D** Risk is increased by hyperkalaemia
- ☑ **E** They occur in 5–15% of alcohol-dependent people

12.22 A 65-year-old lady has reported a number of varied symptoms for which no physical basis has been identified. On further questioning it becomes evident that she is suffering from early morning wakening, increased irritability, loss of appetite, and poor concentration. She has lost interest in gardening, which she had previously enjoyed, and has had a non-specific feeling of guilt. What is the most likely underlying diagnosis?

- ☐ **A** Anaemia
- ☐ **B** Anxiety disorder
- ☑ **C** Chronic major depression
- ☐ **D** Hypothyroidism
- ☑ **E** Moderate depression

12.20   Answer: A

Excessive sweating is a recognised feature, but less specific (eg thyrotoxicosis, alcohol excess). The other stems are more characteristically associated with depressive illness.

12.21   Answer: E

Risk of seizures after alcohol withdrawal is greatest at around 48 h post-withdrawal, and is increased in the setting of hypoglycaemia, hypomagnesaemia, hypokalaemia, subdural haematoma and pre-existing epilepsy.

12.22   Answer: E

Criteria for a moderate depressive episode are: depressed mood most of the day, for most days (at least 2 weeks), diminished interest or pleasure and loss of energy or fatigue. Other features include reduced concentration and attention, reduced confidence and self-esteem, self-reproach or guilt, recurrent thoughts of death or suicide, pessimistic views of the future, and insomnia.

12.23 A single man, aged 24, complains of feeling irritable and dissatisfied with his life. He was made redundant 4 weeks ago, and he broke up with his girlfriend because of debts he had accrued. He now lives with a friend, and binges on alcohol up to 20 units per night. He uses cannabis occasionally. What is the most likely underlying cause of his low mood?

- ☑ **A** Alcohol abuse
- ☐ **B** Drug intoxication
- ☐ **C** Early dementia
- ☐ **D** Korsakoff's psychosis
- ☐ **E** Vitamin B_{12} deficiency

12.24 A 35-year-old woman is admitted to hospital during an acute episode of mania. She has been treated for the past 2 years with lithium and olanzapine for bipolar affective disorder with psychotic symptoms. Which of the following statements is most correct regarding bipolar affective disorder?

- ☐ **A** Almost 40% commit suicide
- ☐ **B** Antidepressant therapy should be stopped during acute mania
- ☒ **C** Auditory hallucinations suggest an alternative diagnosis of schizophrenia
- ☐ **D** Lamotrigine is effective during acute manic episodes
- ☑ **E** Rapid cycling bipolar disorder occurs in 20% of patients

12.25 A 25-year-old woman has recently given birth to her first child, and has been increasingly tearful, not eating or sleeping well, and the midwife has reported that she has failed to bond with her new baby. Which of the following factors most strongly supports the diagnosis of post-natal depression?

- ☒ **A** History of physical abuse
- ☐ **B** Low family income
- ☑ **C** Low level of social support
- ☐ **D** Lower occupational status
- ☐ **E** Obstetric complications

12.23	Answer: A

Depressive symptoms and alcohol abuse are often found together. Treatment includes advice and support regarding alcohol abstinence.

12.24	Answer: E

10–20% commit suicide, mainly during depressive or mixed episodes, and auditory and visual hallucinations are recognised features. Antidepressant cessation during a manic episode should be gradual to avoid side-effects. Rapid cycling disorder occurs in up to 20% of patients: characterised by four or more acute episodes per year.

12.25	Answer: C

Strongest risk factors are past psychiatric illness or psychological disturbance, recent life events, low social support, and poor marital relationship. Other associations are obstetric complications, low family income, history of abuse, and lower occupational status.

12.26 A 35-year-old woman was involved in a road traffic accident 6 weeks ago in which she suffered minor whiplash injuries. Her car was badly damaged. She is referred to the Psychiatry Outpatient Clinic because she has been feeling very anxious, and finds that at times her thoughts are interrupted by vivid and distressing recollection of the accident. During these episodes, she feels that her heart is 'jumping out of her chest' and finds it difficult to breathe calmly. What is the most likely diagnosis?

- [ ] **A** Acute stress disorder
- [ ] **B** Adjustment disorder
- [ ] **C** Mild depressive episode
- [ ] **D** Normal reaction
- [x] **E** Post-traumatic stress disorder (PTSD)

12.27 A 48-year-old man is brought to hospital in a confused state. He appears agitated and is not forthcoming with any history. He requires treatment with haloperidol and lorazepam to control agitation. There is no obvious tremor; plantar responses show bilateral dorsiflexion, and reflexes are brisk and symmetrical. CT head is normal and CSF shows raised protein concentration, normal glucose concentration and a small number of lymphocytes. What is the most likely diagnosis?

- [ ] **A** Acute alcohol intoxication
- [ ] **B** Acute relapse of schizophrenia
- [ ] **C** Catatonic stupor
- [x] **D** HSV encephalitis
- [x] **E** Neurosyphilis

12.28 Which of the following features would be best described as a 'first-rank symptom' in schizophrenia?

- [ ] **A** Aggressive behaviour
- [ ] **B** Low mood
- [ ] **C** Social withdrawal
- [x] **D** Thought broadcasting
- [ ] **E** Visual hallucinations

12.26 Answer: E

PTSD is characterised by intensely intrusive imagery, and recurring distressing dreams; other features include persistent anxiety, irritability, insomnia and poor concentration, avoidance of reminders of the events, detachment, numbness, and diminished interest in activities.

12.27 Answer: D

Agitation and seizures are recognised features, along with hyperreflexia, low-grade fever and cranial nerve abnormalities. HSV is the most commonly identified cause of encephalitis in the UK and should be treated with intravenous aciclovir while awaiting lab confirmation (CSF PCR).

12.28 Answer: D

First-rank symptoms: (i) auditory hallucinations (echo, third person or commentary), (ii) delusions of thought control, (iii) delusions of passivity (eg thought insertion, thought withdrawal, thought broadcast), and (iv) delusional perception.

12.29   You are asked to provide an urgent psychiatric assessment of a
31-year-old man in the Emergency Department, who is very agitated
and becoming increasingly verbally abusive. Which of the following
symptoms is most strongly suggestive of schizophrenia rather than
acute confusional state?

☐ **A**   Delusions of grandeur

☐ **B**   Flat affect

☐ **C**   Nystagmus

☑ **D**   Third-person auditory hallucinations

☐ **E**   Visual hallucinations

12.30   A 24-year-old man is brought to the Emergency Department in a
confused state. There is no reported history of alcohol or illicit drug
use. Which one of the following symptoms would most strongly
suggest a diagnosis of mania?

☐ **A**   Feelings of worthlessness

☐ **B**   Increased attention span

☐ **C**   Low mood

☑ **D**   Over-expansive responses to questions

☐ **E**   Reduced libido

12.31   You review a 68-year-old woman in the Medical Outpatient
Department, who you suspect might have early dementia. Which of
the following features most strongly supports this diagnosis?

☐ **A**   Able to give a coherent and detailed history

☑ **B**   Impairment of recent memory more than memory of past events

☐ **C**   Patient complains of poor memory

☐ **D**   Poor cooperation and effort with psychomotor tests

☐ **E**   Rapid progression over the past 2 months

12.29 Answer: D

Delusions of grandeur might suggest mania, while nystagmus suggests underlying organic disease (eg Wernicke's encephalopathy). Visual hallucinations often indicate an underlying physical cause.

12.30 Answer: D

Features include elevated mood (occasionally depressed mood), pressure of speech, poor attention span, irritability, easily distracted, insomnia, overactivity, risk-taking behaviour and increased libido. Delusions are a recognised feature and are congruent with mood (grandiose or persecutory).

12.31 Answer: B

The other features are more strongly suggestive of underlying depression.

12.32 A 57-year-old woman is taken to the Emergency Department because of apparent weakness affecting her left arm. During initial assessment, she is uncooperative but appears to have normal neurological function in all four limbs. The nursing staff report that she was verbally abusive earlier, but she is now refusing to speak to medical staff. Which of the underlying disorders below is most likely?

- A Alcohol withdrawal
- ☒ B Alzheimer's disease
- ☑ C Depression
- D Generalised anxiety disorder
- E Schizophrenia

12.33 You see a 48-year-old woman in the General Medical Outpatient Clinic who complains of recurrent episodes of extreme anxiety. These have happened on at least six occasions over the past 2 months while she has been shopping and have been associated with nausea, palpitations, sweating and numbness around the fingers. Which of the following disorders would best explain these features?

- A Generalised anxiety disorder
- B Hyperthyroidism
- C Hyperventilation syndrome
- ☑ D Panic attacks
- E Phaeochromocytoma

12.34 A 17-year-old woman is referred to the Medical Outpatient Department for assessment of abdominal bloating symptoms. On examination she appears very thin, and you consider an underlying eating disorder. Which of the following features would most strongly support a diagnosis of anorexia nervosa?

- A BMI 19.4 kg/m²
- ☑ B Extreme avoidance of high-fat foods
- C Guilt about overeating
- D Puberty aged 14 years
- E Regular scanty periods

12.32   Answer: C

Although highly atypical, depression in elderly patients can present in a number of bizarre ways. Hypochondriacal delusions and worries, histrionic behaviour, and pseudodementia are more common features than in younger patients.

12.33   Answer: D

Short-lived episodes of intense fear associated with at least four of the following: palpitations, sweating, fear of loss of control, trembling, choking sensation, fear of dying, abdominal discomfort, chest pain, dizziness, derealisation, numbness around lips and fingers, chills and hot flushes.

12.34   Answer: B

Criteria are (i) loss of > 15% of normal body weight (usually BMI < 17.5 kg/m^2), self-induced by vomiting, purging and exercising, (ii) overvalued ideas and preoccupation about food, morbid fear of fatness, and (iii) amenorrhoea > 3 months or loss of potency in males.

12.35 A 55-year-old man has been attending the General Medical Outpatient Department for investigation of weight loss, apathy and fatigue over the past 6 months. He is taking lisinopril for hypertension, and has no known drug allergies. Thyroid function tests and upper and lower GI endoscopy tests are normal, and a coeliac screen is negative. You consider that his symptoms are due to depression. Which would be the most appropriate initial treatment to consider?

☑ **A** Fluoxetine

☐ **B** Olanzapine

☐ **C** Phenelzine

☐ **D** St John's wort

☐ **E** Venlafaxine

12.36 You are asked to review a 29-year-old man in the Emergency Department who had presented overnight with a short episode of central chest pain. He smells strongly of stale alcohol, cardiovascular examination is normal, and his ECG and chest X-ray are normal. Which of the following features would most strongly suggest a diagnosis of alcohol dependence syndrome?

☒ **A** Family history of heavy alcohol use

☐ **B** Palpable liver edge

☑ **C** Patient wishes to leave the Emergency Department to go to the pub

☐ **D** Sleep disturbance

☐ **E** Spider naevi on the anterior chest wall

12.37 A 41-year-old woman is admitted to hospital after being found collapsed in the street and drowsy. You are called to review her overnight because she has become increasingly agitated and appears confused. On examination, she is sweaty and tachycardic with a coarse tremor in both upper limbs, and she is experiencing vivid visual hallucinations. Which of the following is the most likely cause of her agitation?

☐ **A** Acute schizophrenia

☐ **B** Alcohol withdrawal

☑ **C** Delirium tremens

☐ **D** Pneumonia

☐ **E** Thyroid storm

12.35 Answer: A

Phenelzine (selective monamine oxidase inhibitor, MAOI) is normally reserved for patients who have not responded to SSRI treatment. Venlafaxine is contraindicated in patients with hypertension, angina or ECG abnormalities because of its tendency for cardiotoxicity; it is also more likely to cause seizures and death in overdose.

12.36 Answer: C

Features are sense of compulsion to drink, drink-seeking behaviour, stereotyped drinking pattern and reinstatement after abstinence, increased alcohol tolerance, withdrawal symptoms and drinking to avoid withdrawal symptoms.

12.37 Answer: C

In addition to alcohol withdrawal (tremor, nausea, sweating, anxiety, agitation, tinnitus), there are features of delirium tremens (visual hallucinations, delusion, tremor, agitation, pyrexia, altered conscious level).

12.38 A 55-year-old man is referred to the Outpatient Department for assessment of suspected dementia. Which of the following risk factors would most strongly suggest a diagnosis of Alzheimer's disease?

- [ ] **A** Hypercholesterolaemia
- [ ] **B** Hypertension
- [✓] **C** Normal conscious level
- [ ] **D** Regular smoking
- [ ] **E** Right arm and leg weakness

12.38   Answer: C

Disturbance of multiple cortical functions, but conscious level is not diminished. The other stems listed (A, B, D, E) are risk factors for cerebrovascular disease and multi-infarct dementia (smoking appears protective against Alzheimer's disease and Parkinson's disease).

13. RESPIRATORY

13.1 You are working in the Chemical Pathology Lab and receive a sample for brain natriuretic peptide (BNP) analysis. The only clinical history given is chest pain. In which of the following conditions is BNP most likely to be *normal*?

- A Acute MI
- B Acute mitral valve rupture
- C Left ventricular failure
- ☒ D Pulmonary embolus
- ☑ E Unstable angina

13.2 A 63-year-old man is sent to the Emergency Department with a severe community-acquired pneumonia by his GP. On examination he is pyrexial at 38.6 °C, is very short of breath, and has right-sided inspiratory crackles consistent with infection. Which of the following variables would be associated with increased risk according to the CURB-65 criteria?

- A Age 63
- B Diastolic BP of 75 mmHg
- ☑ C Respiratory rate of 32/min
- D Systolic BP of 105 mmHg
- E Urea of 6.5 mmol/l

13.3 A 60-year-old former boiler-maker who has a history of asbestos exposure presents to the Respiratory Outpatient Department with dull, right-sided chest pain, a cough and weight loss. He has a history of rheumatoid arthritis, for which he was given an anti-TNF preparation a few months earlier. He looks thin and has a BMI of 18 kg/m², and he has an extensive right-sided pleural effusion. Investigations reveal the LDH of the pleural fluid is > 300 IU/l, it contains lymphocytes +++, protein > 30 g/l, and the glucose is 3.4 mmol/l (venous glucose 7.5 mmol/l). Which of the following is the most likely diagnosis?

- A Bronchial carcinoma
- B Inflammatory effusion
- C Lymphoma
- ☒ D Mesothelioma
- ☑ E Tuberculous effusion

13.1 Answer: E

BNP is secreted in response to cardiac volume distension. Clearly, pulmonary embolus, left ventricular failure, valve rupture and acute MI can all lead to volume changes; unstable angina is less likely to cause this.

13.2 Answer: C

The CURB-65 criteria score increases risk if: abbreviated mental test (AMT) score < 9, systolic BP ≤ 90 mmHg, diastolic BP ≤ 60 mmHg, urea > 7 mmol/l, age > 65. The score out of 5 correlates closely with overall mortality.

13.3 Answer: E

Mesothelioma effusions tend to have a normal LDH and no lymphocytosis. The anti-TNF might have triggered the development of TB.

13.4 A 32-year-old woman presents with progressive shortness of breath and decreased exercise tolerance some 10 months after giving birth to her second child. She can no longer walk to work and has difficulty climbing up one flight of stairs. Her BP is 140/80 mmHg, BMI 23 kg/m²; the only abnormal finding of note is a loud P2 on auscultation. What is the most likely diagnosis?

- [ ] **A** Asthma
- [ ] **B** Cryptogenic fibrosing alveolitis
- [ ] **C** Dilated cardiomyopathy
- [ ] **D** Multiple pulmonary emboli
- [x] **E** Primary pulmonary hypertension

13.5 A 58-year-old engineer at a mine project in Africa flies back to the UK because he has had a chronic cough for the last few months, lost 6 kg in weight and has pleuritic chest pain. There is a previous history of rheumatoid arthritis, but this is not currently active. His BP is 135/75 mmHg, his pulse is 70/min and regular. His BMI is 22 kg/m², and there are scattered crackles and wheeze throughout both lung fields. His PaO₂ is 9.2 kPa, PaCO₂ 5.2 kPa, his pulmonary function tests (PFTs) show a mixed picture of obstruction/restriction, and egg-shell calcification is seen on the chest X-ray (CXR). What is the most likely diagnosis?

- [ ] **A** Alveolar cell carcinoma
- [ ] **B** Pulmonary TB
- [ ] **C** Rheumatoid lung disease
- [ ] **D** Sarcoidosis
- [x] **E** Silicosis

13.6 The nurses ask you to see a 76-year-old woman with a BMI of 32 kg/m² who underwent a hemi-arthroplasty for fractured neck of femur 6 days ago. She is short of breath when lying flat. Her BP is 105/70 mmHg, pulse 80/min and regular, and her respiratory rate is 17/min. The chest is clear and her calves are soft and non-tender. Her PaO₂ is 12 kPa on air, her PaCO₂ is 5.2 kPa. Which of the following is the correct course of action?

- [ ] **A** Arrange a chest-X-ray
- [x] **B** Ask the nurses to sit her up
- [ ] **C** Give her intravenous fluids
- [ ] **D** Put her on anticoagulants
- [ ] **E** Put her on oxygen by mask

13.4   Answer: E

The loud P2 and progressive shortness of breath after the birth of her second child raise this as a possibility. Echocardiography and pulmonary angiography are helpful in further elucidating the diagnosis.

13.5   Answer: E

A history of exposure to mineral dusts, coupled with this clinical picture, is typical of silicosis. The key step for management is removal of exposure to mineral dusts.

13.6   Answer: B

This lady has supine hypoventilation, most likely as a result of her obesity and pain from her surgery. Sitting her up will reduce hypoventilation and the risk of subsequent lower respiratory tract infection.

13.7   A 36-year-old man is brought to the Emergency Department by his girlfriend as she is concerned that he is rapidly becoming more poorly. He drank some milk from a bottle on which the seal had been pecked open by the birds a few days ago, had some diarrhoea, and has deteriorated since then. Apart from asthma, there is no other past medical history. He feels more short of breath when you lie him flat, and can hardly sit up after doing this. He has bilateral upper and lower limb power weakness and absent reflexes. His pH is 7.24, PaO_2 9.2 kPa, $PaCO_2$ 6.8 kPa. His bicarbonate is 22 mmol/l. Which of the following is the most likely diagnosis?

- [ ] **A** Acute renal failure
- [ ] **B** Compensated respiratory acidosis
- [ ] **C** Metabolic alkalosis
- [ ] **D** Type 1 respiratory failure
- [x] **E** Type 2 respiratory failure

13.8   A 15-year-old boy presents to the Allergy Clinic for review. He developed oedema and redness of his right foot while standing for a long time at a football match. Most recently he developed swelling around his mouth, facial erythema and stridor at a birthday party. He required corticosteroids, multiple salbutamol nebulisers and antihistamines in the Emergency Department. Routine bloods are normal, C3 is normal, C1 normal, and C4 is low. Which of the following is the most likely diagnosis?

- [ ] **A** Agammaglobulinaemia
- [x] **B** C1-esterase deficiency
- [ ] **C** IgA deficiency
- [ ] **D** IgE deficiency
- [ ] **E** SLE

13.7 Answer: E

This man has a history consistent with Guillain–Barré syndrome. He has respiratory muscle weakness, which has precipitated carbon dioxide retention.

13.8 Answer: B

The presentation with angioedema, and the episode brought on by the pressure of standing on his right foot is typical. The diagnosis often becomes apparent during the teenage years.

13.9 A 50-year-old man comes to the Chest Clinic complaining of worsening shortness of breath. He has a 30 pack-year smoking history, with a number of episodes of bronchiectasis over the years. There is coarse wheeze and occasional crackles throughout both lung fields on auscultation of the chest. Routine bloods look normal, but he is PiMZ genotype, and his FEV_1 is 35% of predicted. The chest X-ray shows predominantly basilar emphysema. Which of the following is likely to be the most significant factor contributing to his shortness of breath?

☑ A Alpha-1-antitrypsin deficiency

☐ B Asthma

☐ C Bronchiectasis

☐ D Pulmonary fibrosis

☒ E Smoking

13.10 A 70-year-old woman with a 60 pack-year smoking history comes to the Respiratory Outpatient Department with shortness of breath. She has been admitted on two occasions in the past year with infectious exacerbations. On examination her BP is 142/78 mmHg, pulse is 81/min with atrial fibrillation, there is peripheral oedema and she has coarse wheeze on auscultation of the lungs. The FEV_1 is 30% of predicted. Which of the following is the most appropriate long-term therapy for her?

☑ A Fluticasone and salmeterol

☐ B Ipratropium

☐ C Low-dose beclometasone

☐ D Salbutamol

☐ E Salmeterol

13.11 A 45-year-old woman with a history of Raynaud's phenomenon and gasto-oesophageal reflux disease (GORD) comes to the clinic with increased shortness of breath. Her BP is elevated at 150/89 mmHg, her pulse is 83/min. There are fine inspiratory crackles throughout both lung fields. Her FEV_1 is 2.1 l, her FVC is 2.3 l. The adjusted KCO is low. Which of the following is the most likely cause of her shortness of breath?

☐ A Asthma

☐ B COPD

☐ C Cryptogenic fibrosing alveolitis

☐ D SLE

☑ E Systemic sclerosis

13.9 Answer: A

The chest X-ray appearance fits with a significant contribution from α_1-antitrypsin deficiency and the PiMZ genotype is associated with a more rapid deterioration in obstructive airways disease, particularly in conjunction with smoking.

13.10 Answer: A

The best evidence for a reduction in exacerbations comes from the TORCH study of high-dose fluticasone and salmeterol.

13.11 Answer: E

Both Raynaud's and GORD fit with the diagnosis of systemic sclerosis, as does the picture of pulmonary fibrosis seen here. Calcium-channel blockers, prostaglandins, PDE-5 inhibitors and cyclophosphamide have all been trialed in an effort to change the prognosis of systemic sclerosis.

13.12 A 68-year-old former plumber comes to the Respiratory Outpatient Department complaining of increased shortness of breath. He is getting increasingly tired walking the dog, which is his main enjoyment. He smokes 5 cigarettes per day. On examination he is clubbed and has fine end-expiratory crackles. Chest radiography reveals bilateral pleural thickening and reticulonodular infiltrates. His FEV_1 is 2.6 l, the FVC is 3.0 l. Which of the following is the most likely diagnosis?

- ☑ **A** Asbestosis
- ☐ **B** Asthma
- ☐ **C** Colophony lung
- ☐ **D** COPD
- ☐ **E** Cryptogenic fibrosing alveolitis

13.13 A 16-year-old boy is admitted with a rapidly worsening exacerbation of his cystic fibrosis, with severe shortness of breath and a cough that is productive of more sputum than usual and marked wheeze. He is losing weight and has a temperature of 37.9 °C. On examination there are coarse crackles and wheeze throughout both lung fields. Gram-negative rods are identified on his sputum sample. Which of the following is the most likely diagnosis?

- ☐ **A** *Bacteroides* infection
- ☐ **B** *Klebsiella* infection
- ☐ **C** *Mycoplasma* infection
- ☑ **D** *Pseudomonas* infection
- ☐ **E** *Staphlococcus* infection

13.14 A 26-year-old woman presents to the Emergency Department with an exacerbation of asthma. Her peak flow on admission is 180 l/min (predicted is 520 l/min). She is given repeated salbutamol and ipratropium nebulisers and intravenous hydrocortisone but fails to improve. Ninety minutes later her peak flow is still only 190 l/min and she is becoming increasingly tired. Which of the following is the most appropriate next step?

- ☐ **A** Intravenous aminophylline
- ☐ **B** Intravenous salbutamol
- ☐ **C** Intravenous antibiotics
- ☑ **D** Intravenous magnesium
- ☐ **E** Oral theophylline

13.12   Answer: A

The clue is his job as a plumber and the X-ray appearance is typical of asbestosis. Unfortunately, corticosteroids and immune modifiers have no impact on the course of the disease.

13.13   Answer: D

Pseudomonas infection is associated with a deterioration in weight and respiratory symptoms. Colonisation is closely correlated with prognosis. Intermittent tobramycin affords symptomatic improvement in colonised patients.

13.14   Answer: D

A Cochrane review and guidelines now recommend intravenous magnesium as the next most appropriate step, and no longer recommend theophylline.

13.15 A 28-year-old woman has suffered a large bleed after a Caesarean section and receives a 4-unit blood transfusion. She suddenly develops shortness of breath, She looks unwell, her BP is 95/60 mmHg, and her pulse is 95/min. On examination she has pulmonary oedema. Her Hb is 9.7 g/dl; other bloods are unremarkable. Which of the following is the most likely diagnosis?

- [ ] **A** ABO incompatibility
- [ ] **B** Anaphylaxis
- [ ] **C** Circulatory overload
- [ ] **D** Rhesus incompatibility
- [✓] **E** Transfusion-associated lung injury (TRALI)

13.16 A 32-year-old postman presents with progressive shortness of breath. He is taking diclofenac for back pain, but no other medications. CXR shows bilateral upper lobe fibrosis. What is the most likely diagnosis?

- [✓] **A** Ankylosing spondylitis
- [ ] **B** Asthma
- [ ] **C** Bronchiectasis
- [ ] **D** Diclofenac-induced pulmonary fibrosis
- [ ] **E** Extrinsic allergic alveolitis

13.17 Which of the following is most likely to be associated with *Mycoplasma pneumoniae* infection?

- [✓] **A** Bullous myringitis
- [ ] **B** Cryoglobulinaemia
- [✗] **C** Eaton–Lambert syndrome
- [ ] **D** Erythema nodosum
- [ ] **E** Warm autoimmune haemolytic anaemia

13.18 Which of these best describes the normal anatomical location of the azygos lobe?

- [ ] **A** Left lower lobe
- [✗] **B** Left upper lobe
- [ ] **C** Right middle lobe
- [ ] **D** Right lower lobe
- [✓] **E** Right upper lobe

13.15　Answer: E

TRALI is non-cardiogenic pulmonary oedema, either due to anti-HLA antibodies in the transfused blood, or to neutrophils from the patient reacting with bioactive substances in the transfused blood.

13.16　Answer: A

The combination of a young male with back pain and upper lobe fibrosis points to a diagnosis of ankylosing spondylitis. Other causes of upper lobe fibrosis include pneumoconiosis, allergic bronchopulmonary aspergillosis, post-radiotherapy, TB, extrinsic allergic alveolitis and sarcoidosis.

13.17　Answer: A

Other recognised associations are Guillain–Barré syndrome, autoimmune haemolytic anaemia, aseptic meningitis, hepatitis, pancreatitis, erythema multiforme. Cryoglobulinaemia can be a feature of infection with hepatitis C.

13.18　Answer: E

The azygous lobe is a normal variant, seen as the 'inverted comma sign' on the chest X-ray near the right hilum. It is not a true lobe, as it does not have its own bronchus, it is produced by an invagination of the azygos vein.

13.19 A 45-year-old male smoker is diagnosed with α_1-antitrypsin deficiency. Which of the following statements is most correct regarding this condition?

- [ ] **A** Administration of α_1-antitrypsin is an effective treatment
- [ ] **B** Genetic counselling is not required
- [✓] **C** Pulmonary function tests show an obstructive defect and reduced KCO
- [✗] **D** Pulmonary function tests show a restrictive defect and reduced KCO
- [ ] **E** Smoking cessation will not alter the prognosis

13.20 A 36-year-old factory worker is a lifelong non-smoker, and presents with shortness of breath and wheeze. Symptoms generally worsen throughout the week and improve over the weekends. Which test would be most appropriate for establishing the underlying diagnosis?

- [ ] **A** Bronchial provocation testing
- [ ] **B** Full pulmonary function tests (with reversibility)
- [✓] **C** PEFR monitoring both at work and at home
- [ ] **D** Total IgE levels
- [ ] **E** Tryptase levels

13.21 A patient presents to you with an exacerbation of COPD. At discharge you are asked about the possibility of oxygen at home. Which of the following most strongly indicates a need for long-term oxygen therapy?

- [ ] **A** $FEV_1 < 3.0$ l
- [✗] **B** $PaO_2 < 8.0$ kPa on air
- [ ] **C** $PaO_2 < 10$ kPa on 28% oxygen
- [✓] **D** PaO_2 7.3–8.0 kPa with evidence of nocturnal hypoxaemia
- [ ] **E** Raised $PaCO_2$ on air

13.19   Answer: C

Alpha-1-antitrypsin deficiency is a hereditary condition accounting for 2% of all cases of emphysema, and genetic counselling should be offered. Neutrophil elastase (protease) activity is increased, resulting in destruction of alveolar cell walls.

13.20   Answer: C

Over 200 materials have been identified to cause occupational asthma (eg isocyanates, flour, wood dust, pharmaceuticals, stainless steel). It is often justification for industrial compensation. PEFR monitoring will confirm an association and the offending agent can then be identified using *specific* IgE levels or bronchial provocation testing.

13.21   Answer: D

The patient *must* have stopped smoking. They must have PaO_2 of 7.3–8.0 kPa and evidence of either pulmonary hypertension/peripheral oedema or nocturnal hypoxaemia, or $PaO_2 < 7.3$ kPa on air, with either a normal or elevated $PaCO_2$ and an $FEV_1 < 1.5$ l.

13.22 A 42-year-old intravenous drug abuser presents with shortness of breath. On examination he is thin and pyrexial with a temperature of 39.3 °C. Blood tests show: Hb 10.0 g/dl, WCC 3.5×10^9/l, neutrophils 2.0×10^9/l, platelets 165×10^9/l, CD4 count 50/mm³ (normal: 600–1200/mm³). What is the most likely cause?

- [ ] **A** CMV pneumonitis
- [✓] **B** *Pneumocystis carinii* pneumonia
- [ ] **C** Pneumothorax
- [ ] **D** Pulmonary embolus
- [ ] **E** Staphylococcal pneumonia

13.23 A 57-year-old woman presents to the Asthma Clinic complaining of foot drop. She has a past history of allergic rhinitis, asthma and depression. Investigations show: Hb 14.6 g/dl, WCC 6.2×10^9/l (eosinophils 2.1×10^9/l), urea 7.0 mmol/l, creatinine 136 µmol/l, glucose 9.3 mmol/l, ESR 49 mm/h and CRP < 5 mg/l. What is the most likely diagnosis?

- [ ] **A** Allergic bronchopulmonary aspergillosis
- [✓] **B** Churg–Strauss syndrome
- [ ] **C** Sarcoidosis
- [ ] **D** Steroid-induced neuropathy
- [ ] **E** Wegener's granulomatosis

13.24 A 40-year-old man with a BMI of 36 kg/m² presents with daytime somnolence and poor concentration. He has been trying to lose weight over the past 12 months with little success. His wife has complained to him about excessive snoring at night. A sleep study indicates significant periods of oxygen desaturation. Which is the next best management step?

- [ ] **A** Advise weight loss diet
- [✓] **B** Continuous positive airways pressure
- [ ] **C** ENT referral
- [ ] **D** Polysomnography
- [ ] **E** Uvulopalatopharyngoplasty

13.22   Answer: B

The low CD4 count indicates susceptibility to opportunistic infections. Desaturation on minimal exertion and pyrexia suggest the diagnosis; this is an AIDS-defining illness. CXR is normal in 25%. Cytomegalovirus more commonly presents with ocular or gastrointestinal infection.

13.23   Answer: B

Triad of rhinitis, asthma and vasculitis, with an associated eosinophilia; p-ANCA is often positive; usually responds well to corticosteroid treatment.

13.24   Answer: B

Obstructive sleep apnoea is more common in obese males. Weight loss is the first step in management. Continuous positive airways pressure (CPAP) improves quality of life. ENT referral is appropriate if mandibular positioning or tonsillectomy is required. Uvulopalatopharyngoplasty is of little benefit.

13.25   A patient presents with shortness of breath, and plain chest X-ray shows patchy pulmonary infiltrates. He has been taking medications for long-term treatment of atrial fibrillation, hypertension, and ischaemic heart disease. Which of the following drugs might be most likely to contribute to his current presentation?

 A Amiodarone

☐ **B** Atenolol

☐ **C** Digoxin

☐ **D** Glyceryl trinitrate

☐ **E** Simvastatin

13.26   A 46-year-old male lifelong smoker is found to have an abnormal chest X-ray during a routine health screen. Subsequent investigations confirmed the presence of lung cancer. Which of the following findings would most strongly contraindicate surgical resection?

☐ **A** Abnormal liver biochemistry

☐ **B** Background history of asthma

☑ **C** $FEV_1 < 1.0$ l

☐ **D** Haemoptysis

☐ **E** Pleural effusion

13.27   A 37-year-old woman who is taking the oral contraceptive pill has just returned from New Zealand by long-haul flight. She presents to you with tachypnoea and tachycardia, and is complaining of right-sided pleuritic chest pain. What is the definitive investigation of choice to confirm pulmonary embolus?

☐ **A** Arterial blood gases

☑ **B** CT pulmonary angiogram

☐ **C** Echocardiogram

☐ **D** Lung perfusion scan

☐ **E** Plain chest X-ray

13.25 Answer: A

Amiodarone is a recognised cause of reversible and irreversible lung fibrosis and pneumonitis. Both dose-dependent and idiosyncratic pulmonary complications are recognised.

13.26 Answer: C

Other contraindications to surgical resection include: stage IIIB and above, malignant pleural effusion (rather than other causes of effusion, eg pneumonia), phrenic/recurrent laryngeal nerve involvement, SVC obstruction, involvement of mediastinum or contralateral hilar or mediastinal nodes, and distant metastases.

13.27 Answer: B

Pulmonary angiography is the gold standard in the investigation for pulmonary embolus, now superseded by CTPA. Echocardiogram may be used as an immediate bedside tool in severe cases where the patient shows signs of haemodynamic compromise.

13.28 Which of the following organisms would be *least* likely to cause extrinsic allergic alveolitis?

- ☒ **A** *Aspergillus clavatus*
- ☑ **B** *Aspergillus fumigatus*
- ☐ **C** *Chlamydia psittaci*
- ☐ **D** *Micropolyspora faeni*
- ☐ **E** Thermophilic *Actinomycetes*

13.29 A 38-year-old schoolteacher presents with recurrent haemoptysis over the past 2 weeks, and intermittent symptoms of wheeze, headache and flushing. She is a non-smoker and denies weight loss. Chest X-ray shows right lower lobe collapse. Which of the following investigations would be most appropriate?

- ☑ **A** Bronchoscopy
- ☐ **B** CT-guided lung biopsy
- ☐ **C** CT thorax
- ☐ **D** Pulmonary function tests (with reversibility)
- ☐ **E** V/Q scan

13.30 A 41-year-old man of Afro-Caribbean descent presents with erythema nodosum overlying both shins. Investigations show hypercalcaemia and normal renal function. What chest X-ray findings most strongly support a diagnosis of sarcoidosis?

- ☑ **A** Bilateral hilar lymphadenopathy
- ☐ **B** Cavity in the upper lobe
- ☐ **C** Pleural calcification
- ☐ **D** Pleural effusion
- ☐ **E** Widened mediastinum

13.31 A 58-year-old ex-smoker presents to you in the Chest Clinic. He has recently been started on inhaled tiotropium and enquires about its mechanism of action. Which of the following best describes this?

- ☑ **A** Antimuscarinic
- ☐ **B** Combination of corticosteroid and anticholinergic
- ☐ **C** Inhaled corticosteroid
- ☐ **D** Long-acting β_2 agonist
- ☐ **E** Short-acting β_2 agonist

13.28 Answer: B

Extrinsic allergic alveolitis is a hypersensitivity pneumonitis, usually IgG-mediated. The offending agent is usually some form of organic dust. Examples include: farmer's lung (*M. faeni* and *Thermoactinomyces vulgaris*), pigeon-fancier's lung (*C. psittaci*), malt-worker's lung (*A. clavatus*) and bagasossis (*T. sacchari*).

13.29 Answer: A

The scenario points to a diagnosis of bronchial carcinoid. Bronchoscopy would best identify a centrally placed lesion in a main bronchus proximal to the lung collapse.

13.30 Answer: A

Staging of pulmonary sarcoidosis, based on chest X-ray appearances:

0 normal chest X-ray
1 bilateral hilar lymphadenopathy (BHL)
2 BHL + interstitial infiltrates
3 interstitial infiltrates only
4 diffuse fibrosis

13.31 Answer: A

Tiotropium is used in maintenance of COPD remission. It is long-acting, allowing once daily administration.

13.32 An analysis of pleural fluid shows: pH 7.67, neutrophils < 1/mm³, lymphocytes 34/mm³, total protein 63 g/l, glucose 2.3 mmol/l, LDH 665 IU/l, triglycerides < 0.1 mmol/l, amylase not detected. What is the most likely explanation?

- ☐ **A** Liver cirrhosis
- ☑ **B** Lung carcinoma
- ☒ **C** Pneumonia
- ☐ **D** Rheumatoid arthritis
- ☐ **E** SLE

13.33 An 84-year-old man presents with an episode of collapse; on examination he is hypoxic with chest signs. You request a chest X-ray which shows evidence of calcification. Which of the following is this patient most likely to have had in the past?

- ☐ **A** Aspergillosis
- ☐ **B** Berylliosis
- ☐ **C** Coxsackievirus
- ☐ **D** Shingles
- ☑ **E** Tuberculosis

13.34 A 29-year-old man is referred for further investigation of wheeze, eosinophilia and abnormal chest X-ray. Which of the following diagnoses best explains these features?

- ☑ **A** Aspergillosis
- ☐ **B** Asbestosis
- ☐ **C** Extrinsic allergic alveolitis
- ☐ **D** Sarcoidosis
- ☐ **E** Tuberculosis

13.32   Answer: B

The findings indicate an exudate; absence of neutrophils makes
infection less likely. Low glucose can be seen in effusions associated
with infection, malignancy, rheumatoid.

13.33   Answer: E

Other causes of pulmonary calcification on plain chest X-ray include
sarcoidosis, asbestos, previous varicella pneumonia, silicosis, previous
empyema or haemothorax, and carcinoid tumours.

13.34   Answer: A

Other causes of eosinophilia with an abnormal chest X-ray include:
eosinophilic pneumonia, Churg–Strauss syndrome, tropical
pulmonary eosinophilia and eosinophilic leukaemia.

13.35 A patient presents with sudden exacerbation in shortness of breath. Examination reveals stony dullness and decreased air entry at the left base. Transthoracic aspiration of fluid shows a haemorrhagic effusion. Which of the following conditions is most likely to be associated with aspiration of clear fluid with a protein concentration of 12 g/l?

- ☑ **A** Heart failure
- ☐ **B** Lung carcinoma
- ☐ **C** Parapneumonic effusion
- ☐ **D** Pulmonary infarction
- ☐ **E** Tuberculosis

13.36 A middle-aged woman presents to the Emergency Department with breathlessness. Blood gases on air are as follows: pH 7.52, $PaCO_2$ 3.0 kPa, PaO_2 12.6 kPa, bicarbonate 22 mmol/l. What is the most likely explanation for these results?

- ☐ **A** Acute asthma
- ☑ **B** Hyperventilation syndrome
- ☐ **C** Lactic acidosis
- ☐ **D** Pulmonary embolus
- ☐ **E** Pulmonary oedema

13.37 A 56-year-old man presents with a large left-sided pleural effusion. You insert a chest drain, and send fluid for analysis. Laboratory results indicate an abnormally high LDH concentration. What is the most likely explanation?

- ☐ **A** Malnutrition
- ☒ **B** Myxoedema
- ☐ **C** Nephrotic syndrome
- ☐ **D** Sarcoidosis
- ☑ **E** Sjögren syndrome

13.35   Answer: A

The other listed conditions more typically cause exudative effusions; malignancy and pulmonary infarction are more commonly associated with a haemorrhagic pleural effusion.

13.36   Answer: B

There is respiratory alkalosis but no hypoxia, suggesting hyperventilation. An alternative explanation might be early salicylate toxicity, which produces respiratory alkalosis before metabolic acidosis.

13.37   Answer: E

High LDH concentration (> 250 IU/l) is suggestive of an exudate, often accompanied by a high protein concentration (typically > 30 g/l). The other listed conditions typically cause a transudate pleural effusion.

13.38 A patient with major burns is admitted to Intensive Care with a suspected diagnosis of adult respiratory distress syndrome. Which of the following most strongly supports this diagnosis?

- [ ] **A** Bilateral fluffy infiltrates on chest film
- [ ] **B** Ejection fraction < 50% on echocardiogram
- [ ] **C** PaO_2 of < 7.5 kPa on FiO_2 of 0.5
- [ ] **D** Pulmonary artery capillary wedge pressure 34 mmHg
- [x] **E** Reduced lung compliance during mechanical ventilation

13.39 A 35-year-old woman with long-standing SLE complains of reduced exercise capacity and breathlessness. Which of the following pulmonary complications is most likely to be responsible?

- [ ] **A** Bronchiectasis
- [ ] **B** Caplan syndrome
- [x] **C** Obliterative bronchiolitis
- [ ] **D** Rheumatoid nodules
- [x] **E** Shrinking lung syndrome

13.40 A 72-year-old male smoker presents with gradually declining exercise tolerance limited by shortness of breath. A chest X-ray shows diaphragmatic calcification. Which of the following is the most likely diagnosis?

- [x] **A** Asbestos-related lung disease
- [ ] **B** Miliary tuberculosis
- [ ] **C** Pneumoconiosis
- [ ] **D** Sarcoidosis
- [ ] **E** Silicosis

13.41 Which of the following anti-tuberculous treatments is most likely to cause irreversible visual impairment?

- [x] **A** Ethambutol
- [ ] **B** Isoniazide
- [ ] **C** Pyrazinamide
- [ ] **D** Rifampicin
- [ ] **E** Streptomycin

13.38 Answer: E

ARDS involves non-cardiogenic pulmonary oedema, and LV systolic function is preserved. Reduced ejection fraction and increased pulmonary capillary wedge pressure suggest cardiogenic shock. Recognised causes of ARDS are trauma, sepsis, DIC, pancreatitis, drugs, inhalation injury and near-drowning.

13.39 Answer: E

Shrinking lung syndrome is a feature of SLE that arises through abnormally poor movement of the diaphragm. The other options are more characteristic complications of rheumatoid arthritis.

13.40 Answer: A

This is the only one likely to cause diaphragmatic calcification. All of the listed conditions are associated with an increased risk of pulmonary fibrosis.

13.41 Answer: A

Ethambutol can cause a dose-related retrobulbar neuritis, and visual acuity should be documented before treatment starts. Isoniazid is known to cause a peripheral neuropathy which may be prevented by co-administration of pyridoxine (vitamin B_6). Pyrazinamide, rifampicin and isoniazid can cause hepatotoxicity and liver function tests should be monitored. Streptomycin can potentially cause irreversible vestibular nerve damage.

13.42 Regarding atypical mycobacteria, which of the following is true?

- ☑ **A** Contact tracing is not normally required in confirmed cases
- ☐ **B** Extrapulmonary disease is not a recognised feature
- ☒ **C** *M. avium* complex is most common in HIV-infected patients, causing 50% of mycobacterial infections
- ☐ **D** *M. kansasii* is the most common atypical infection in immunocompromised patients in the UK
- ☐ **E** Treatment is as for typical mycobacterial tuberculosis

13.43 In which one of the following conditions is chest drain insertion normally *avoided*?

- ☐ **A** Empyema
- ☐ **B** Malignant pleural effusion
- ☑ **C** Rheumatoid pleural effusion
- ☒ **D** Secondary pneumothorax
- ☐ **E** Traumatic haemopneumothorax

13.44 A 69-year-old regular smoker presents with weight loss, shortness of breath and haemoptysis. A chest X-ray reveals a spiculated opacification, and blood tests show anaemia and hypercalcaemia. A bone scan is normal. What is the most likely underlying diagnosis?

- ☐ **A** Adenocarcinoma
- ☐ **B** Bronchogenic carcinoma with bony metastases
- ☐ **C** Sarcoidosis
- ☒ **D** Small-cell lung cancer
- ☑ **E** Squamous cell lung cancer

13.45 A 78-year-old lifelong smoker presents with shortness of breath. On examination he is clubbed. A chest X-ray reveals a cavitating mass, and you suspect cancer. Which of the following is the most likely type?

- ☐ **A** Adenocarcinoma
- ☐ **B** Alveolar cell carcinoma
- ☐ **C** Large-cell carcinoma
- ☐ **D** Small-cell lung carcinoma
- ☑ **E** Squamous cell carcinoma

13.42   Answer: A

Atypical person-to-person transmission is not a recognised feature, even in sputum smear-positive individuals. *M. kansasii* is the most common atypical affecting the immunocompetent in the UK. *M. avium* complex is common in HIV patients, causing over 90% of opportunistic mycobacterial infections.

13.43   Answer: C

Rheumatoid-associated effusions are normally small, and tend not to reaccumulate if disease-modifying treatment is administered. Malignant pleural effusions reaccumulate quickly so chest drain insertion reduces the risk of infection associated with repeated aspiration.

13.44   Answer: E

Absence of bone metastases suggests paraneoplastic hypercalcaemia. Squamous cell carcinoma is associated with production of parathyroid hormone-related protein (PTHrP). Neuroendocrine associations with small-cell lung cancer include SIADH and Cushing syndrome due to ACTH.

13.45   Answer: E

This is the most common type of lung cancer, and shows the greatest tendency to cavitate. Clubbing is a recognised paraneoplastic feature.

13.46 Which of the following gastrointestinal disorders is most likely to be associated with fibrosing alveolitis?

- ☐ **A** Coeliac disease
- ☒ **B** Crohn's disease
- ☐ **C** Hepatitis B
- ☐ **D** Portal hypertension
- ☑ **E** Ulcerative colitis

13.47 A young adult presents with acute epiglottitis. Which organism is most likely to be isolated from blood cultures?

- ☐ **A** Adenovirus
- ☐ **B** *Haemophilus influenzae* type A
- ☑ **C** *Haemophilus influenzae* type B
- ☐ **D** Respiratory syncytial virus
- ☐ **E** Rhinovirus

13.48 A 26-year-old bakery assistant is diagnosed with Lofgren syndrome. What feature would you be most likely to identify on a plain chest X-ray?

- ☒ **A** Apical fibrosis
- ☑ **B** Bilateral hilar lymphadenopathy
- ☐ **C** Cardiomegaly
- ☐ **D** Pleural calcification
- ☐ **E** Pleural effusion

13.49 Which of the following tests is most helpful in establishing a diagnosis of asthma?

- ☐ **A** Peak flow monitoring for 2 weeks at work and away from work
- ☐ **B** Spirometry testing after methacholine challenge test
- ☑ **C** Spirometry testing before and after bronchodilators
- ☐ **D** Spirometry testing before and after exercise
- ☐ **E** Spirometry testing during exercise

13.46 Answer: E

Crohn's disease is known to produce large-airway stenosis and bronchiectasis, while ulcerative colitis is known to do the same with added fibrosing alveolitis.

13.47 Answer: C

Epiglottitis is a potentially life-threatening illness. Intravenous cefuroxime would provide appropriate antibiotic cover.

13.48 Answer: B

Features include erythema nodosum, bilateral hilar lymphadenopathy on chest X-ray and arthralgia. It is a self-limiting form of sarcoidosis. Prognosis is excellent.

13.49 Answer: C

Asthma is a reversible airways disease; patients normally show improvement of 15% or more in the FEV_1 post-bronchodilator therapy. Spirometry testing before and after exercise may be useful in exercise-induced asthma, and regular peak flow monitoring can be useful in diagnosing occupation-related asthma.

13.50 Which of the following is the most likely explanation for a posterior mediastinal mass identified on a CT thorax investigation?

- ☐ A Dermoid cyst
- ☑ B Oesophageal carcinoma
- ☒ C Retrosternal goitre
- ☐ D Teratoma
- ☐ E Thymoma

13.51 A 24-year-old man complains of bloodstained nasal discharge, and is found to have: Hb 9.9 g/l, WCC 7.8 × 10⁹/l, platelets 255 × 10⁹/l, urea 20.2 mmol/l, creatinine 458 μmol/l. A renal ultrasound scan shows hyperechoic lesions throughout the renal cortices but no evidence of obstructive uropathy. Which of the following tests would be most helpful in confirming the underlying diagnosis?

- ☐ A ANA
- ☐ B Anti-basement membrane antibody
- ☐ C Anti-Jo antibodies
- ☑ D c-ANCA
- ☒ E p-ANCA

13.52 Which of the following would be the best initial management in treatment of acute-phase Goodpasture syndrome?

- ☐ A Cyclophosphamide
- ☐ B Interferon
- ☑ C Plasma exchange
- ☐ D Prednisolone
- ☐ E Treat underlying infection

13.53 A 22-year-old woman presents with sore throat, cervical lymphadenopathy and rash. She has received a week's course of amoxicillin with no improvement. Blood count reveals thrombocytopenia. Which of the following investigations would be most helpful?

- ☐ A ASO titres
- ☐ B HIV testing
- ☑ C Monospot test
- ☐ D *Mycoplasma pneumoniae* titres
- ☐ E Streptococcal challenge test

13.50 Answer: B

The other listed stems would be expected to be found in the anterior mediastinum. Middle mediastinum: aortic aneurysm, pericardial cyst, hilar lymphadenopathy. Posterior mediastinum: oesophageal cyst, neural lesions.

13.51 Answer: D

The combination of upper airways and renal involvement and likely glomerulonephritis are highly suggestive of Wegener's granulomatosis. Treatment is with a combination of corticosteroids and cyclophosphamide.

13.52 Answer: C

Goodpasture syndrome is an autoimmune condition, p-ANCA positive in 30%, due to deposition of anti-glomerular basement membrane antibodies in the lungs and kidneys. Treatment is with immunosuppression. Goodpasture's can be precipitated by infection, but treatment of the infection will not affect outcome.

13.53 Answer: C

History suggestive of glandular fever; rash typically worsens following broad-spectrum antibiotics. Other features include petechiae, thrombocytopenia and atypical lymphocytes on the blood film.

13.54 A 54-year-old woman is being investigated for fever associated with a dry cough. Which of the following organisms is responsible for development of Q fever?

- A *Bordetella pertussis*
- B *Chlamydia pneumoniae*
- ☑ C *Coxiella burnetii*
- D *Coxsackievirus*
- E *Nocardia mycetoma*

13.55 Which of the following is the most characteristic feature of Pontiac fever?

- A It is a common cause of pulmonary fibrosis
- ☑ B It is caused by *Legionella pneumophila*
- C It is caused by *Mycoplasma pneumoniae*
- ☒ D It presents with massive haemoptysis
- E Treatment is with benzylpenicillin

13.56 Which of the following groups of viruses is the most commonly recognised cause of severe acute respiratory distress syndrome (SARS)?

- A Arbovirus
- ☒ B Avian influenza
- C *Bartonella henselae*
- ☑ D Coronavirus
- E Ebola virus

13.57 A patient presents to you with a diagnosis of primary ciliary dyskinesia. Which of the following is most commonly associated with this condition?

- ☒ A Cilia in the retina may be affected
- ☑ B Dextrocardia
- C Hypogammaglobulinaemia
- D Inheritance is sporadic
- E Patient fertility is unaffected

13.54 Answer: C

Q fever is a zoonosis caused by *Coxiella burnetii*. Farmers, abbatoir workers and vets are predominantly affected. The illness starts with fever, myalgia, pneumonia can develop in up to 30%, hepatosplenomegaly in up to 50%. Chronic Q fever should be suspected in all culture negative cases of endocarditis. Tetracycline is the drug of choice.

13.55 Answer: B

Pontiac fever is caused by a hypersensitivity reaction to *L. pneumophila*. It presents with severe influenza-like symptoms with limited chest signs but extensive involvement on chest X-ray. Extra-pulmonary features of diarrhoea, abdominal pain, renal failure and haematuria are recognised and, rarely, pulmonary fibrosis. Clarithromycin is the antibiotic of choice.

13.56 Answer: D

An acute viral respiratory tract infection, first identified in 2003. Transmission is mainly via the respiratory route, though faeco-oral is also possible. Features include high fever, myalgia and dry cough. Diagnosis can be established by PCR testing. At present there is no effective antiviral treatment.

13.57 Answer: B

Found in up to 50% of cases. Other recognised features are situs inversus, male and female infertility, and autosomal recessive inheritance. Kartagener syndrome is ciliary dyskinesia with situs inversus.

13.58 Which of the following investigations would be most helpful in establishing the underlying cause of secondary bronchiectasis?

- ☑ A Bronchoscopy
- ☐ B CT thorax
- ☒ C Lung function tests
- ☐ D Skin-prick testing
- ☐ E Sputum cytology

13.59 Which of the following is most likely to cause a leftward shift of the oxygen dissociation curve?

- ☐ A Acidosis
- ☐ B Carbon dioxide concentration
- ☐ C 2,3-diphosphoglycerate
- ☑ D High haemoglobin concentration
- ☒ E Temperature increase

13.60 Which of the following features is most closely associated with a diagnosis of Goodpasture syndrome?

- ☐ A Cavitation on chest X-ray
- ☐ B Gas transfer is reduced
- ☐ C Haematemesis as a presenting symptom
- ☑ D Renal biopsy demonstrating crescentic glomerulonephritis
- ☐ E Women are more often affected than men

13.61 You receive a call about a patient in the wards who has become more breathless than normal. He has background COPD, and his current oxygen saturation is only 77% on 24% inhaled oxygen by Venturi mask. Which one of the following arterial blood gas descriptions most strongly suggests a severe exacerbation of existing COPD?

- ☐ A Low $PaCO_2$, low PaO_2, normal bicarbonate, normal pH
- ☐ B Normal $PaCO_2$, low PaO_2, low bicarbonate, alkalosis
- ☑ C Raised $PaCO_2$, low PaO_2, high bicarbonate, acidosis
- ☐ D Raised $PaCO_2$, low PaO_2, high bicarbonate, picture of alkalosis
- ☒ E Raised $PaCO_2$, low PaO_2, low bicarbonate, picture of acidosis

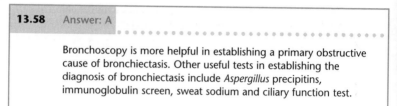

13.58 Answer: A

Bronchoscopy is more helpful in establishing a primary obstructive cause of bronchiectasis. Other useful tests in establishing the diagnosis of bronchiectasis include *Aspergillus* precipitins, immunoglobulin screen, sweat sodium and ciliary function test.

13.59 Answer: D

The oxyhaemoglobin dissociation curve describes the relationship between the saturation of haemoglobin and the partial pressure of oxygen in the blood. The other factors cause a rightward shift, and therefore bind oxygen less tightly so as to liberate more oxygen to the tissues.

13.60 Answer: D

Goodpasture syndrome typically affects young adult males, and is usually preceded by an upper respiratory tract infection. It is associated with pulmonary haemorrhage (causing haemoptysis and raised KCO) and renal failure.

13.61 Answer: C

COPD results in a type 2 respiratory failure with respiratory acidosis. Bicarbonate is raised due to renal retention, and is a chronic feature.

13.62 A 61-year-old previously healthy man presents with a large pleural effusion. You insert a chest drain and aspirate milky effusion. Biochemistry confirms high lipid concentration in the effusion fluid. What is the most likely diagnosis?

- [ ] **A** Autoimmune disease
- [ ] **B** Bronchial carcinoma
- [ ] **C** Hepatocellular carcinoma
- [✓] **D** Lymphoma
- [ ] **E** Myeloma

13.63 Arterial blood gas analysis shows: pH 7.47, PaO_2 8.0 kPa, $PaCO_2$ 3.42 kPa, bicarbonate 23 mmol/l and base excess –3.5 mmol/l. What is the most likely explanation for these findings?

- [ ] **A** Anxiety state
- [ ] **B** Exacerbation of COPD
- [ ] **C** Pneumonia
- [✓] **D** Pulmonary embolus
- [ ] **E** Renal failure

13.64 Which of the following ECG findings is most commonly associated with a diagnosis of acute pulmonary embolus?

- [ ] **A** Frequent ventricular ectopic beats
- [ ] **B** Prolonged PR interval
- [ ] **C** Prolonged QT interval
- [ ] **D** Right bundle branch block
- [✓] **E** Sinus tachycardia

13.65 Which of the following statements most closely describes the features of cryptogenic fibrosing alveolitis?

- [ ] **A** CT scan with contrast is the investigation of choice
- [ ] **B** Immunosuppression shows improvement in 90% patients
- [✗] **C** Oxygen therapy improves prognosis
- [ ] **D** Peak flows should be maintained regularly
- [✓] **E** Pulmonary function tests show decreased lung and residual volumes

13.62   Answer: D

Lipaemic fluid indicates a chylothorax, suggesting thoracic duct infiltration. Commonest causes are lymphoma and tuberculosis, but it can be seen with other infiltrative lung disease.

13.63   Answer: D

The patient is hyperventilating (raised pH, low $PaCO_2$) in response to hypoxaemia. This is characteristic of a type 1 respiratory failure pattern.

13.64   Answer: E

Other features include small QRS complexes in anterior leads, T-wave inversion in the anterior leads, and the ECG can be normal in around 30%.

13.65   Answer: E

High-resolution CT scan is the investigation of choice. Peak flows are more indicative of airflow obstruction, whereas fibrosis is a restrictive defect. Oxygen offers symptomatic relief only, and up to 50% of patients will respond to steroids.

13.66 A patient presents with sudden onset of pleuritic chest pain and breathlessness. A chest X-ray reveals a pneumothorax with a 2-cm gap between the pleural edge and costal margin. There is no significant past medical history. What is the management of choice?

- ☑ **A** Aspiration
- ☐ **B** Discharge home with advice
- ☐ **C** Inpatient observation with serial chest X-rays
- ☐ **D** Intercostal drain insertion
- ☐ **E** Outpatient follow-up with repeat chest X-ray in 6 weeks

13.67 A patient with known cystic fibrosis presents to you unwell with wheeze, eosinophilia, fever and increased plasma IgE. Chest X-ray shows diffuse opacification. Which of the following would you consider the most likely diagnosis in this scenario?

- ☑ **A** Allergic bronchopulmonary aspergillosis
- ☐ **B** Asthma
- ☒ **C** Bronchiectasis
- ☐ **D** Exacerbation of cystic fibrosis
- ☐ **E** Pneumococcal pneumonia

13.68 Regarding treatment of malignant mesothelioma, which of the following is most appropriate?

- ☐ **A** Chemotherapy alone
- ☒ **B** Chemotherapy and radiotherapy combined
- ☐ **C** Lung resection alone
- ☑ **D** Radiotherapy alone
- ☐ **E** Radiotherapy followed by lung resection

13.69 A normally independent 87-year-old lady presents to you with breathlessness due to florid pulmonary oedema. You have treated her with furosemide and high-flow oxygen. She is currently on a nitrate infusion, but her condition is deteriorating. Which of the following forms of ventillatory support would be most appropriate?

- ☒ **A** BiPAP
- ☐ **B** Bronchodilators
- ☑ **C** CPAP
- ☐ **D** Endotracheal intubation
- ☐ **E** Intravenous furosemide infusion

13.66 Answer: A

In a patient with a simple pneumothorax (first time presentation, with no known chronic lung disease), BTS guidelines suggest serial chest X-ray follow-up as outpatient if patient is symptom-free and rim less than 2 cm. If symptomatic and rim less than 2 cm, pleural aspiration, chest X-ray and discharge home with advice. If > 2 cm, for aspiration initially and consideration of intercostal chest drain.

13.67 Answer: A

Allergic bronchopulmonary aspergillosis is encountered in approximately 20% of patients with cystic fibrosis. Treatment is with high-dose corticosteroids.

13.68 Answer: D

Commonly associated with asbestos. Poor prognosis (with estimated maximum 12-month survival).

13.69 Answer: C

Continuous positive airways pressure works by recruiting alveoli and so improving oxygenation, useful in pictures of type 1 respiratory failure. Trials have shown that patients with pulmonary oedema in the acute setting respond well to CPAP.

13.70 A 67-year-old businessman has recently flown back to the UK from Thailand. He presents with sudden onset of shortness of breath and right leg swelling. Which of the following statements best describes investigation of thromboembolic disease?

- [ ] A DVT is demonstrable in 50% patients with pulmonary embolism
- [ ] B Low-probability perfusion scan would exclude pulmonary embolism
- [x] C Spiral CT can detect segmental artery clot
- [ ] D Ultrasound of leg should be conducted before a V/Q scan
- [ ] E V/Q scan is the gold standard in patients with pre-existing lung disease

13.71 Which statement is most accurate regarding asbestos exposure?

- [x] A Around 90% of people exposed to asbestos develop pleural plaques
- [ ] B Benign pleural plaques require annual chest X-ray follow-up
- [ ] C Chest X-ray is the most sensitive way of detecting pleural plaques
- [x] D Compensation is available in the form of a disability benefit
- [ ] E Pleural biopsy is required to make a definitive diagnosis

13.72 A 47-year-old Afro-Caribbean woman presents with polydipsia and a nodular rash on the lower limbs. Which of the following would be the best test to confirm an underlying diagnosis?

- [x] A Chest X-ray
- [ ] B Plasma and urine osmolalities
- [x] C Serum calcium
- [ ] D Serum glucose
- [ ] E Thick and thin blood films

13.73 A 35-year-old man presents with weight loss, night sweats and fever. On examination there is a widened mediastinum. Which investigation would be most helpful to confirm the diagnosis?

- [x] A CT thorax with contrast
- [ ] B Gallium uptake scan
- [x] C Mediastinoscopy
- [ ] D Positron emission tomography (PET)
- [ ] E Single-photon emission computed tomography (SPECT)

13.70 Answer: C

Spiral CT can detect clot from pulmonary trunk to the segmental arteries. V/Q is an alternative that can be used if there is no underlying lung defect. DVT is demonstrable in about 10% of cases of pulmonary embolism.

13.71 Answer: D

Patients with pleural plaques only are not entitled to compensation. Those with asbestos-related fibrotic lung disease or mesothelioma of course are. Around 50% develop plaques after exposure; high-resolution CT scan is more sensitive than plain chest X-ray, and benign plaques require no follow-up.

13.72 Answer: A

The clinical scenario suggests sarcoidosis complicated by erythema nodosum and thirst due to hypercalcaemia or diabetes insipidus.

13.73 Answer: C

This is the only investigation which will allow histopathological confirmation of diagnosis, although CT scanning would normally be undertaken in the first instance.

13.74 An 86-year-old lady presents with respiratory distress 4 days after surgical repair of her fractured neck of femur. Respiratory rate is 45/min, temperature is 38 °C, Glasgow Coma Scale score is 9, and there is a petechial rash over her lower limbs. Which of the following would best explain the above findings?

- ☐ **A** Acute respiratory distress syndrome
- ☒ **B** Disseminated intravascular coagulation
- ☑ **C** Fat emboli
- ☐ **D** Meningococcal meningitis
- ☐ **E** Pulmonary embolus

13.75 Your colleague calls you for advice about a patient with very advanced rheumatoid arthritis who has developed breathlessness. Which of the following patterns of lung function test abnormalities would be most consistent with a diagnosis of bronchiolitis obliterans?

- ☐ **A** Raised FEV_1
- ☑ **B** Reduced FEV_1
- ☐ **C** Reduced residual volume
- ☐ **D** Reduced total lung volume
- ☐ **E** Reduced vital capacity

13.74 Answer: C

ARDS and DIC can be the result of a fat embolus but do not offer the most precise underlying explanation. Fat embolus most commonly occurs 3–10 days post-fracture.

13.75 Answer: B

Bronchiolitis obliterans is a picture of progressive small distal airways inflammation, resulting in an obstructive picture (reduced FEV_1) with raised residual volume.

14. RHEUMATOLOGY

14.1 A 60-year-old man with a history of rheumatoid arthritis comes to the Rheumatoloty Outpatient Department complaining of tiredness. He takes NSAIDs, prednisolone and methotrexate, and amlodipine for hypertension. His Hb is 11.1 g/dl, MCV 87 fl, ferritin is 410 µg/l, and his iron is low at 8 g/dl. The differential diagnosis is between anaemia of chronic disease and iron deficiency anaemia. Which of the following is the most appropriate investigation?

- [ ] **A** Barium enema
- [✓] **B** Bone marrow biopsy
- [ ] **C** Erythropoeitin levels
- [ ] **D** Small-bowel follow-through
- [✗] **E** Upper GI endoscopy

14.2 A 68-year-old woman who lives alone has misread the directions for taking her methotrexate therapy and has been taking it every day. As a consequence she presents with glossitis, mouth ulcers and severe anaemia. She has been taking around 40 mg per week (she should have been taking 7.5 mg). Her Hb is 9.6 g/dl, MCV 108 fl, WCC 2.1 × 10⁹/l, platelets 90 × 10⁹/l. Which of the following is the most appropriate rescue therapy for her?

- [ ] **A** B_{12}
- [✓] **B** Folinic acid
- [ ] **C** Multivitamins
- [ ] **D** Niacin
- [ ] **E** Thiamine

14.3 A 29-year-old man returns from a safari with rapidly worsening psoriasis and a symmetrical small-joint polyarthritis. He normally has mild disease with no joint component at all. He took antimalarials and antibiotics during his trip. On examination he has widespread psoriasis and pain and swelling over the small joints of his hands and feet, his wrists and ankles. Which of the following is the most likely drug to be responsible?

- [✓] **A** Chloroquine
- [ ] **B** Ciprofloxacin
- [ ] **C** Co-amoxiclav
- [ ] **D** Metronidazole
- [ ] **E** Oxytetracycline

14.1 Answer: B

If the iron content of bone marrow on biopsy is normal, then it rules out iron deficiency anaemia.

14.2 Answer: B

Medication errors are quite common in the treatment of rheumatoid. Calcium folinate is a potent antagonist of the effects of methotrexate and is the drug of choice.

14.3 Answer: A

While definitively establishing the link from clinical trials is difficult, a significant number of adverse event reports on worsening psoriasis have resulted from chloroquine studies.

14.4 A 77-year-old woman presents with shoulder- and hip-girdle pain, and increasing headaches. Most recently she suffered transient loss of vision in her right eye. She has a history of hypertension, for which she takes ramipril. Bloods are normal apart from an ESR of 78 mm/h. Which of the following is the most appropriate treatment?

- ☐ **A** Aspirin
- ☐ **B** Aspirin and dypridamole
- ☐ **C** Clopidogrel
- ☐ **D** Prednisolone 10 mg daily
- ☑ **E** Prednisolone 60 mg daily

14.5 A 34-year-old man who is undergoing treatment for acute leukaemia asks to see you because he has acute swelling, pain and erythema over his right great toe. On examination this looks consistent with gout. You check his bloods and see that his creatinine has deteriorated from 112 µmol/l to 182 µmol/l over the past 48 h. How would you best manage him?

- ☐ **A** Allopurinol
- ☒ **B** Colchicine
- ☐ **C** Ibuprofen
- ☐ **D** Prednisolone
- ☑ **E** Rasburicase

14.6 A 57-year-old man presents with a history of dysphagia, first to liquids, then to solids; now it varies from day to day. He also feels tired all the time and has had to be moved from his delivery job out in the van to a computer-based one. On examination he has a purple-red rash on his face, his BMI is 31 kg/m² and his BP is normal. You have to help him out of the chair into the consultation room. His bloods are normal apart from positive anti-nuclear antibodies. Which of the following is the most likely diagnosis?

- ☑ **A** Dermatomyositis
- ☐ **B** Oesophageal carcinoma
- ☐ **C** Reflux oesophagitis
- ☐ **D** SLE
- ☐ **E** Scleroderma

14.4   Answer: E

The symptoms are suggestive of giant-cell arthritis, for which high-dose prednisolone is the treatment of choice. Failure of symptoms to respond rapidly to high-dose steroids would suggest another diagnosis.

14.5   Answer: E

Rasburicase is licensed for the prophylaxis and treatment of urate nephropathy, which can occur as a result of tumour lysis syndrome. It accelerates the metabolism of uric acid to allantoin.

14.6   Answer: A

The variable dysphagia and proximal weakness stopping him getting out of the chair, coupled with the rash, point towards dermatomyositis. Anti-nuclear antibodies are not specific, but are often positive.

14.7 A 36-year-old woman who has been suffering from recurrent sinusitis over the past few months presents to her GP with shortness of breath and haemoptysis. She has been feeling increasingly tired over the past few months and has been held up for a performance review at work. She is hypertensive on examination, with a BP of 178/94 mmHg. She appears to have collapse of her nasal bridge and there is bilateral wheeze and inspiratory crackles on auscultation of the chest. She is anaemic, with an Hb of 10 g/dl, and her WCC is slightly elevated at 11.2 × 10⁹/l. Her creatinine is 185 µmol/l and there are bilateral hazy pulmonary opacities on the chest X-ray. Which of the following antibodies is most likely to be positive?

- [ ] **A** Anti-centromere
- [x] **B** Anti-myeloperoxidase
- [x] **C** Anti-serine protease 3
- [ ] **D** Anti-thyroid
- [ ] **E** Rheumatoid factor

14.8 A 50-year-old man has a 2-year history of burning pain and loss of sensation in his hands and feet. He has a problem with alcohol and drinks 10 bottles of wine per week, and he has pain from severe rheumatoid arthritis. His BP is 135/72 mmHg, he has a raised JVP and pitting oedema. Bloods reveal macrocytic anaemia, an elevated creatinine of 155 µmol/l and marked proteinuria. What is the most likely diagnosis?

- [ ] **A** Alcoholic cardiomyopathy
- [ ] **B** Amyloid neuropathy
- [x] **C** B₁₂ deficiency
- [ ] **D** Chronic inflammatory demyelinating polyradiculoneuropathy (CIDP)
- [x] **E** Uraemic neuropathy

14.7 Answer: C

This patient has a history that fits perfectly with Wegener's granulomatosis. Biopsy diagnosis is made from an active lesion, be it in the nasal mucosa, lung or kidney.

14.8 Answer: E

Of course, he could have developed peripheral neuropathy just from the alcohol abuse. However, his significant proteinuria and the history of rheumatoid arthritis point to the possibility of systemic amyloidosis.

14.9 A 60-year-old man on long-term sulfasalazine therapy for rheumatoid is referred to the Medical Outpatient Department with painless haematuria. He is also hypertensive, for which he takes amlodipine. His BP is 155/92 mmHg. Examination reveals obvious signs of rheumatoid. Bloods reveal mild anaemia, his ESR is 13 mm/h, and his U&Es are actually relatively normal; the creatinine is 130 μmol/l. He has significant haematuria and proteinuria. Which of the following is the most appropriate investigation?

 A Cystoscopy

 B Rectal biopsy

 ☑ C Renal biopsy

 D Renal ultrasound

 E Urinary cytology

14.10 A 72-year-old man has been taking twice the recommended dose of diclofenac for controlling pain from his rheumatoid for the past few months. Additional medication includes low-dose prednisolone and bendroflumethiazide for hypertension. He now has lethargy, daily nausea, and flank pain. His BP is 151/92 mmHg. Abnormalities in his bloods include anaemia with an Hb of 10.0 g/dl, a potassium of 6.0 mmol/l and a creatinine of 250 μmol/l. His urine contains excessive protein, and renal CT shows bilateral small kidneys, medullary ring shadows and pelviceal filling defects. Which of the following is the most likely diagnosis?

 ☒ A Acute tubular necrosis

 B Interstitial nephritis

 C Membranous glomerulonephritis

 D Minimal-change disease

 ☑ E Papillary necrosis

14.9   Answer: C

The presence of haematuria and proteinuria on sulfasalazine therapy raises the possibility of drug-induced lupus. Marked proteinuria in the absence of haematuria could be a pointer to amyloidosis.

14.10   Answer: E

Diuretic use with NSAID excess can be associated with this problem, and the renal CT appearance is typical of papillary necrosis. Stenting of an obstruction, withdrawal of the offending agent, and adequate hydration is the standard treatment.

14.11 A 40-year-old woman is experiencing cognitive decline, as exhibited by the fact most recently she was unable to find her way home from the supermarket, and has been mis-arranging various objects around the kitchen. Her husband is very worried about her. She has hypertension, treated with ramipril, and has had three episodes of mononeuritis over the past year. On examination she is hypertensive and has livedo reticularis. Her FBC is abnormal (Hb 10.1 g/dl, WCC 11.5 × 10⁹/l, platelets 50 × 10⁹/l). Her creatinine is 185 μmol/l, she is Hep B surface antigen positive, and has haematuria and proteinuria. Which of the following antibodies is most likely to be positive?

A Anti-cardiolipin

B Anti-GBM

C Anti smooth muscle

D c-ANCA

E p-ANCA

14.12 A 70-year-old man presents with acute significant haemoptysis, nausea and lethargy. Hypertension managed with amlodipine is his only past history of note. His BP is elevated at 180/100 mmHg, there are widespread inspiratory crackles, and he looks short of breath at rest. He is anaemic with an Hb of 10.2 g/dl, and he has a raised WCC of 12.0 × 10⁹/l. His creatinine is over 200 μmol/l and he has haematuria and proteinuria. Renal biopsy shows necrotising glomerulonephritis. Which of the following antibodies is most likely to be positive?

A Anti-GBM

B Anti-mitochondrial

C Anti smooth muscle

D c-ANCA

E p-ANCA

14.11   Answer: E

This clinical picture, including the neurological symptoms, raises the possibility of polyarteritis nodosa. Up to 30% of cases are associated with hepatitis B and as a consequence are managed with antiviral therapy.

14.12   Answer: A

This patient has Goodpasture syndrome. Prednisolone and cyclophosphamide are the treatments of choice for remission induction, but mortality in this age group is high.

14.13 A 30-year-old woman with a history of poorly controlled asthma now presents with abdominal pain and diarrhoea, weight loss and a petechial skin rash. She has become particularly unwell with increasing nausea over the past week. Other history of note includes an episode of common peroneal mononeuritis in the past year. Her Hb is 11.0 g/dl, and she has a WCC of 10.0 × 10⁹/l with marked eosinophilia. Her creatinine is 244 µmol/, the ESR is 76 m/h and rheumatoid factor is positive. There is haematuria and proteinuria on urine screening. Chest radiography reveals bilateral pulmonary infiltrates. Which of the following autoantibodies is most likely to be positive in this case?

- A Anti-cardiolipin
- B anti-GBM
- ☑ C Anti-myeloperoxidase
- D Anti smooth muscle
- ☒ E c-ANCA

14.14 A 50-year-old woman complains that her fingers go white and blue and are excrutiatingly painful when she goes out in cold weather. Her GP has also given her an asthma inhaler for shortness of breath and omeprazole for reflux. She admits to using ibuprofen for multiple joint pains. On examination she is hypertensive and has telengiectasia. There is soft-tissue calcification and sclerodactyly on hand examination. The FBC is normal; the creatinine is elevated at around 140 µmol/l. Which of the following autoantibodies is most likely to be found in this patient?

- ☑ A Anti-centromere
- B Anti smooth muscle
- C c-ANCA
- D p-ANCA
- E Rheumatoid factor

14.15 You are reviewing research on denosumab, a new RANK-ligand inhibitor for the treatment of osteoporosis. Which one of the following correctly describes the action of the RANK ligand?

- A It down-regulates osteoblast activity
- B It down-regulates osteoclast activity
- ☒ C It promotes osteoblast activity
- ☑ D It promotes osteoclast activity
- E It promotes osteoblast activity and osteoclast activity

14.13 Answer: C

The history of severe asthma, with marked peripheral eosinophila and neurological symptoms is very typical of Churg–Strauss syndrome. Skin biopsy is the diagnostic investigation of choice, with methylprednisolone and cyclophosphamide the preferred treatment.

14.14 Answer: A

This patient has the features of CREST syndrome (**c**alcinosis, **R**aynaud's, o**e**sophageal dysmotility, **s**clerodactyly, **t**elangiectasia), in which over 90% of cases are associated with anti-centromere antibodies. Patients are managed symptomatically, but PDE-5 inhibitors and endothelin-receptor antagonists are an important part of the management of pulmonary hypertension.

14.15 Answer: D

The RANK ligand induces differentiation of pre-osteoclasts into osteoclasts and so promotes bone resorption. Denosumab inhibits RANK-ligand activity.

14.16 Which of the following statements most correctly describes the clinical features of osteoarthritis?

- [ ] **A** Characteristic distribution is asymmetrical
- [ ] **B** It is more common in Afro-Caribbean populations
- [x] **C** Radiological features are present in most people aged > 60 years
- [ ] **D** The prevalence is gradually declining
- [ ] **E** There are no effective interventions to delay disease progression

14.17 Which of the following is most likely to predispose to the development of generalised osteoarthritis?

- [ ] **A** Atrophy and loss of peri-articular bone
- [ ] **B** Decreased local production of interleukin 1 (IL-1)
- [x] **C** Inhibition of matrix metalloproteinases
- [ ] **D** Irregular cartilage surface due to disordered osteoblast function
- [x] **E** Repetitive jogging in youth

14.18 A 56-year-old woman is referred to the General Medical Outpatient Department for review of joint deformity affecting both hands. On examination, there are painless bony swellings affecting the distal and proximal interphalangeal joints of both hands. Which of the following is the most likely explanation?

- [ ] **A** Acute osteoarthritis
- [x] **B** Nodal osteoarthritis
- [ ] **C** Psoriatic arthropathy
- [x] **D** Rheumatoid arthritis
- [ ] **E** Systemic lupus erythematosus

14.19 Which of the following factors is most likely to be associated with significant pain in patients with osteoarthritis affecting the knee?

- [ ] **A** Cartilage abnormalities shown on MRI scan
- [ ] **B** Depression
- [ ] **C** Family history of joint disease
- [x] **D** Fissures and surface erosion seen on arthroscopy
- [x] **E** Loss of joint space on plain X-ray

14.16   Answer: C

Clinical features are less prevalent, most common in white and Western populations. Weight loss can delay disease progression in certain patients.

14.17   Answer: E

Repetitive joint use, trauma (particularly involving articular discontinuity), obesity and joint hypermobility predispose to osteoarthritis. Increased metalloproteinase activity contributes to cartilage destruction. Chondrocyte activity is often disordered.

14.18   Answer: B

This is associated with Bouchard's nodes (PIP joints) and Heberden's nodes (DIP joints). Often associated with carpometacarpal and metacarpophalangeal osteoarthritis of the thumb.

14.19   Answer: E

Other factors include the extent of disability and quadriceps femoris weakness. Clinical features of osteoarthritis do not correlate well with investigation findings.

14.20 A 54-year-old man presents to the local Emergency Department with spontaneous onset of acute pain and swelling of his left knee. On examination, there is local erythema and limitation of movement. Plain X-ray appearances are normal. Which of the following diagnoses is most likely?

- [ ] **A** Acute osteoarthritis
- [ ] **B** Haemarthrosis
- [ ] **C** Reactive arthritis
- [ ] **D** Rheumatoid arthritis
- [✓] **E** Septic arthritis

14.21 Which of the following statements is correct in relation to rheumatoid arthritis?

- [ ] **A** Affects around 10% of adults
- [ ] **B** HLA-DR4 phenotype is found in 98% of patients
- [✓] **C** Incidence in post-menopausal women is similar to age-matched men
- [ ] **D** Most cases present at 50–60 years of age
- [ ] **E** Oral contraceptive pill use provokes earlier disease onset

14.22 Which of the following factors is most relevant to the development and progression of joint abnormalities in patients with rheumatoid arthritis?

- [ ] **A** Development of anti-TNFα antibodies
- [ ] **B** Impaired secretion of IL-1 and IL-8
- [ ] **C** Production of autoantibodies directed at the Fab portion of IgG
- [ ] **D** Synovial atrophy and thinning
- [✓] **E** TNFα-mediated bony erosion

14.23 A 38-year-old woman attends the Rheumatology Outpatient Department for assessment of symmetrical joint pains and stiffness affecting both wrist and hands, for around 8 weeks. Which of the following most strongly indicates a diagnosis of rheumatoid arthritis?

- [✓] **A** Characteristic radiographic changes
- [ ] **B** Morning stiffness
- [ ] **C** Raised ESR
- [ ] **D** Rheumatoid factor positive
- [ ] **E** Subcutaneous nodules

14.20 Answer: E

Haemarthrosis is less likely in the absence of trauma; acute psoriatic arthritis should also be considered. The other disorders listed typically present as an inflammatory polyarthritis.

14.21 Answer: C

Affects 1–2% of the population, and the commonest age of onset is 30–50 years. OCP use appears to delay disease onset, and incidence is 2- to 3-fold higher in pre-menopausal women than in age-matched men. HLA-DR4 is found in 60–70% of patients.

14.22 Answer: E

Rheumatoid factor is present in around 70% of patients, which is an autoantibody directed at the Fc portion of IgG, and stimulates cytokine release by macrophages.

14.23 Answer: A

American College of Rheumatology criteria are four or more of:

Morning stiffness > 1 h (> 6 weeks)
Arthritis affecting more than two joints (> 6 weeks)
Arthritis of hand and wrists (> 6 weeks)
Symmetrical arthritis (> 6 weeks)
Positive rheumatoid factor
Subcutaneous nodules
Typical radiological changes

14.24 A 56-year-old woman with long-standing rheumatoid arthritis presents with progressive breathlessness. Which of the following disorders is most likely to be an extra-articular manifestation of rheumatoid arthritis?

- ☐ **A** Emphysema
- ☑ **B** Fibrosing alveolitis
- ☒ **C** Pleural effusion
- ☐ **D** Streptococcal pneumonia
- ☐ **E** Tuberculosis

14.25 A 42-year-old man with long-standing rheumatoid arthritis is referred to the Medical Outpatient Department for assessment of progressive peripheral sensory loss affecting both upper and lower limbs. Which of the following should be considered the most likely diagnosis?

- ☐ **A** Addisonian crisis
- ☒ **B** Atlanto-axial subluxation
- ☐ **C** Mononeuritis multiplex
- ☐ **D** Sulfasalazine toxicity
- ☑ **E** Vasculitis affecting the vasa nervorum

14.26 A 51-year-old woman has been suffering from rheumatoid arthritis for the past 3 years. Recently, she has been experiencing increasing pain and stiffness of her left shoulder despite persisting with regular analgesia. Which of the following statements regarding local intra-articular corticosteroid administration is correct?

- ☐ **A** Avoids systemic adverse effects of corticosteroids
- ☐ **B** Injections should be repeated at regular intervals
- ☑ **C** Semi-crystalline preparations are commonly used
- ☐ **D** Symptom relief is usually sustained for 4–6 months
- ☐ **E** They are generally less effective than high-dose oral corticosteroids

14.24 Answer: B

Other manifestations include pleural nodules and obstructive bronchiolitis. Effusion is less specific but it can be a complication of rheumatoid-mediated pleural serositis.

14.25 Answer: E

Mononeuritis multiplex and compression neuropathies (eg carpal tunnel syndrome) are also recognised.

14.26 Answer: C

These provide effective symptom relief, but it is often short-lived. They may be associated with fewer systemic complications but do not avoid them completely. They should only be used where other treatments are ineffective.

14.27 A 43-year-old man is referred to the Outpatient Department for assessment of pain and stiffness affecting the sacro-iliac joints and lower back. On examination, there is severe limitation of lumbar spine movement. The GP letter states that 'rheumatoid factor is negative'. Which of the following disorders is most likely to account for his symptoms?

- ☒ **A** L4–L5 disc prolapse
- ☐ **B** Osteoarthritis
- ☐ **C** Polymyositis
- ☑ **D** Psoriatic arthropathy
- ☐ **E** Rheumatoid arthritis

14.28 A 37-year-old man has a past history of psoriasis, which has been quiescent for several years. He presents to the Rheumatology Outpatient Department with a symmetrical polyarthropathy affecting both hands and wrists. Which of the following statements is correct regarding treatment of this condition?

- ☐ **A** Ciclosporin is the initial treatment of choice
- ☐ **B** Intra-articular corticosteroids are ineffective
- ☐ **C** Methotrexate controls skin lesions but not joint involvement
- ☐ **D** NSAIDs prevent future relapses
- ☑ **E** Sulfasalazine delays progression of joint disease

14.29 A 22-year-old man attends the Rheumatology Outpatient Department with back pain and stiffness and a diagnosis of reactive arthritis is considered. Which of the following factors would most strongly suggest an *alternative* diagnosis?

- ☐ **A** Conjunctivitis
- ☐ **B** Exfoliative rash on soles
- ☐ **C** Involvement of MTP joints
- ☐ **D** Nail dystrophy
- ☑ **E** Syndesmophytes on lumbar spine X-ray

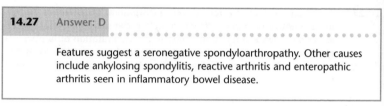

14.27 Answer: D

Features suggest a seronegative spondyloarthropathy. Other causes include ankylosing spondylitis, reactive arthritis and enteropathic arthritis seen in inflammatory bowel disease.

14.28 Answer: E

NSAIDs and analgesics are effective for symptomatic relief. Methotrexate and ciclosporin delay progression of both skin and joint involvement in psoriasis.

14.29 Answer: E

This is strongly suggestive of ankylosing spondylitis. Other features of reactive arthritis include circinate balanitis, large-joint effusion and heel pain.

14.30 A 56-year-old man attends the Emergency Department with a sudden onset of pain and swelling of the first metacarpophalangeal joint of his left foot. Which of the following would most strongly suggest a diagnosis of acute gout?

- ☑ **A** Demonstration of urate crystals in joint fluid
- ☐ **B** Normal appearance of plain X-ray
- ☐ **C** Previous acute gout 1 year before
- ☐ **D** Raised circulating neutrophil count
- ☐ **E** Serum uric acid 520 µmol/l

14.31 A 56-year-old woman presents to the Emergency Department with a hot, swollen and painful left knee. Joint aspiration reveals a watery yellow fluid, which is cloudy, but no crystals are seen on microscopy, and the neutrophil count is 5200/mm³. Which of the following is the most likely diagnosis?

- ☐ **A** Acute gout
- ☐ **B** Chondrocalcinosis
- ☐ **C** Pseudogout
- ☐ **D** Rheumatoid arthritis
- ☑ **E** Septic arthritis

14.32 A 52-year-old man is referred to the Rheumatology Outpatient Department with sudden onset of pain in his left knee. On examination, the joint is swollen and red, with limited movement due to pain. Aspiration of joint fluid reveals a turbid, bloodstained yellow fluid, and microscopy shows a neutrophil count of 85 000/mm³. Which of the following is the most likely diagnosis?

- ☐ **A** Acute gout
- ☐ **B** Chondrocalcinosis
- ☐ **C** Pseudogout
- ☐ **D** Rheumatoid arthritis
- ☑ **E** Septic arthritis

14.30 Answer: A

Serum urate concentrations are poor indicators: majority of patients with acute gout have 'normal' serum values at presentation. Fewer than 10% of patients with chronic hyperuricaemia ever develop an episode of acute gout.

14.31 Answer: D

Presents acutely in around 15% of cases. Typically, white cell count is increased to 2000–40 000/mm^3 and rheumatoid factor may be positive.

14.32 Answer: E

Such a high white cell count is highly suggestive of infection. Diagnosis might be confirmed by Gram stain and culture of aspirated fluid, and there might be a raised systemic WCC and positive blood cultures.

14.33 A 59-year-old woman presents to the Emergency Department with an acutely swollen and tender right knee. Microscopy of aspirated joint fluid shows a neutrophil count of 3280/mm³ and the presence of rhomboid crystals that are weakly positively birefringent. Which of the following is the most likely diagnosis?

- A Acute gout
- B Chondrocalcinosis
- ☑ C Pseudogout
- D Rheumatoid arthritis
- E Septic arthritis

14.34 A 70-year-old woman is referred to the Rheumatology Outpatient Department with progressive pain in her left knee, which has begun to limit the distance she can walk. Plain X-rays of both knee joints show narrowing of the joint space, predominantly affecting the left side. In addition, there is patchy linear calcification within the joint-space cartilage. Which of the following is the most likely diagnosis?

- A Acute gout
- ☑ B Chondrocalcinosis
- C Pseudogout
- D Rheumatoid arthritis
- E Septic arthritis

14.35 A previously well 17-year-old girl presents with sudden onset of a painful and swollen right knee. The joint appears diffusely swollen and red, and a diagnosis of septic arthritis is suspected. Which of the following is the most appropriate initial step in her management?

- A Blood cultures
- ☑ B Intravenous antibiotics before undertaking other investigations
- ☒ C Joint aspiration and urgent microscopy
- D Peripheral blood count
- E X-ray of the right knee

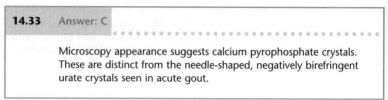

14.33   Answer: C

Microscopy appearance suggests calcium pyrophosphate crystals. These are distinct from the needle-shaped, negatively birefringent urate crystals seen in acute gout.

14.34   Answer: B

Condition characterised by calcium pyrophosphate deposition in the cartilage; can manifest as pseudogout, osteoarthritis-like features or a rapidly destructive arthritis.

14.35   Answer: B

This should be given immediately on diagnosis, even before other investigations have been performed.

14.36 A 42-year-old man presents to the local Emergency Department with severe pain affecting his left knee joint. The joint appears red and swollen, and a suspected diagnosis of septic arthritis is made. Which of the following would be the most appropriate initial treatment?

☑ **A** Intravenous high-dose flucloxacillin

☐ **B** Intravenous high-dose benzylpenicillin

☐ **C** Intravenous ciprofloxacin

☐ **D** Oral co-amoxiclav

☐ **E** Oral erythromycin

14.37 A 45-year-old farmer is referred to you because of recent symptoms suggesting arthritis of his knees and wrists. He had been treated several months earlier for a febrile illness associated with headache and an unusual rash. You suspect a diagnosis of Lyme disease. Which of the following tests would be most appropriate for confirming this?

☐ **A** Detection of *Borrelia burgdorferi* in blood culture

☐ **B** Detection of *Borrelia burgdorferi* in joint aspirate

☐ **C** IgE antibodies to *Borrelia burgdorferi*

☑ **D** IgM antibodies to *Borrelia burgdorferi*

☐ **E** Peripheral eosinophilia

14.38 Which of the following confers the greatest likelihood of developing SLE?

☑ **A** Affected first-degree relative

☐ **B** Age > 50 years

☐ **C** Male gender

☐ **D** HLA-B27 genotype

☐ **E** Suppressed B-lymphocyte function

14.36   Answer: A

The most common organism is *Staphylococcus aureus*; an alternative to flucloxacillin is high-dose intravenous erythromycin or clarithromycin. Oral fucidic acid is often co-administered. Gonococcal arthritis is a common cause in young patients.

14.37   Answer: D

Around 25% of cases develop oligoarthritis; 20% of these progress to a chronic arthritis. Treatment with antibiotics is effective for early disease, and prolonged therapy may be effective in chronic arthritis.

14.38   Answer: A

Around 3% risk; 25% concordance in monozygotic twins. Risk greater in females, those aged 20–40 years and with the HLA-B8 and -DR3 genotypes.

14.39 A 56-year-old man is treated with hydralazine and nitrate therapy for heart failure. Three months after commencing treatment, he complains of aches and pains across many joints. Examination shows an erythematous scaly rash and lymphadenopathy, and a plain chest X-ray shows diffuse pulmonary infiltration. Which one of the following statements regarding hydralazine-induced lupus is correct?

- **A** Corticosteroid treatment is contraindicated
- **B** People with HLA-B27 antigen are at significantly greater risk
- ☒ **C** Rapid acetylators are at greatest risk
- ☑ **D** Remission usually occurs after drug withdrawal
- **E** Renal involvement is a characteristically prominent feature

14.40 A 28-year-old woman is referred to the Rheumatology Outpatient Department for assessment of chronic inflammatory symptoms affecting the joints of both hands, wrists and shoulders. Which of the following features would be most strongly suggestive of SLE as the underlying diagnosis?

- ☑ **A** Alopecia with scarring
- **B** Nail-bed infarcts
- **C** Negative rheumatoid factor
- **D** Positive anti-nuclear antibody
- **E** Scaly, erythematous skin rash overlying both knees

14.41 A 38-year-old woman attends the General Medical Outpatient Department with a suspected diagnosis of Raynaud's disease. She describes blanching and pain of her extremities following exposure to cold weather. Which of the following is most likely to be an effective treatment?

- **A** Atenolol
- **B** Clopidogrel
- **C** Misoprostol
- ☑ **D** Nicardipine
- **E** Sumatriptan

14.39   Answer: D

HLA-DR4 and slow acetylator phenotype are risk factors. Unlike SLE, renal and CNS involvement is uncommon. Treatment with corticosteroids may be helpful.

14.40   Answer: A

Present in around 50% of cases. Positive ANA test in SLE, rheumatoid arthritis and other conditions. Nail-bed infarction is non-specific, and occurs after trauma and in patients with vasculitis of any origin.

14.41   Answer: D

Dihydropyridine calcium-channel blockers cause smooth muscle relaxation and oppose the vasoconstriction in Raynaud's disease (eg nifedipine). Beta-blockers (eg atenolol) tend to cause peripheral vasoconstriction and reduced cardiac output, which might exacerbate the condition.

14.42 A 52-year-old woman is referred to the Rheumatology Outpatient Clinic with shiny and atrophic skin overlying her fingers, with ulceration of a number of her fingertips. She is noted to have facial telangiectasia. Which of the following diagnoses is most likely to account for these features?

- [ ] **A** Discoid lupus
- [ ] **B** Pseudogout
- [ ] **C** Psoriatic arthropathy
- [✓] **D** Scleroderma
- [ ] **E** SLE

14.43 A 52-year-old woman with long-standing systemic sclerosis presents with progressive breathlessness over the past 4 months. Which of the following investigations would be most helpful in establishing the cause of her breathlessness?

- [ ] **A** Arterial blood gas analysis
- [✓] **B** High-resolution CT thorax
- [ ] **C** Measurement of anti-topoisomerase I titres
- [✗] **D** Plain chest X-ray
- [ ] **E** Pulmonary function tests

14.44 Which of the following statements is correct with regard to Paget's disease of the bone?

- [ ] **A** Affects around 10% of patients over the age of 50 years
- [ ] **B** Diagnosis is unlikely if serum calcium concentration is normal
- [ ] **C** High serum phosphate is a characteristic finding
- [✓] **D** It confers a 30-fold increased risk of osteosarcoma
- [ ] **E** Plain X-ray investigations are usually normal

14.45 A 72-year-old woman is referred to the Medical Outpatient Clinic for investigation of progressive breathlessness. She has been diagnosed with Paget's disease several years before. Which of the following diagnoses is most likely to account for her current symptoms?

- [✓] **A** High-output cardiac failure
- [ ] **B** Hypercalcaemia
- [ ] **C** Myocardial ischaemia
- [ ] **D** Phrenic nerve compression
- [ ] **E** Pulmonary fibrosis

14.42 Answer: D

Typically presents between 30 and 50 years. May also be calcinosis, and erythema and dilated capillaries in the proximal nail folds.

14.43 Answer: B

Pulmonary fibrosis occurs in many patients with systemic disease. Presence of anti-topoisomerase I (anti-Scl 70) antibody is suggestive of pulmonary involvement. Recurrent infection is a recognised complication, particularly in patients with significant gastro-oesophageal reflux.

14.44 Answer: D

Occurs in 0.5–1.0% of cases. Serum calcium and phosphate are typically normal, while alkaline phosphatase is significantly raised. X-ray changes can show lytic lesions or sclerotic lesions and thickening of bony trabeculae.

14.45 Answer: A

Myocardial ischaemia is a less common but recognised complication.

14.46 A 56-year-old man is referred to the General Medical Outpatient Department with a 4-month history of progressive lower limb weakness and vague hip and knee pains. Examination shows proximal muscle weakness and tenderness, and investigations show corrected calcium 1.98 mmol/l, phosphate 0.8 mmol/l, alkaline phosphatase 230 IU/l and alanine transferase 24 IU/l. Which of the following is the most likely diagnosis?

☑ A Osteomalacia

☐ B Osteoporosis

☐ C Paget's disease

☒ D Polymyalgia rheumatica

☐ E Polymyositis

14.47 A 65-year-old woman is referred to the General Medical Outpatient Department following a recent traumatic hip X-ray. Plain X-rays showed marked osteopenia, and reports suggested osteoporosis. Which of the following is the strongest risk factor for osteoporosis?

☐ A Alcohol excess

☐ B Cigarette smoking

☐ C Diabetes mellitus

☑ D Female gender

☐ E Low dietary calcium intake

14.48 A 48-year-old man is admitted to the Medical Assessment Unit with an 8-week history of fever, weight loss and generalised myalgia. On examination, blood pressure is 186/94 mmHg. Investigations show ESR 52 mm/h, WCC 13.2 × 10⁹/l and dipstick urinalysis shows proteinuria ++ and haematuria +++. Which of the following is the most likely underlying diagnosis?

☐ A Paraneoplastic myopathy

☐ B Phaeochromocytoma

☑ C Polyarteritis nodosa

☐ D Polymyalgia rheumatica

☐ E Polymyositis

14.46 Answer: A

Raised alkaline phosphatase (ALP) is the characteristic finding in this condition, secondary to raised PTH. Calcium is low to normal.

14.47 Answer: D

The others are also important risk factors; others include early menopause, family history and advancing age.

14.48 Answer: C

Can also involve CNS, abdominal viscera, heart and skin. Angiography demonstrates pathognomonic multiple microaneurysms.

14.49 A 56-year-old woman is undergoing inpatient investigations of weight loss, fever and rash. Skin biopsy of an affected site shows inflammation consistent with a small-vessel vasculitis. ANCA test is negative. Which of the following is the most likely explanation for these findings?

- ☐ **A** Churg–Strauss granulomatosis
- ☑ **B** Henoch–Schönlein purpura
- ☐ **C** Kawasaki's disease
- ☒ **D** Microscopic polyangiitis
- ☐ **E** Wegener's granulomatosis

14.50 A 60-year-old man is referred to the General Medical Outpatient Clinic with a short history of severe pain and stiffness affecting both shoulder girdles, lumbar spine and hips. His symptoms are usually worst in the mornings. Which of the following is the most likely diagnosis?

- ☐ **A** Cushing syndrome
- ☐ **B** Graves' disease
- ☐ **C** Osteomalacia
- ☑ **D** Polymyalgia rheumatica
- ☐ **E** Polymyositis

14.51 A 64-year-old woman is referred to the General Medical Outpatient Clinic with suspected polymyalgia rheumatica. Which of the following investigations is most useful in confirming this diagnosis?

- ☐ **A** Alkaline phosphatase
- ☐ **B** Creatinine kinase
- ☑ **C** ESR
- ☐ **D** Serum calcium
- ☐ **E** Temporal artery biopsy

14.49 Answer: B

Kawasaki's disease is associated with medium- to large-vessel vasculitis. The others are typically associated with positive c-ANCA (Wegener's) or p-ANCA (Churg–Strauss and microscopic polyangiitis).

14.50 Answer: D

Although some features overlap with the other conditions, the symptoms and diurnal variation make polymyalgia rheumatica the most likely.

14.51 Answer: C

Invariably high, and can be used to monitor response to treatment. Temporal artery biopsy shows giant-cell arteritis in only 20–30% of cases.

14.52 You review a 71-year-old woman in the Medical Assessment Unit, who presents with new onset of left-sided headache associated with blurred vision. Neurological examination of her limbs is normal. ESR is 68 mmol/l. Which of the following is the best initial treatment?

- [ ] **A** Amitriptyline
- [ ] **B** Co-amoxiclav
- [✓] **C** High-dose prednisolone
- [ ] **D** Intramuscular morphine
- [ ] **E** Nimodipine

14.53 A previously well 38-year-old man presents with 12-week history of progressively worsening dry eyes and dry mouth. He is taking no regular medications. Which of the following is the most likely diagnosis?

- [ ] **A** Allergic conjunctivitis
- [ ] **B** Hypothyroidism
- [ ] **C** Rheumatoid arthritis
- [✓] **D** Sjögren syndrome
- [ ] **E** Stevens–Johnson syndrome

14.54 A 42-year-old woman is admitted with sudden onset of left arm weakness and left homonymous hemianopia. On examination, she has a soft systolic murmur. ESR and full blood count are normal. Which of the following tests would best establish an underlying cause for stroke?

- [ ] **A** Anti-dsDNA antibody
- [✓] **B** Anti-cardiolipin antibodies
- [✗] **C** Coagulation screen
- [ ] **D** Coombs' test
- [ ] **E** Lupus anticoagulant

14.52 Answer: C

These features suggest giant-cell arteritis. Ophthalmic artery involvement is associated with the risk of permanent blindness and urgent corticosteroid treatment is required, eg prednisolone 60–100 mg daily.

14.53 Answer: D

Xerostomia and dry eyes (keratoconjunctivitis sicca), in the absence of rheumatoid arthritis or autoimmune disease. Can be associated with Raynaud's phenomenon, arthralgia, neuritis and renal tubular defects.

14.54 Answer: B

Diagnostic for antiphospholipid syndrome, which accounts for a quarter of strokes < 45 years. May be associated with lupus anticoagulant antibodies and positive Coombs' test.

14.55 A 34-year-old woman is admitted via the Emergency Department with sudden onset of left leg pain, 6 weeks after a spontaneous abortion. On examination, the leg is cold and pale with absent pulses beyond the popliteal artery. Which of the following disorders is most likely to be responsible?

- [ ] **A** Addison's disease
- [x] **B** Antiphospholipid syndrome
- [ ] **C** Disseminated intravascular coagulation (DIC)
- [ ] **D** Polycythaemia rubra vera
- [ ] **E** SLE

14.56 A 43-year-old woman is referred to the Outpatient Department with pain and stiffness of her joint associated with a facial rash. The GP letter has suggested a diagnosis of SLE. Which of the following would most strongly suggest an alternative diagnosis?

- [ ] **A** Cranial nerve palsy
- [x] **B** Finger clubbing
- [ ] **C** Normocytic anaemia
- [ ] **D** Pleural effusion
- [ ] **E** Raynaud's phenomenon

14.57 A 31-year-old woman attends the Medical Outpatient Department for investigation of exertional breathlessness. She has recently been diagnosed with SLE, and has a characteristic facial rash. Which of these investigations would most strongly suggest pulmonary involvement?

- [x] **A** Anti-Jo1 antibody
- [x] **B** ESR > 45 mm/h
- [ ] **C** High anti-nuclear antibody titres
- [ ] **D** PEFR 85% of predicted
- [ ] **E** Rheumatoid factor positive

14.55   Answer: B

Arterial and venous thrombosis; 30% of woman with recurrent miscarriages have antiphospholipid antibody syndrome. May also be associated with migraine, thrombocytopenia, livedo reticularis and valvular heart disease.

14.56   Answer: B

The others are characteristic findings, along with vasculitis and skin, pulmonary and cardiac involvement.

14.57   Answer: A

Around 60% of patients have lung involvement: pleurisy, pleural effusion, pneumonitis and restrictive lung defect with reduced lung volumes.

14.58 A 49-year-old woman is referred for measurement of bone mineral density. Which of the following clinical factors most strongly suggests underlying osteoporosis?

☐ **A** Alcoholism

☐ **B** Long-standing asthma

☐ **C** Obesity

☑ **D** Prolonged corticosteroid treatment

☐ **E** Regular cigarette smoking

14.59 A previously well 64-year-old woman presents to the Emergency Department with sudden onset of lumbar back pain. Plain X-rays of the lumbar spine indicate wedge-type fractures affecting L3 and L4 vertebrae. Which of the following statements is correct regarding her management?

☑ **A** Bisphosphonate therapy will reduce her long-term fracture risk

☐ **B** Bone biopsy should be performed

☐ **C** Constipation is most likely due to hypercalcaemia

☐ **D** Hormone replacement therapy should be commenced

☐ **E** Radiotherapy of the lumbar spine should be arranged

14.60 A 34-year-old woman with long-standing asthma is referred to the General Medical Outpatient Department for investigation of pulmonary infiltrates noted on a recent chest X-ray. Full blood count shows a raised eosinophil count; the ESR is normal. Which of the following diagnoses is most likely?

☐ **A** Acute exacerbation of COPD

☐ **B** Chronic lymphocytic leukaemia

☑ **C** Churg–Strauss syndrome

☐ **D** Goodpasture syndrome

☐ **E** Pneumoconiosis

14.58 Answer: D

Other risk factors include inflammatory bowel disease, coeliac disease, lack of physical exercise, immobility, female gender and advanced age.

14.59 Answer: A

Osteoporotic crush fracture is the most likely cause. Underlying metastases or myeloma important but uncommon. Transient constipation is common, due to entrapment of parasympathetic nerves.

14.60 Answer: C

Characteristic features also include allergic rhinitis and cardiac involvement; often p-ANCA positive.

14.61 A 46-year-old patient is admitted to the Emergency Department with breathlessness. He has a history of asthma and allergic rhinitis, and his plain chest X-ray shows diffuse pulmonary infiltration. Which of these findings would most strongly support a diagnosis of Churg–Strauss syndrome?

- [ ] **A** Anti-dsDNA antibody positive
- [ ] **B** Anti-nuclear antibody positive
- [ ] **C** c-ANCA positive
- [✓] **D** p-ANCA positive
- [ ] **E** Raised blood lymphocyte count

14.62 A 59-year-old man is referred for investigation of pain and swelling of his nose associated with significant tenderness. There is no history of trauma. Investigations show ESR 45 mm/h, and urinalysis shows protein ++ and blood ++. Which of the following diagnoses best explains these findings?

- [ ] **A** Dermatomyositis
- [ ] **B** Polymyalgia rheumatica
- [ ] **C** Polymyositis
- [✓] **D** Relapsing chondritis
- [ ] **E** SLE

14.63 A 54-year-old woman is referred to the General Medical Outpatient Department for investigation of proximal muscle weakness and facial rash. The GP letter suggests a diagnosis of dermatomyositis. Which of the following features would most strongly suggest an alternative diagnosis?

- [✓] **A** Electromyography shows delayed axonal conduction
- [ ] **B** Heliotropic rash over the upper eyelids
- [ ] **C** Peri-orbital oedema
- [ ] **D** Positive rheumatoid factor
- [ ] **E** Raised anti-nuclear antibody titres

14.61 Answer: D

Also associated with high eosinophil count. c-ANCA more strongly suggestive of Wegener's granulomatosis.

14.62 Answer: D

Classically involves relapsing course with inflammation of the pinna or nasal cartilage. Can result in permanent damage, eg saddle-nose deformity. Associated with anti-type II collagen antibody.

14.63 Answer: A

This suggests a peripheral neuropathy.

14.64 A 56-year-old woman has recently been diagnosed with dermatomyositis. Which of the following statements is most accurate regarding the clinical course in this condition?

- [ ] **A** A relapsing–remitting pattern is most common
- [✓] **B** Corticosteroids are an effective treatment
- [ ] **C** Joints are typically spared
- [ ] **D** The ESR is elevated in around two-thirds of patients
- [✗] **E** There is a 10-fold increased risk of underlying malignancy

14.65 A 55-year-old man has been diagnosed with asymptomatic hyperuricaemia. Which of the following factors is most likely to predispose to high serum urate concentrations?

- [✓] **A** Bendroflumethizide
- [ ] **B** Ibuprofen
- [ ] **C** Sedentary lifestyle
- [ ] **D** Triamterene
- [ ] **E** Type 1 diabetes

14.66 A 45-year-old man is referred to the General Medical Outpatient Department because of progressive pain in both knees, which is limiting mobility. On examination, his weight is 108 kg, blood pressure is 176/92 mmHg, there is mild swelling of both knee joints and there are active striae across the abdominal wall. Which of the following is most likely to account for his joint pains?

- [ ] **A** Avascular necrosis
- [ ] **B** Chondrocalcinosis
- [ ] **C** Haemarthrosis
- [✓] **D** Osteoarthritis
- [ ] **E** Psoriatic arthropathy

14.64 Answer: B

Long-term, there may be muscle contractures and a 2- to 3-fold increased risk of underlying malignancy. The ESR is high in only around 5%.

14.65 Answer: A

Type 1 diabetes typically associated with hypouricaemia, whereas type 2 diabetes, hypertension, renal impairment are associated with hyperuricaemia.

14.66 Answer: D

The clinical features suggest Cushing's syndrome and obesity; the latter is a major risk factor for premature osteoarthritis.

14.67 A 34-year-old man is referred to the Rheumatology Outpatient Department because of a symmetrical arthropathy involving the knees, ankles and wrists. You note the presence of dusky-coloured raised plaques over both shins. Which of the following is the most likely underlying diagnosis?

- A Dermatomyositis
- B Psoriatic arthropathy
- **[X] C Rheumatoid arthritis**
- **[✓] D Sarcoidosis**
- E Tuberculous arthritis

14.68 A 48-year-old man has received immunosuppressive treatment for severe rheumatoid arthritis. Which of the following best describes the pharmacological action of these drugs?

- A Azathioprine is a pyrimidine analogue
- **[✓] B Azathioprine is metabolised to 6-mercaptopurine**
- C Ciclosporin A increases IL-1 activity
- D Cyclophosphamide acts by inhibiting folate dehydrogenase
- E Methotrexate is an alkylating agent

14.69 A 62-year-old woman presents to the General Medical Outpatient Clinic for assessment of easy bruising. She has had rheumatoid arthritis for more than 30 years, but this has been asymptomatic recently. On examination, the skin is dry and thin and there is purpura overlying the forearms and lower limbs. Which of the following is most likely to account for her symptoms and signs?

- **[X] A Autoimmune thrombocytopenia**
- **[✓] B Cushing syndrome**
- C Immunosuppression secondary to sulfasalazine
- D Impaired liver function
- E Lupus anticoagulant antibodies

14.67   Answer: D

Also associated with bilateral hilar lymphadenopathy, and there may be raised serum calcium and ACE concentrations. The rash distribution is characteristic of erythema nodosum.

14.68   Answer: B

Azathioprine is a pro-drug; both are purine analogues and are also useful in Crohn's disease. Cyclophosphamide is an alkylating agent, ciclosporin is a lymphocyte calcineurin inhibitor, and methotrexate is a folate antagonist.

14.69   Answer: B

Other features include truncal obesity, hirsutism, impotence, acne, striae, hypertension and diabetes mellitus.

14.70 A 49-year-old woman has had rheumatoid arthritis for 8 years, and is complaining of a recent exacerbation of pain and stiffness affecting her hands and wrists. Which of the following factors would most strongly suggest the need for systemic corticosteroid therapy?

- [ ] **A** Effective symptom relief after previous corticosteroid administration
- [X] **B** ESR > 60 mm/h
- [✓] **C** Lack of response to sulfasalazine
- [ ] **D** Raised blood leukocyte count
- [ ] **E** Rheumatoid factor very strongly positive

14.71 A 50-year-old woman has had diffuse muscle pain and stiffness for more than 8 months. She is found to have local tenderness overlying both biceps muscles. Serum creatinine kinase, ESR, full blood count and EMG studies are normal, and rheumatoid factor is negative. Which of the following is the most likely diagnosis?

- [✓] **A** Fibromyalgia
- [ ] **B** Polymyalgia rheumatica
- [ ] **C** Polymyositis
- [ ] **D** Rhabdomyolysis
- [ ] **E** Rheumatoid arthritis

14.72 A 45-year-old labourer is complaining of lumbar back pain. He had fallen from a ladder at work 2 months earlier. Which of the following features would most strongly support the diagnosis of functional low back pain?

- [ ] **A** Documented history of malignant disease
- [ ] **B** Loss of bladder control
- [ ] **C** Night sweats
- [✓] **D** Tenderness on superficial palpation over the lumbar spine
- [ ] **E** Weight loss

14.73 A 56-year-old woman is complaining of progressively worsening lumbar back pain. There is no history of trauma. Which of the following features indicate the need for urgent investigation?

- [✓] **A** Limited straight-leg raising
- [X] **B** Loss of bowel and bladder continence
- [ ] **C** Pain aggravated by lumbar spine movements
- [ ] **D** Severe pain not relieved by simple analgesia
- [ ] **E** Recurrent episodes

14.70 Answer: C

Lack of pain relief with rest, NSAIDs, disease-modifying anti-rheumatic agents or local corticosteroids, or if there is life-threatening visceral disease (eg severe pericarditis) or sight-threatening ocular involvement.

14.71 Answer: A

Affects around 2% of GP attenders, 10 times more common in women. Often associated with features of anxiety and depression. Management involves exclusion of more serious pathology, reassurance and physiotherapy.

14.72 Answer: D

The other features should prompt more urgent investigation.

14.73 Answer: A

Other signs indicating a need for urgent/emergency investigation include saddle-area sensory loss, loss of sphincter tone, bilateral leg pain and neurological deficit and finding a discrete sensory level.

14.74 A 52-year-old woman complains of aching and stiffness affecting both hands and wrists for the past 6 weeks. Rheumatoid factor is positive. Which of the following conditions is most likely to account for the presence of this antibody?

- ☐ A Achalasia of the oesophagus
- ☐ B Polyarteritis nodosum
- ☑ C Tuberculosis
- ☐ D Viral meningitis
- ☐ E Wegener's granulomatosis

14.75 Which of the following statements related to bone turnover is most accurate?

- ☐ A Bone remodelling is inhibited by thyroxine
- ☐ B IL-1 inhibits bone remodelling
- ☑ C Osteoblasts lay down unmineralised 'osteoid' material
- ☐ D Osteoclasts stimulate new bone formation
- ☐ E Osteocytes are anuclear and cannot multiply by meiosis

14.76 A 30-year-old woman is suspected of having SLE. Detection of which of the following antibodies most strongly suggests an alternative diagnosis?

- ☐ A Anti-dsDNA antibody
- ☐ B Anti-histone antibody
- ☐ C Anti-nuclear antibody
- ☐ D Anti-ribonuclear protein antibody
- ☑ E Anti-topoisomerase I antibody

14.74 Answer: C

Other non-articular causes of a false-positive test include Epstein–Barr virus infection, endocarditis, hepatitis and syphilis.

14.75 Answer: C

Parathyroid hormone, active vitamin D, thyroid hormone, growth hormone and IL-1 (rheumatoid arthritis) stimulate bone remodelling, whereas oestrogen, androgen and calcitonin can inhibit it. Osteoclasts are active in bone resorption.

14.76 Answer: E

This is more suggestive of systemic sclerosis. Anti-histone antibody is found in SLE (H1, H3, H4) and drug-induced lupus (H2), while anti-ribonuclear protein antibody is found also in mixed connective tissue disease.

INDEX

ABO blood groups 7.38
ACE inhibitors 2.40, 2.51, 9.39
acid–base balance 2.50, 2.63, 3.21
acromegaly 5.29
acute coronary syndrome 1.29
Addison's disease 5.57
Adie's pupil 11.2
adrenal adenoma 5.56
adult respiratory distress syndrome
    (ARDS) 13.38
adverse drug effects 2.99, 4.31
agonists, partial 2.96
AIDS *see* HIV/AIDS
alcohol abuse 7.62, 12.23, 12.36
alcohol withdrawal 2.67, 12.21, 12.37
alkaptonuria 3.53, 5.47
allergic bronchopulmonary
    aspergillosis 13.67
allergy 2.34, 3.114–3.116, 4.39
alopecia 4.5
α-1 antitrypsin deficiency 13.9, 13.19
α-fetoprotein (AFP) 3.76, 3.117
α-galactosidase A deficiency 3.30
Alport syndrome 9.42, 9.43
Alzheimer's disease 10.58, 12.38
amenorrhoea 5.61
amine hormones 3.77
amino acids, essential 3.107
aminosalicylates 2.23, 2.56
amiodarone 1.22, 1.23, 13.25
amoebiasis, hepatic 8.64
amoebic dysentery 8.63
amyloid-related diseases 3.86, 9.25
    light-chain amyloidosis 7.58
    reactive amyloidosis 9.47
    systemic amyloidosis 7.64, 14.8
amyotrophic lateral sclerosis 10.70
anaemia 7.19, 7.62
    deficiency (iron and/or B_{12}) 6.41,
        7.16–7.18, 7.21, 7.51, 7.59
    drug-induced 2.92
    haemolytic 2.92, 7.22, 7.40, 7.69
    investigations 6.36, 7.23, 14.1
anaerobic metabolism 3.108
analgesia 2.48, 2.64, 2.83, 2.94, 7.8,
    7.50
anaphylactic reactions 3.114

angioedema 4.30
angioplasty 1.29
angular cheilitis 4.37
anion gap 3.80
ankylosing spondylitis 13.16
anorexia nervosa 12.34
anterior circulation stroke
    partial 10.17, 10.25
    total 10.20
anterior uveitis 11.15
antibiotics
    adverse effects/interactions 2.12,
        2.16, 2.82, 2.84, 2.85, 2.87,
        2.102, 13.41
    C. difficile risk 8.3
    choosing 1.13, 2.69, 2.70, 8.6,
        8.11, 8.41, 8.53, 14.36
anti-centromere antibodies 14.14
anti-epileptic drugs 2.3, 2.14, 10.47
anti-GBM antibodies 9.66, 14.12
antihistamines 2.27
anti-mitochondrial antibodies 6.66
anti-myeloperoxidase antibodies
    14.13
anti-neutrophil cytoplasmic antibodies
    (ANCA) 3.84, 4.2, 9.69, 13.51,
    14.11, 14.61
antiphospholipid syndrome 14.54,
    14.55
antipsychotic drugs 2.38, 2.66
anti-Ro antibodies 3.68
anti-serine protease 3 antibodies 14.7
anti-thyroid antibodies 5.18
antiviral agents 8.14
anti-Yo antibodies 10.76
anxiety disorders 2.37, 2.61, 12.16,
    12.20, 12.26, 12.33
aortic aneurysm 1.47
aortic coarctation 1.49, 1.63
aortic dissection 1.64
aortic stenosis 1.37, 1.67
aortic valve disease, mixed 1.38
apoptosis 3.44
Argyll Robertson pupil 10.63
arterial blood gases 3.21, 13.36,
    13.61, 13.63
arthroplasty 8.4

asbestos-related diseases 13.12, 13.40, 13.68, 13.71
aspergilloma 8.1
aspergillosis, pulmonary 8.57, 8.58, 13.34, 13.67
aspirin 2.71, 7.1
asthma 2.57, 3.126, 7.27, 13.14, 13.20, 13.49
atheroembolism 3.83, 9.1
atopic dermatitis 4.25
atrial fibrillation 1.5
atrial septal defect 1.26, 1.74
atropine 2.52
autoantibodies 3.73, 14.76
  see also specific antibodies
autoimmune polyglandular syndrome type 1 (APS-1) 5.58
autonomic neuropathy 5.73
azygous lobe 13.18

back pain 14.27, 14.59, 14.72, 14.73
bacteriuria, asymptomatic 9.56
basal cell papilloma 4.17
BCR-ABL gene 3.25
Becker's muscular dystrophy 3.61
Behçet's disease 3.31
Bence Jones protein 9.25, 9.26
beta-blockers 2.15
biceps muscle injuries 3.87
bile salt malabsorption 6.64
bipolar affective disorder 12.24
bitemporal hemianopia 10.1, 10.61
blood transfusions 7.13, 7.28, 7.35, 8.23
  reactions to 7.29, 7.30, 7.37, 13.15
blue vision 2.8, 11.1
body dysmorphia 12.3
bone turnover 14.75
borderline personality disorder 12.1
Bordetella pertussis 8.45
bowel ischaemia 6.10, 6.46
brachial plexus injuries 3.93
brain natriuretic peptide (BNP) 13.1
breast cancer 7.46–7.48
breastfeeding 2.70, 2.71
bronchial cancer see lung cancer
bronchiectasis 13.58
bronchiolitis obliterans 13.75
bronchospasm 3.126

brucellosis 8.49
bruising 7.1, 7.6, 7.32
bulbar palsy 10.60
bullous pemphigoid 4.18
buprenorphine 2.97

C1-esterase deficiency 13.8
C1-esterase inhibitor deficiency 4.40
CA-125 6.4
calcium
  hypercalcaemia 3.57, 5.40–5.44, 6.58, 9.64
  urinary 3.120, 9.64
calcium-channel blockers 2.6, 10.23, 14.41
Campylobacter jejuni 8.47
carbamazepine 2.33, 2.36, 10.65
carcinoid tumours 6.47, 7.7, 13.29
cardiac failure see heart failure
cardiac rehabilitation 1.20
cardiac tamponade 1.43
cardiogenic shock 1.34
cardiomyopathy 1.30–1.32, 3.70
cataracts 11.11, 11.20
cavernous sinus lesions 3.52
CD3 receptors 3.9
celcoxib 2.59
cerebellar lesions 7.44, 10.19, 10.59, 10.76
cerebral metastases 10.49
cerebrospinal fluid (CSF), Ig in 3.119
cerebrovascular disease see stroke
Charcot's arthropathy 3.1, 5.66
chest drains 13.43
chickenpox 8.5, 8.14
Chlamydia trachomatis 8.37, 8.72, 9.55
chloasma 4.11
cholera 8.50, 8.51
cholesterol embolism 3.83, 9.1
chondrocalcinosis 14.34
chromosomal disorders 3.40, 3.82
chronic lymphocytic leukaemia 7.5, 7.71, 9.62
chronic obstructive pulmonary disease (COPD) 1.12, 13.21, 13.61
Churg–Strauss syndrome 10.11, 13.23, 14.13, 14.60, 14.61
ciclosporin 9.13
cirrhosis 6.66, 6.71

clinical trials 2.88–2.90
Clostridium difficile 8.3
Clostridium perfringens 3.69
cluster headaches 2.95, 10.41
cocaine 2.44
coeliac disease 3.39, 6.5, 6.8, 6.16,
  6.35, 6.38, 7.63
coital cephalgia 10.42
colchicine 2.10, 5.9
colonic carcinoma 6.9, 6.63
common peroneal nerve 3.63, 3.95
complement 3.58, 3.112, 3.113, 4.40,
  13.8
Conn syndrome 5.12, 5.55
consciousness
  GCS 10.56
  loss of 10.16, 10.18
constipation 2.100, 6.57–6.60
continuous positive airways pressure
  (CPAP) 13.24, 13.69
Coombs' test 7.23
coronary artery bypass grafting 1.60
coronary artery disease 1.28, 1.29,
  1.36, 1.62, 1.67
coronary microangiopathy 1.39
corticosteroids 2.57, 3.78, 4.27, 5.26,
  6.14, 10.67, 14.4, 14.26, 14.70
cortisol 2.5
cough, drug-induced 2.40
Coxiella burnetii 8.39, 13.54
cranial nerve III 3.96, 10.62
cranial nerve IV 11.5
CREST syndrome 14.14
Crohn's disease 6.13, 6.14, 6.43, 6.54
cryoglobulins 3.111
Cryptococcus spp. 3.66, 8.59
cryptogenic fibrosing alveolitis 13.65
Cryptosporidium 6.15, 8.15
CURB-65 criteria 13.2
Cushing syndrome 5.30, 14.69
cyclophosphamide 2.65
cystic fibrosis 3.125, 8.11, 13.13,
  13.67
cysticerosis 8.67
cystitis 9.21
cytomegalovirus (CMV) 7.13, 8.8,
  8.26, 11.4

deafness 10.8

deep vein thrombosis 7.36, 13.70
delirium tremens 12.37
dementia 10.58, 12.2, 12.19, 12.31,
  12.38
Dengue fever 8.18
depression 12.7, 12.10, 12.12, 12.22,
  12.23, 12.25, 12.32, 12.35
dermatitis herpetiformis 4.10, 4.19,
  6.39, 6.40
dermatomyositis 6.11, 14.6, 14.63,
  14.64
dexamethasone suppression test 5.31
diabetes insipidus 2.16
  cranial 5.33, 9.16
  nephrogenic 7.11
diabetes mellitus 5.8, 5.37, 5.70
  complications 5.68, 9.6, 9.7, 11.9,
    11.10
  treatment 1.9, 2.1, 2.18, 5.5, 5.6,
    5.36
diabetic ketoacidosis 5.38, 5.67, 5.69
dialysis 2.46, 9.36–9.38
diaphragmatic calcification 13.40
diarrhoea, infective 2.24
DiGeorge syndrome 3.50
digoxin 2.35, 2.72, 2.91, 9.2
diphtheria 8.43, 8.44
dissociative disorder 12.17
disulfiram 2.39
diverticulitis 6.61
dopamine 3.106
dressings 4.3
driving 10.45
Drug and Therapeutics Committees
  2.98
drug-induced lupus 14.9, 14.39
drugs of abuse 2.44, 2.101
dyaesthesia 10.65
dysarthria 10.59, 10.60
dysphagia 6.11, 6.17, 6.20, 6.25,
  6.28, 10.60
dysphasia 3.94, 10.57

Ebola virus 8.16
ecstasy 2.101
Edwards syndrome 3.82
efficacy 2.19, 2.93, 2.98
Ehlers–Danlos syndrome 4.15
Eisenmenger syndrome 1.50

elbow movement 3.87, 3.89, 3.92
elderly patients
    drugs 2.75, 2.76
    vitamin B_{12} deficiency 7.65
electrocardiograms (ECGs) 1.18, 1.21,
    1.28, 1.39, 1.48, 13.64
electroconvulsive therapy 12.12
electroencephalograms (EEGs) 10.34
encephalitis 8.8, 12.27
endocarditis 1.13, 1.58, 1.59, 8.7
enterovirus meningitis 10.26
eosinophilia 7.27, 8.68, 13.34
epidemiological research 2.11
epiglottitis 13.47
epilepsy 10.16, 10.33, 10.45–10.48,
    10.73
ErbB2 inhibitors 3.4
erysipelas 8.40
erythrocytosis 7.45
erythropoietin (EPO) 9.11
Escherichia coli O157 8.13, 8.75
ethylene glycol 2.63
extraocular muscles 11.5
extrinsic allergic alveolitis 13.28

faecal occult blood test 6.31
Fallot's tetralogy 1.24, 1.25, 1.73
Fanconi syndrome 5.65
fasciculations 10.9
fat embolism 13.74
fat malabsorption 6.37
Felty syndrome 7.9
fibromyalgia 14.71
fibrosing alveolitis 13.46, 13.65, 14.24
fine-needle aspiration cytology 5.19
fragile X syndrome 3.24
Friedreich's ataxia 3.43, 3.71
fruit juices 2.4

G-protein defects 3.79
γ-amino butyric acid (GABA) 3.100,
    10.33
gas gangrene 3.69
gastric carcinoma 6.6
gastric emptying 3.99, 6.33, 6.34
gastrin 3.18, 3.98, 3.99, 6.32
gastroenteritis 2.24, 6.44, 8.46–8.48
gastrointestinal haemorrhage 6.30,
    6.72

generalised anxiety disorder 2.61,
    12.20
genetic anticipation 3.43
gentamicin-related neuromuscular
    blockade 10.13
giant-cell (temporal) arteritis 10.10,
    14.4, 14.52
giardiasis 6.45, 8.65
glandular fever 13.53
Glasgow Coma Scale (GSC) 10.56
glaucoma 2.9, 11.19
glomerulonephritis 2.51, 9.44, 9.46
glucagon-like peptide 1 (GLP-1) 3.10
glucose-6-phosphate dehydrogenase
    deficiency 3.64
glue solvents 2.58
glyceryl trinitrate 2.60
glycosuria 9.52
goitre 5.22
gonorrhoea 8.10, 8.70
Goodpasture syndrome 9.66, 9.67,
    13.52, 13.60, 14.12
gout 2.10, 2.26, 5.9, 5.49, 14.5,
    14.30
graft-versus-host disease 7.70
granulocyte colony-stimulating factor
    7.56
Graves' ophthalmopathy 5.20, 11.17
'Group and Save' 7.28
growth hormone 5.24, 5.27, 5.29
gum hypertrophy 2.6
gynaecomastia 1.51, 5.39

haematemesis 6.30, 6.72
haemochromatosis 3.8, 5.10, 5.51,
    5.52, 6.3
haemodialysis 2.46, 9.37
haemoglobin
    methaemoglobinaemia 7.60, 7.61
    and oxygen 3.109, 13.59
    S variant 7.20
haemoglobinuria 3.121
haemolytic anaemia 2.92, 7.22, 7.40,
    7.69
haemolytic uraemic syndrome 9.70
haemophilia A 3.22, 3.23, 7.33
hair loss 4.5
Hashimoto's thyroiditis 5.21
HDL cholesterol 5.11

headaches 2.45, 2.94, 2.95, 3.119, 10.15, 10.36–10.42

hearing loss 10.8

heart block 1.10, 1.27, 1.53, 10.18

heart failure 1.6, 1.7, 1.12, 1.19, 1.45, 1.46, 13.35, 14.45

heart murmurs 1.69

Helicobacter pylori 6.6, 6.26

HELLP syndrome 7.68

hemorrhagic fever 8.16, 8.18

Henoch–Schönlein purpura 9.68, 14.49

hepatic amoebiasis 8.64

hepatitis A 6.67

hepatitis B 6.68, 9.5

hepatitis (drug-induced) 2.85

hepatocellular carcinoma 3.76, 3.117

hepatopulmonary syndrome 6.7

hepcidin 3.26

hereditary spherocytosis 7.3

herpes simplex virus (HSV) 4.33, 8.34, 12.27

hip movement 3.90

hirsutism 4.20

histology 3.66

HIV/AIDS

    disorders associated with 4.4, 8.15, 8.25–8.31, 8.59, 10.72, 10.74, 12.6, 13.22

    tests 8.73

    transmission risks 8.22–8.24

HLA (human leukocyte antigen) 3.13

Hodgkin's disease 7.72

homocystinuria 11.12

hormone replacement therapy (HRT) 5.62

Huntington's disease 3.122, 12.5

hydrocortisone 2.57

hypercalcaemia 3.57, 5.40–5.44, 6.58, 9.64

hyperkalaemia 1.48, 2.42, 5.35, 9.10

hyperosmolar non-ketotic (HONK) syndrome 5.8

hyperparathyroidism 5.3, 5.40, 5.43, 5.44, 5.64, 9.8

hypersensitivity 2.34, 3.114–3.116, 4.39

hypertension 1.3, 2.6, 2.13, 2.41, 5.55, 5.56, 9.40, 10.64

    pulmonary 3.19, 13.4

hyperthyroidism 4.9, 5.1, 5.2, 5.7, 5.16, 5.17, 5.54, 5.71

hypertriglyceridaemia 3.12, 4.32

hypertrophic cardiomyopathy 1.31, 1.32, 3.70

hyperuricaemia 14.65

hyperventilation 13.36

hypoglycaemia 2.62, 5.70, 5.74

hypokalaemia 2.72, 5.12

hypoparathyroidism 3.79

hypopituitarism 5.25–5.27

hypotension 2.15, 3.102

    postural 5.4

hypothyroidism 5.18, 5.21

hypoventilation 13.6

IgA nephropathy 9.12, 9.22, 9.45

ileostomy 6.43

imatinib 7.2

imipramine 2.30

immune thrombocytopenic purpura 3.42

immunodeficiency, post-splenectomy 7.15

immunoglobulins 3.16, 3.59

immunosuppressant drugs 9.13, 14.68

infectious mononucleosis 13.53

infertility 2.49, 5.14, 5.61, 8.72

inflammatory bowel disease 6.13, 6.14, 6.43, 6.49–6.56, 13.46

inheritance patterns 3.43, 3.124, 3.125

    see also X-linked disorders

insulin sensitivity 5.75

insulinoma 5.74, 7.42

interleukin 1 (IL-1) 3.103

intestinal bacterial overgrowth 6.41, 6.42

intra-aortic balloon pumps 1.52

intracranial pressure, raised 10.74, 11.14

iron

    deficiency 4.36, 4.37, 7.17, 7.18, 7.21, 7.51, 7.59, 7.62

    overload (haemochromatosis) 3.8, 5.10, 5.51, 5.52, 6.3

    in pregnancy 7.52

irritable bowel syndrome 6.65

ischaemic bowel 6.10, 6.46

isoniazid 2.31

jaundice, drug-induced 2.84, 6.73
jugular venous pressure (JVP) 1.27,
    1.61, 1.68

Kaposi's sarcoma 4.4, 8.30
kidney *see entries at* renal
knee movement 3.91
Kussmaul's sign 1.68

labyrinthitis 10.44
lactate 3.108
larynx 3.17
lateral medullary syndrome 10.24
laxatives 2.100, 6.59, 6.60
    abuse 12.4
left bundle branch block 1.53
Legionnaire's disease 8.12
lens dislocation 11.12
leprosy 8.52, 8.53
leptospirosis (Weil's disease) 8.6, 8.54
leukaemia 7.5, 7.71, 9.62
leukocytoclastic vasculitis 4.31
Lewy body dementia 12.2
lichen planus 4.38
lisinopril 2.51
lithium 1.3, 7.26
liver cancer 3.76, 3.117
liver function test abnormalities 6.70,
    6.73
    antibiotics and 2.84, 2.85
liver transplantation criteria 6.69
Lofgren syndrome 13.48
lumbar puncture 10.36
lung cancer 7.14, 13.26, 13.32
    carcinoid 7.7, 13.29
    non-small-cell 7.43
    small-cell 7.41, 7.44
    squamous cell 13.44, 13.45
lung injury, transfusion-related 7.37,
    13.15
Lyme disease 8.55, 14.37
lymphoma 7.4, 7.72, 7.73, 8.31,
    13.62

macrocytosis 3.45, 3.46, 7.62
magnesium 5.46
malabsorption 6.37, 6.64
malaria 8.60–8.62
mammography 7.47

mania 12.9, 12.30
mast cells 3.41
McArdle syndrome 3.62
measles 8.19, 8.20
median nerve 3.92
mediastinal masses 13.50
mediastinal widening 13.73
meningitis 8.59, 10.26–10.30, 10.37
meningococcal meningitis 10.28
mesothelioma 13.68
metabolic acidosis 2.50, 2.63
methaemoglobinaemia 7.60, 7.61
methotrexate 14.2
microscopic polyangiitis 9.41, 9.69
midbrain lesions 10.55
migraine 2.45, 10.15, 10.39, 10.40
mitral stenosis 1.54
molluscum contagiosum 8.36
morphine 2.55
motilin 6.33
motor neurone disease 3.65
multiple endocrine neoplasia I (MEN I)
    3.32
multiple endocrine neoplasia II (MEN
    II) 3.33
multiple sclerosis 10.65–10.68
mumps 8.21
muscular dystrophy 1.21, 3.61
myasthenia gravis 10.14, 10.50, 10.71
mycobacteria, atypical 13.42
Mycobacterium avium intracellulare 8.28
Mycobacterium tuberculosis 8.27
Mycoplasma pneumoniae 13.17
myeloma 7.74, 9.26
myocardial infarction (MI) 1.11, 1.20,
    1.35, 1.44
myotonic dystrophy 3.60
myxoma 1.40

NAC (*N*-acetylcysteine) 2.54, 2.86
nails
    brittle 4.36
    fungal infections of 4.34
narcolepsy 10.7
necrobiosis lipoidica 4.35
needlestick injuries 8.24
nephritis
    acute interstitial 9.48, 9.49
    chronic tubulo-interstitial 9.72

nephrocalcinosis 9.73
nephrolithiasis 3.15, 5.48, 9.61, 9.62, 9.65
nephropathy, contrast-mediated 9.71
nephrotic syndrome 3.2, 3.28, 9.5, 9.28–9.31
nerve root lesions 3.88–3.91, 3.93
neurofibromatosis 3.123, 10.75
neurotransmitters 3.100, 10.33
neutropenia 7.31, 7.56
neutrophilia 7.26
nitric oxide 3.101
non-alcoholic steatohepatitis 6.70
non-Hodgkin's lymphoma 7.4, 7.73, 8.31
non-steroidal anti-inflammatory drugs (NSAIDs) 2.21, 2.59

obesity 1.9, 5.31
obstructive sleep apnoea 13.24
obstructive uropathy 9.53, 9.58, 9.59
odynophagia 6.21, 6.22
oesophageal cancer 6.23–6.25, 6.27, 6.28, 13.50
oesophageal dysphagia 6.17, 6.25, 6.28
oesophageal spasm 6.18
oesophageal stricture 6.20
oesophagitis 6.21, 6.22
oligospermia 2.49
omeprazole 6.19, 6.29
optic chiasm lesions 10.1, 10.61
optic disc swelling (papilloedema) 10.64, 11.14
optic nerve compression 11.17
optic neuritis 11.13
organophosphates 2.52
osmolarity 3.81
osteoarthritis 14.16–14.19, 14.66
osteodystrophy, renal 9.34, 9.35
osteomalacia 14.46
osteoporosis 2.2, 5.15, 5.45, 14.15, 14.47, 14.58, 14.59
osteoprotogenerin 3.7
overdoses, diagnosis 2.28, 2.30, 2.33, 2.44, 2.62, 2.101
oxygen
   in the blood 3.109, 3.110, 13.59
   long-term therapy 13.21

Paget's disease of bone 14.44, 14.45
pain relief see analgesia
pancreatic disease 6.1
   insulinoma 5.74, 7.42
   pancreatitis 2.3, 2.18, 6.12, 6.74, 6.75
panic attacks 2.37, 12.33
papillary necrosis 14.10
papilloedema 10.64, 11.14
paracetamol
   mechanism of action 3.104
   overdose 2.29, 2.53, 2.54, 2.62, 2.68, 2.86
paraneoplastic syndrome 7.44, 7.45, 10.76
parathyroid disease 3.49, 3.79, 5.3, 5.40, 5.43, 5.44, 5.64, 9.8
parietal lobe 3.94
parkinsonism 2.78, 10.53
Parkinson's disease 2.77, 2.79, 3.5, 10.5, 10.51
paroxysmal nocturnal haemoglobinuria 7.25
parvovirus B19 8.35
pemphigoid 4.6, 4.18
penis, pearly penile papules 4.7
peptic ulcers 3.18, 5.42
pericarditis 1.4, 1.42, 1.65, 8.9
peritoneal dialysis 9.38
Peutz–Jeghers syndrome 3.38, 4.13, 6.48
phaeochromocytoma 2.13, 5.59, 5.60, 5.72
pharmacogenetics 2.32
pharmacokinetics 2.22, 2.46, 2.55, 2.96
phenylketonuria 3.56
phenytoin 4.20, 4.39
phosphate 2.7
phosphodiesterase 5 inhibitors 2.8, 5.63, 11.1
pituitary apoplexy 10.2
pituitary gland
   hormone production 3.51, 5.24
   hypopituitarism 5.25–5.27
   tumours 5.23, 5.29, 5.30
Plasmodium falciparum 8.61, 8.62
platelet disorders 7.6, 7.39, 7.55

pleural effusions 13.3, 13.32, 13.35, 13.37, 13.62
pneumatosis cystoides intestinalis 6.62
pneumococcal infections 7.15, 10.29
Pneumocystis carinii pneumonia 8.25, 8.74, 13.22
pneumonia 8.25, 8.74, 13.2, 13.22
pneumothorax 13.66
polyarteritis nodosa 4.14, 14.11, 14.48
polycystic kidney disease 9.50, 9.51
polycystic ovarian syndrome (PCOS) 5.13, 5.14
polymyalgia rheumatica 14.50, 14.51
polyps, intestinal 6.48, 6.63
polyuria 7.11, 9.14, 9.16
Pontiac fever 13.55
pontine haemorrhage 10.3
porphyria, acute intermittent 3.55, 5.53
porphyria cutanea tarda 3.54
post-cranial irradiation somnolence syndrome 10.6
post-herpetic neuralgia 2.25
post-natal depression 12.25
post-traumatic stress disorder 12.26
posterior circulation stroke 10.19
potassium *see* hyperkalaemia; hypokalaemia
pregnancy
    drugs and 2.14, 2.41, 2.69, 2.73, 2.74, 5.2, 6.14
    haemodynamics 1.33
    HIV and 8.22
    iron supplements 7.52
pressure sores 4.3
pretibial myxoedema 4.9
primary biliary cirrhosis 6.66, 6.71
primary ciliary dyskinesia 13.57
progressive multifocal leukoencephalopathy 10.72, 12.6
prolactin 5.28, 5.32
prolonged QT interval 1.17, 1.71
Propionibacterium acnes 8.4
prostate cancer 7.49
prostate specific antigen (PSA) 3.118
prosthetic valves 1.14
proteinuria 9.6, 9.23, 9.24, 9.27–9.30, 9.47
proton pump inhibitors 6.19, 6.29

pseudogout 14.33
pseudohypoparathyroidism 3.49
Pseudomonas spp. 3.72, 13.13
pseudoxanthoma elasticum 4.16
psoriasis 4.28, 14.3, 14.28
psoriatic arthropathy 14.27
pulmonary calcification 13.33
pulmonary embolism 1.56, 1.57, 13.27, 13.63, 13.64
pulmonary hypertension 3.19, 13.4
pulmonary oedema 9.15, 13.69
pulsus paradoxus 1.66
pupillary defects 10.63, 11.2
pyelonephritis 3.113, 9.57

Q fever 8.39, 13.54
quinine 2.47

radial nerve 3.75
radiotherapy
complications 6.44, 10.6
    contraindications 7.14
    radioiodine 5.7, 5.54
RANK ligand 2.2, 14.15
rasburicase 7.10, 14.5
Raynaud's disease 14.41
re-feeding syndrome 2.7
reactive arthritis 14.29
recreational drugs 2.44, 2.101
red eye 11.15
relapsing (poly)chondritis 3.27, 14.62
renal artery disease 9.4, 9.15, 9.40
renal biopsy 9.17–9.19
renal calculi 3.15, 5.48, 9.61, 9.62, 9.65
renal cell carcinoma 9.63
renal conditions, microscopy 3.85
renal failure
    acute 9.37, 9.39, 9.49, 9.60
    cancer and 9.53
    chronic 9.11, 9.34–9.36, 9.46
    drugs and 2.1, 2.80, 2.81, 9.39, 9.49
    end-stage 9.38, 9.42, 9.43
    pre-renal 9.33
renal function
    aquaporin channels 9.14
    in the elderly 2.75
    glomerular filtration pressure 9.32

glycosuria 9.52
  protein excretion 9.23, 9.27–9.30
renal transplants 9.13, 9.43
renal tubular acidosis 9.7, 9.73
research studies 2.11, 2.88–2.90
respiratory failure type 1 13.63
respiratory failure type 2 13.7
retinal artery occlusion 11.7, 11.16
retinal vein occlusion 10.4, 11.3, 11.6
retinitis, CMV 8.26, 11.4
retinoids 4.22
retinopathy
  diabetic 5.68, 11.9, 11.10
  hypertensive 11.8
retrobulbar neuritis 10.35
rhabdomyolysis 9.3
rheumatic fever 1.55
rheumatoid arthritis 14.2,
  14.21–14.26, 14.31, 14.68, 14.70
rheumatoid factor 14.74
Rickettsia 8.38
ringworm 8.56
rituximab 3.6
rubella 8.32, 8.33

sarcoidosis 4.21, 9.64, 11.18, 13.30,
  13.72, 14.67
'Saturday night palsy' 3.75
schistosomiasis 8.66
schizophrenia 2.38, 2.66, 12.8,
  12.13–12.15, 12.28, 12.29
scleroderma 14.42
seizures 10.16, 10.33, 10.45–10.48,
  10.73, 12.21
self-harm 12.1, 12.11, 12.18
sepsis 3.102
septic arthritis 14.20, 14.32, 14.35,
  14.36
severe acute respiratory distress
  syndrome (SARS) 13.56
shingles 10.32
shortness of breath, treatment 13.10,
  13.69
shoulder injuries 3.88
shrinking lung syndrome 13.39
sickle cell disease 7.20
sildenafil 2.8, 5.63, 11.1
silicosis 13.5
Sipple syndrome 3.33

Sjögren syndrome 13.37, 14.53
sleep disorders 10.6, 10.7, 13.24
solvent abuse 2.58
spasticity 10.66
splenic atrophy 7.39
Staphylococcus aureus 8.2, 8.41, 8.46,
  8.69, 10.27
Staphylococcus epidermidis 8.42
statins, antibiotics and 2.12, 2.102
steatorrhoea 6.35, 6.37
stem cell transplantation, autologous
  7.57
stents 1.8
Stevens–Johnson syndrome 4.23
Still's disease 3.74
streptococcal skin infections 3.112
Streptococcus pneumoniae 7.15, 10.29
stroke 14.54
  prophylaxis 10.21, 10.23
  see also specific areas
strongyloidiasis 8.68
struma ovarii 5.1
subdural empyema 10.73
suicide risk 12.11, 12.18
sulfasalazine 2.23, 2.49, 2.56, 14.25
sunlight 4.29
supraventricular tachycardia 1.15
swallowing, problems with *see*
  dysphagia; odynophagia
syncope 10.18
syndrome of inappropriate ADH
  secretion (SIADH) 2.36, 5.34,
  10.12
syphilis 3.67, 8.71
systemic lupus erythematosus (SLE)
  3.48, 3.58, 3.68, 13.39, 14.38,
  14.40, 14.56, 14.57, 14.76
systemic sclerosis 13.11, 14.43

tachycardia 1.15, 1.16, 1.70
tacrolimus 4.26
tamoxifen 7.48
target cells 7.18
temporal (giant-cell) arteritis 10.10,
  14.4, 14.52
temporal lobe lesions 3.97, 10.57
tension headaches 10.38
tetralogy of Fallot 1.24, 1.25, 1.73
thalassaemia trait 7.19

theophylline 2.39, 2.43, 2.87, 10.54
therapeutic drug monitoring 2.20
thoracic spine compression 10.52
thrombocythaemia 7.39
thrombocytopenia 7.55
thromboembolism 7.36, 13.70
    see also pulmonary embolism
thrombophilia screening 7.66, 7.67
thrombotic thrombocytopenic purpura
    (TTP) 7.24
thyroid disease 4.9, 5.1, 5.2, 5.7,
    5.16–5.22, 5.54, 5.71
tiotropium 13.31
torsades de pointes 1.2, 1.17, 1.72
toxic shock syndrome 8.69
Toxoplasma gondii 8.29
trachoma 8.37
transfusions *see* blood transfusions
transtuzumab 1.7
transverse myelitis 10.31
tremor 10.54
trigeminal neuralgia 10.43
troponin 3.20
tuberculosis 8.9, 8.27, 13.3, 13.33,
    14.74
    anti-TB drugs 13.41
tuberous sclerosis 3.37
tumour lysis syndrome 7.10, 14.5
tumour markers 3.76, 3.117, 6.4
tumour necrosis factor (TNF) 3.3,
    3.105, 4.1
Turner syndrome 3.40
typhus fever 8.38
Tzanck test 4.33

ulcerative colitis 6.52, 6.55, 6.56,
    13.46
^{13}C-urea breath test 6.26
urethritis 9.55
urinary calculi 3.15, 5.48, 9.61, 9.62,
    9.65
urinary tract infections 9.21, 9.54–9.56
urine, dark colour 5.53, 9.20
urticaria 2.27, 4.40

v-waves 1.61
vaccination (meningitis) 10.29

vasculitis
    small-vessel 9.41, 9.69, 14.49
    temporal arteritis 10.10, 14.4, 14.52
ventricular septal defect 1.1
ventricular tachycardia 1.16, 1.70
verapamil 1.2, 2.91
vertebral artery dissection 10.22
vertebral fractures 14.59
vesico-ureteric junction obstruction
    9.58
viral meningitis 10.30, 10.37
visual disturbances
    drug-induced 2.8, 2.9, 11.1, 13.41
    neurological 3.96, 3.97, 10.1,
        10.25, 10.61, 10.62
vitamin B_{12} 7.53
    deficiency 3.47, 6.41, 7.16, 7.17,
        7.59, 7.65
vitamin D 9.34
vitiligo 4.12, 4.24
volume of distribution (V_d) 2.22
von Hippel–Lindau syndrome 3.36
von Willebrand's disease 3.29, 7.12,
    7.34

Waldenström's macroglobulinaemia
    7.75
warfarin 1.5, 2.4, 2.17, 2.82
    reversal of anticoagulation 7.54
Wegener's granulomatosis 4.2, 9.9,
    13.51, 14.7
Weil's disease 8.6, 8.54
Werner syndrome 3.32
Whipple's disease 6.2
whooping cough 8.45
Wilson's disease 3.34, 3.35, 5.50,
    10.69
Wiskott–Aldrich syndrome 3.11
Wolff–Parkinson–White syndrome 1.18

X-linked disorders 3.14, 3.22–3.24,
    3.124
xanthomata 4.32
ximelagatran 1.41

yaws 4.8
yellow fever 8.17